Biomedical Applications of Metals

Mahendra Rai · Avinash P. Ingle
Serenella Medici
Editors

Biomedical Applications of Metals

Springer

Editors
Mahendra Rai
Nanobiotechnology Laboratory
Department of Biotechnology
Sant Gadge Baba Amravati University
Amravati, Maharashtra
India

Serenella Medici
Departmento Di Chimica Farmacia
University of Sassari
Sassari
Italy

Avinash P. Ingle
Nanobiotechnology Laboratory
Department of Biotechnology
Sant Gadge Baba Amravati University
Amravati, Maharashtra
India

ISBN 978-3-030-09081-4 ISBN 978-3-319-74814-6 (eBook)
https://doi.org/10.1007/978-3-319-74814-6

Printed on acid-free paper

This Springer imprint is published by the registered company Springer International Publishing AG part of Springer Nature
The registered company address is: Gewerbestrasse 11, 6330 Cham, Switzerland

Foreword

Metals play a pivotal role in the biomedical field, either as poisons or remedies. They can even be both things at the same time. Some metals are essential to organic life as cofactors in enzymes called metalloproteins and mediate a number of biological processes. For this reason, their homeostasis must be strictly regulated, and in case of deficiency the organism develops a series of pathologies so that these inorganic elements have to be reintegrated with dietary supplements. Metal overload can also cause damage to the body and results in serious poisoning, even in the case of essential elements. The so-called chelation therapy helps remove the excess metals and re-establish a healthy condition.

Metals are also used in medicine for diagnosis and therapy with an impressive number of applications, ranging from imaging techniques to cancer treatment, radiation therapy, mammographic and radiographic analysis, bone replacements or prosthetics, manic-depression behaviour prophylaxis, rheumatoid arthritis treatment, burn wounds healing, antibacterial surfaces and layers in hospital devices, etc.

Together with such consolidated medical practices, a series of new potential applications are emerging, which are capturing the interest of numerous researchers all over the world. Thus, novel non-platinum drugs for cancer treatment continuously appear in the literature, often with better performances with respect to the lead compound—Cisplatin; silver regained popularity as an antimicrobial agent, due to its high efficiency in killing germs and almost no tendency to induce resistance in bacteria, but it also seems to possess anticancer and antiprotozoan properties with low toxicity in humans; rhodium and iridium complexes showed to be potential agents for imaging, tracking of small biological molecules, and sensors; gold exhibited anti-HIV effects in preliminary tests; and many other metal compounds demonstrated to be effective against several other diseases or pathogens. The success of metals in medical applications is probably due to the variety of forms in which they can be used, such as salts, complexes, nanoparticles, just to quote some, that offer a virtually infinite range of compositions and combinations, with the possibility of finely tuning their properties and characteristics. Nevertheless, the intrinsic toxicity of metals cannot be neglected, as it generates most of the drawbacks evidenced in metallodrugs, which limit their safety and spectrum of applications.

The dual nature of metals in biomedical treatment have been thoroughly examined and discussed in this valuable book, where both their applications and toxicity issues have been described. The recent advances in this field are also explored, in order to give a complete overview on the latest research trends and the most interesting results reported in the literature. In this way, the present book represents a reference point for both researchers and students but also for neophytes who wants to delve into these fascinating topics.

The chapters of the book highlight the sophisticated understanding of the role of the metals in medicine but they also hint at the many aspects still to be discovered, ranging from the novel applications of noble metals as theranostics, with special attention to their anticancer and antibiotic properties, to the toxicity of metallodrugs, the impact of heavy metals on human health and their biological targets, and finally the health implications of a traditional ayurvedic practice, the use of Bhasmas, thus providing a complete and integrated picture of the role of metals in the biomedical applications.

This book would open up new avenues for research and future development in the field of the clinical uses of metals in medicine.

Sardinia, Italy

Dr. Guido Crisponi
Professor of Analytical Chemistry
University of Cagliari

Preface

Metals dominate the inorganic side of the universe. In fact, out of the 98 naturally occurring elements identified so far, 71 are metals and the rest are non-metals or metalloids. Nevertheless, they also play a fundamental role in biological systems, where they accomplish both structural and catalytic functions. Metals, in their cationic forms, are often active sites in enzymes or cofactors in the so-called metalloproteins. It is estimated that approximately half of all proteins contain a metal centre and that about 25–30% of all proteins need metals to carry out their functions. Thus, metals are involved in numerous biological functions such as enzyme reactions, signal transduction, storage and transport processes. For instance, haemoglobin is an iron-containing oxygen carrier, while ferritin stores iron(III) ions and transferrin transports them where needed. Cobalt is contained in vitamin B12, preferentially called cobalamin. Some biologically relevant metals (e.g. iron, copper and manganese) can assume different oxidation states, so that they are involved in cellular redox mechanisms. The role of the essential metals is so utterly important that their homeostasis must be strictly regulated: any imbalance or depletion can lead to pathological conditions, such as anemia (iron deficiency), impaired body growth (zinc deficiency) and heart diseases in infants (copper deficiency). The reverse is also true: metal excess too can result in pathological conditions, so that proper antidotes or metal chelators should be used to treat these disorders.

The capability of metals to extensively interact with numerous biological components has been unintentionally exploited in the biomedical field since very old times, when gold, silver and copper were used to keep water and other drinks pure and to treat wounds, burns and other diseases. Following these ancient practices, several new medical and pharmacological concepts evolved in modern days, leading to the development of metal-based anticancer drugs, antibacterial agents, sedatives, antacid or antirheumatic remedies. Successful therapeutic and diagnostic metallodrugs include platinum compounds in the treatment of tumours, while approved metal-based radiopharmaceuticals are employed as a measure of last resort in advanced stages of cancer, or in the so-called brachytherapy. Contrast agents containing radioactive metal isotopes are produced and administered daily in single-photon emission computed tomography (SPECT) scans of the human body.

Magnetic resonance imaging (MRI) contrast techniques employ other metal ions. Finally, biocompatible and light metals like titanium, aluminium and their alloys are used in prosthesis and bone implants.

The extremely versatile biological and pharmaceutical properties of metals have quickly imposed them as prominent research targets in the field of theranostics, so that their applications in medicine and related topics are countless. In this book, we have given an account of the most recent trends in the exploration of their characteristics, which can be exploited to prepare novel metallodrugs, biosensors and imaging reagents. The pharmacological and therapeutic properties of selected metals (platinum, copper, silver and selenium) have been discussed, with particular attention to their mechanisms of action, drawbacks and limitations. The applications of metal compounds against bacteria and other pathogens have been discussed, in particular the latest results against malaria disease. The aspects of metal toxicity will be finally addressed in a special section, since the dual nature of metals not only makes them valuable resources in the treatment of many pathological conditions but unfortunately it also causes severe side effects especially in the case of heavy metal poisoning. Thus, their biochemical and molecular targets will be discussed, together with the effects of such noxious interactions.

All the chapters of this book have been written by one or more specialists, experts in the concerned topic, and are highly informative and detailed. In this way, we would like to offer a rich guide to both biomedical applications and limitations of metals in the therapeutic practice, together with other key aspects such as toxicological issues and safety concerns, which will be particularly useful to researcher in this field, undergraduate or graduate students of chemistry, biochemistry, pharmacology, microbiology, biotechnology and allied subjects, facing the topic of metals in medicine and metal toxicity, and also to readers simply interested in understanding the main aspects of metal interactions with the human body.

Amravati, India Mahendra Rai
Amravati, India Avinash P. Ingle
Sassari, Italy Serenella Medici

Contents

Editors and Contributors

About the Editors

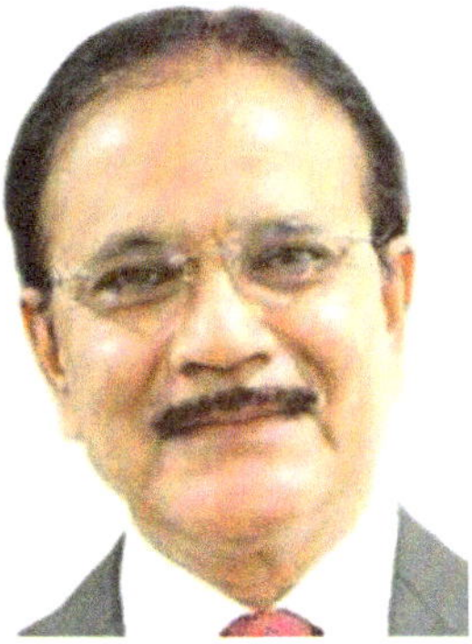

Mahendra Rai is a Senior Professor at the Department of Biotechnology, Sant Gadge Baba Amravati University at Amravati, Maharashtra, India. He was a Visiting Scientist at the Department of Bioenergetics, University of Geneva, Switzerland in 2004 and at the Department of Plant Protection of Debrecen University, Debrecen, Hungary in 2005 and 2008. He visited Department of Chemical Biology, University of Campinas, Brazil under Indo-Brazil Research Programme (DST-CNPq collaboration) in 2009, 2011 and 2012. In 2012, he was Visiting Professor in Nicolaus Copernicus University, Torun, Poland. In 2013, he was Visiting Scientist at State University of Campinas, Brazil. He was also Visiting Professor in 2015 in Ostrava, Czech Republic and in 2016 in National University of Rosario, Argentina. His area of expertise includes microbial biotechnology and nanobiotechnology. His present research interest includes application of nanobiotechnology in medicine with particular reference to development of nanoantimicrobials. He has published more than 380 research papers in national and international journals. In addition, he has edited/authored more than 44 books and 7 patents. Recently, he has been awarded Basic Science Research Faculty Fellowship by University Grants Commission, New Delhi, Government of India.

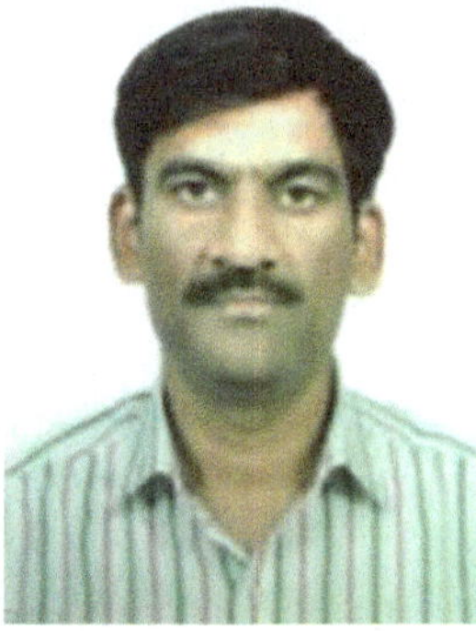

Dr. Avinash P. Ingle has completed his doctoral degree in Department of Biotechnology, Sant Gadge Baba Amravati University, Amravati, Maharashtra (India) in 2012. Further, he worked as research scientist in the same department from 2013–2016. He has more than 55 research publications, 26 book chapters and 1 book to his credit. He has been awarded travel grants from different funding/sponsoring agencies to present his research work in international conferences held at Malaysia, China, Spain and France. His area of research mainly includes microbial biotechnology, nanobiotechnology and biofuel technology. Currently, he is working as Post-Doctoral Fellow at Department of Biotechnology, Engineering School of Lorena, University of São Paulo, Brazil and he is actively engaged in development of nanotechnology-based methods for the efficient production of biofuels.

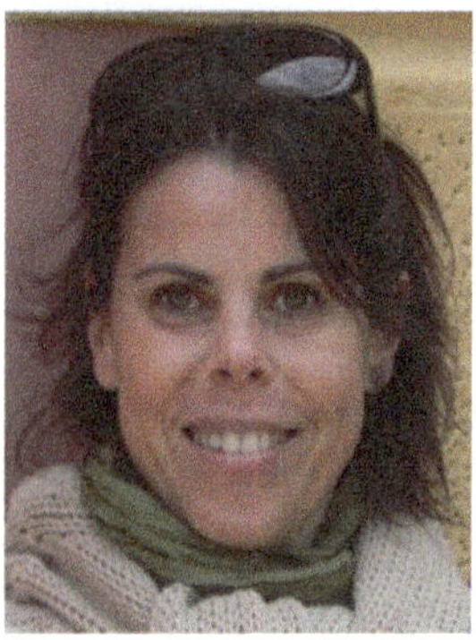

Serenella Medici is currently working as Assistant Professor of General and Inorganic Chemistry at the University of Sassari, Italy, and after receiving her Ph.D. in Chemistry in Sassari, she worked as a Post-Doctoral Fellow at the Debye Institute, University of Utrecht (the Netherlands), and was a Visiting Researcher at the Rovira i Virgili University (Tarragona, Spain) and Cerm (Centre for Magnetic Resonances, University of Florence, Italy). Her research interests include the study of organometallic complexes, metal ion–protein interactions, toxicity mechanisms and carcinogenesis of heavy metals, NMR applications and archaeometry.

Contributors

Blair S. Ashley Department of Orthopaedic Surgery, University of Pennsylvania, Philadelphia, PA, USA

Jayanta Kumar Biswas Pollution, Ecotoxicology and Ecotechnology Research Unit, Department of Ecological Studies, University of Kalyani, Kalyani, Nadia, West Bengal, India; International Centre for Ecological Engineering, University of Kalyani, Kalyani, West Bengal, India

Anand Chaudhary Department of Rasa Shastra and Bhaishjya Kalpana, Faculty of Ayurveda, Institute of Medical Sciences, Banaras Hindu University, Varanasi, India

Júlia Helena da Silva Martins Faculty of Electrical Engineering, Federal University of Pará—UFPA, Belém, Pará, Brazil

Luiza Helena da Silva Martins Center of Natural Sciences and Technology, State University of Pará, UEPA, Belém, Pará, Brazil

Silvio Silvério da Silva Department of Biotechnology, Engineering School of Lorena, São Paulo University, Lorena, Brazil

Paulo Weslem Portal Gomes Center of Social Sciences and Education, State University of Pará—UEPA, Salvaterra, Pará, Brazil

Natalie Gugala Biofilm Research Group, University of Calgary, Calgary, Canada

Indarchand Gupta Department of Biotechnology, Institute of Science, Aurangabad, Maharashtra, India

Vivek Kumar Gupta Department of Biochemistry, University of Allahabad, Allahabad, Uttar Pradesh, India

William M. Hardaker Department of Orthopaedic Surgery, University of Pennsylvania, Philadelphia, PA, USA

Avinash P. Ingle Nanobiotechnology Laboratory, Department of Biotechnology, SGB Amravati University, Amravati, Maharashtra, India

Abhishek Kumar Department of Biochemistry, University of Allahabad, Allahabad, Uttar Pradesh, India

Talita Martins Lacerda Department of Biotechnology, Engineering School of Lorena, São Paulo University, Lorena, Brazil

Abbas Ali Mahdi Department of Biochemistry, King George's Medical University, Lucknow, Uttar Pradesh, India

Paulo Ricardo Franco Marcelino Department of Biotechnology, Engineering School of Lorena, São Paulo University, Lorena, Brazil

Serenella Medici Department of Chemistry and Pharmacy, University of Sassari, Sassari, Italy

Carmen Mejía Facultad de Ciencias Naturales, Universidad Autónoma de Querétaro, Avenida de las Ciencias S/N Juriquilla, Delegación Santa Rosa Jáuregui, Querétaro, México

Sanjay Mishra Laboratory of Biochemistry, Department of Biotechnology, IFTM University, Moradabad, Uttar Pradesh, India

Monojit Mondal Pollution, Ecotoxicology and Ecotechnology Research Unit, Department of Ecological Studies, University of Kalyani, Kalyani, Nadia, West Bengal, India

Mariete Barbosa Moreira Department of Biotechnology, Engineering School of Lorena, São Paulo University, Lorena, Brazil

João Moreira Neto School of Chemical Engineering, University of Campinas—UNICAMP, Campinas, São Paulo, Brazil

Alexander L. Neuwirth Department of Orthopaedic Surgery, University of Pennsylvania, Philadelphia, PA, USA

Said Ortega-Rosales Departamento de Química Inorgánica y Nuclear, Laboratorio de Química Inorgánica Medicinal. Facultad de Química, Universidad Nacional Autónoma de México, Mexico City, Mexico

Rukmani Pandey Developmental Toxicology Laboratory, Systems Toxicology and Health Risk Assessment Group, CSIR-Indian Institute of Toxicology Research (CSIR-IITR), Lucknow, Uttar Pradesh, India

Shruti Pandey Department of Rasa Shastra and Bhaishjya Kalpana, Faculty of Ayurveda, Institute of Medical Sciences, Banaras Hindu University, Varanasi, India

Raksha Pandit Nanobiotechnology Research Lab, Department of Biotechnology, SGB Amravati University, Amravati, Maharashtra, India

Priti Paralikar Nanotechnology Laboratory, Department of Biotechnology, SGB Amravati University, Amravati, Maharashtra, India

Massimiliano Francesco Peana Department of Chemistry and Pharmacy, University of Sassari, Sassari, Italy

Mahendra Rai Nanobiotechnology Laboratory, Department of Biotechnology, SGB Amravati University, Amravati, Maharashtra, India

Lena Ruiz-Azuara Departamento de Química Inorgánica y Nuclear, Laboratorio de Química Inorgánica Medicinal. Facultad de Química, Universidad Nacional Autónoma de México, Mexico City, Mexico

Bechan Sharma Department of Biochemistry, University of Allahabad, Allahabad, Uttar Pradesh, India

Sudhir Shende Nanotechnology Laboratory, Department of Biotechnology, SGB Amravati University, Amravati, Maharashtra, India

Neil P. Sheth Department of Orthopaedic Surgery, University of Pennsylvania, Philadelphia, PA, USA

Nitika Singh Department of Biochemistry, University of Allahabad, Allahabad, Uttar Pradesh, India

Reetika Singh Department of Biochemistry, University of Allahabad, Allahabad, Uttar Pradesh, India

Olga Sinitsyna Laboratory for Physical Chemistry of Polymers, A.N. Nesmeyanov Institute of Organoelement Compounds of Russian Academy of Sciences, Moscow, Russia; Department of Chemistry, Moscow State University, Moscow, Russia

Amit Kumar Mani Tiwari Laboratory of Biochemistry, Department of Biotechnology, IFTM University, Moradabad, Uttar Pradesh, India

Raymond J. Turner Biofilm Research Group, University of Calgary, Calgary, Canada

Maria Antonietta Zoroddu Department of Chemistry and Pharmacy, University of Sassari, Sassari, Italy

Abbreviations and Acronyms

2-hepy	2-(2-hydroxyethyl)pyridine
AMPZ	$[\{cis\text{-Pt}(NH_3)_2\}_2(\mu\text{-OH})(\mu\text{-pyrazolate})]^{2+}$
Auranofin	(1-thio-beta-d-glucopyranosato)-(triethylphosphine) goldI-2,3,4,6-tetraacetate
bipy	2,2′-bipyridine
Carboplatin	*cis*-diammine(1,1-cyclobutanedicarboxylato)platinum(II)
Cisplatin	*cis*-diamminedichloroplatinum(II)
COX-2	Cyclooxygenase-2
dmf	Dimethylformamide
dmso	Dimethylsulfoxide
EDTA	Ethylenediamine tetraacetic acid
en	Ethylenediamine
GSH	Glutathione
HeLa	Henrietta Lacks cancer cells
HIV	Human immunodeficiency virus
Hptab	*N,N,N′,N′,N″,N″*-hexakis(2-pyridylmethyl)-1,3,5-tris(aminomethyl) benzene
IL-6	Interleukin-6
Iproplatin	Dichlorodihydroxybis(2-propanamine)platinum
KP1019	*trans*-[tetrachlorobis(1H-indazole)ruthenate(III)]
Lobaplatin	1,2-diammino-methyl-cyclobutaneplatinum(II)-lactate
MMP-3	Metalloproteinase-3
MRI	Magnetic resonance image
mtDNA	Mitochondrial DNA
NAMI-A	*trans*-[tetrachloro(DMSO)(imidazole)ruthenate(III)]
Nedaplatin	Diammine[(hydroxy-κO)acetato(2-)-κO]platinum
NHC	N-Heterocyclic carbene
Oxaliplatin	[(1*R*,2*R*)-cyclohexane-1,2-diamine](ethanedioato-*O,O′*)platinum(II)
p53	Tumour protein p53
Picoplatin	*cis*-amminedichloro(2-methylpyridine) platinum(II)

PL	Permitting limit
PPh_3, tpp	triphenylphosphine
PTA	1,3,5-triaza-7-phosphatricyclo-[3.3.1.1]decane
RAPTA-C	$[(\eta^6$-p-cymene)Ru(II)(PTA)$Cl_2]$
ROS	Reactive oxygen species
Satraplatin	Bis(acetato)amminedichloro(cyclohexylamine)platinum(II)
SOD	Superoxide dismutases
terpy	2,2′;6′,2″-terpyridine
Transplatin	*trans*-diamminedichloroplatin
TrxR	Thioredoxin reductase
TSC	Thiosemicarbazone

Part I
Applications of Metals in Medicine

Chapter 1
Noble Metals in Pharmaceuticals: Applications and Limitations

Serenella Medici, Massimiliano Francesco Peana and Maria Antonietta Zoroddu

Abstract Metal-based drugs like Cisplatin are still the most widely employed therapeutics in the treatment of cancer. Nevertheless, due to their severe drawbacks, such as extended toxicity, scarce bioavailability and drug resistance, the need of a valid alternative to Cisplatin and its derivatives has led to the synthesis and assessment as therapeutical agents of a series of complexes based on platinum and other noble metals, which showed not only anticancer activity but also antibacterial and antiprotozoal action with outstanding results. Here, the most used metals are discussed, together with their applications in medicine and limitations.

Keywords Noble metals · Chemotherapeutics · Anticancer · Antibacterial Toxicity

1.1 Introduction

The medical properties of noble metals have been recognized and applied since very ancient times. Their antibacterial action was not understood but yet exploited by early civilizations. Copper and silver vessels, for instance, were employed by the Egyptians to keep water pure, a habit which was also common among the Greeks, as reported by Herodotus, or the Romans, who stored wine in silver urns to prevent spoilage. In more recent times, a similar trick was exploited by settlers and pioneers in both Australia and the American West, who suspended silverware or put silver or copper coins into their water tanks or milk casks for the same reason. Moreover, the empiric observation that such practice could avoid rottenness and corruption may have led to the habit of using silverware and cutlery by rich families throughout time.

S. Medici (✉) · M. F. Peana · M. A. Zoroddu
Department of Chemistry and Pharmacy, University of Sassari, 07100 Sassari, Italy
e-mail: sere@uniss.it

M. Rai et al. (eds.), *Biomedical Applications of Metals*,
https://doi.org/10.1007/978-3-319-74814-6_1

The use of metals as remedies and drugs is also very ancient: medical applications of gold can be dated back to 2500 B.C. in China; silver foils were employed in the treatment of wounds and ulcers, as documented by the Greek physician Hippocrates, a therapeutic practice maintained up to the early 1800s when silver wires were used to seal surgical wounds, and during World War I when a silver leaf was applied against infections in wounded soldiers. The use of silver nitrate, $AgNO_3$ (*lapis infernalis*, or lunar caustic, as it was later called by the alchemists), was reported as early as 69 B.C. in the Roman Pharmacopeia (Hill and Pillsbury 1939) and continued until modern days as a bland antibiotic for topical applications. Other silver-based drugs, mainly containing this metal under the form of colloidal solutions, Ag(I) proteinates (Vaupel 2005), silver salts and silver sulfadiazine, have been widely used during the twentieth century for their bactericidal properties, before the advent of antibiotics decreased their applications against infections. Nevertheless in the past few years, as the phenomenon of antibiotic resistance became more and more alarming, such compounds regained popularity, since silver does not induce resistance, except in rare or transient cases. Gold salts and arsenic compounds, on the other hand, have already been in use for decades in the treatment of rheumatoid arthritis and syphilis.

The real breakthrough of metal-based drugs occurred in the 1960s when Cisplatin demonstrated to inhibit cellular division in *E. coli*, leading to the first studies on its antitumour activity in rats and its assessment as one of the most powerful chemotherapeutics ever. After nearly 50 years, and although many other novel metal-based compounds exhibited a high potential as antitumor agents, Cisplatin and a few other derivatives of this complex are still the lead drugs for the treatment of several kinds of cancer, in spite of their toxicity and severe drawbacks, with rare contenders. Nonetheless, the astounding success of Cisplatin drew the attention of the scientific community on the impressive biomedical features shown by coordination compounds so that also gold, silver, ruthenium, palladium and the rest of the so-called noble elements became the topic of intensive investigation. Within a few years after Cisplatin discovery, a large assortment of metal complexes had been synthesized and tested in the pharmacological field, mostly as anticancer, but also as anti-inflammatory, antibacterial, anti-rheumatic and antimalarial drugs. Still, their applications against tumours are the most desirable and numerous (Medici et al. 2015).

Besides complexes, the colloidal state is another form in which noble metals can exert their biological action, as in the case of silver and gold nanoparticles. Although the efficacy of metal nanoparticles against cancer and bacteria or as theranostics has been thoroughly demonstrated, there is still debate about their safety. Nevertheless, colloidal gold, silver, iridium, ruthenium and rhodium are commonly sold as dietary supplements, and claims have been made by 'alternative' medicine they can be effective remedies against many diseases, free radicals and bacteria, or to prevent ageing and mental decay.

1.2 Platinum

Although gold salts had been tested against tuberculosis and were employed as antirheumatics as early as 1929 (Healy et al. 2009), Cisplatin (*cis*-diamminedichloroplatinum(II), *cis*-$[PtCl(NH_3)_2Cl_2]$) (Rosenberg et al. 1965, 1969) is considered the forerunner of modern noble metal applications in medicine, and the design of novel chemotherapeutics was, and still is, often inspired by its structural features. The fortuitous discovery of its properties in 1965 led to one of the main innovations in the treatment of cancer, nearly nullifying the mortality for testicular tumours with about 98% of survival rate, and bringing impressive improvements also against ovarian, bladder, neck and small cell lung cancer. In spite of the fact that Cisplatin activity is limited to a small range of tumours and it exhibits numerous and severe drawbacks, so that several derivatives have been prepared in order to overcome these problems (Bruijnincx and Sadler 2008; Gabano et al. 2009; Lovejoy and Lippard 2009; Harper et al. 2010; Wang 2010; Komeda and Casini 2012, Wang and Guo 2013), Cisplatin is still the lead compound and extensively used against various types of cancer. Among the platinum derivatives, Carboplatin and Oxaliplatin are globally diffused and applied in the medical practice, and Nedaplatin, Lobaplatin and Heptaplatin are more used in Asia, while Satraplatin and Picoplatin are still under trial (Fig. 1.1).

Cisplatin mechanism of action is based on the interaction with the DNA double strand of the two aqua species, *cis*-$[PtCl(NH_3)_2(H_2O)]^+$ and *cis*-$[Pt(NH_3)_2(H_2O)_2]^{2+}$, obtained through the successive displacement of two chloride ions by water molecules via a process called aquation within the cellular environment. One of the two water ligands can be in turn displaced by a DNA base, normally a guanine. The second water molecule can be finally replaced by another nucleotide to form cross-links. DNA platination leads to adducts which are mainly 1,2-intrastrand cross-links of adjacent deoxyguanosines with platinum binding to the N7 positions of the bases. Minor adducts include 1,2-intrastrand cross-links of adenine–guanine pairs and longer range intra- and interstrand cross-links involving guanine bases (Dasari and Tchounwou 2014).

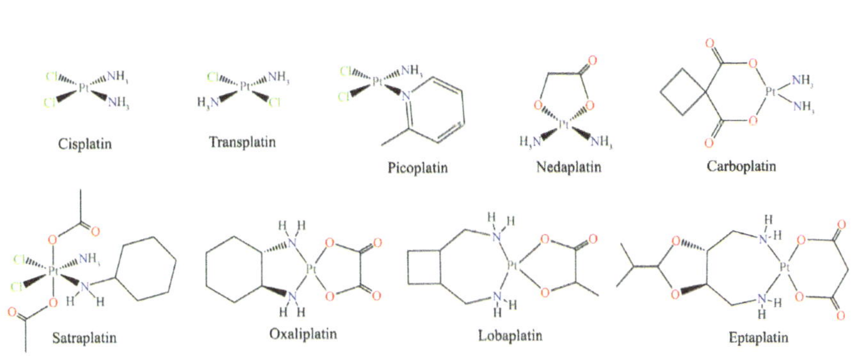

Fig. 1.1 Platinum complexes admitted to the medical practice

Cisplatin binding to DNA can induce cytotoxicity by interfering with transcription and/or DNA replication mechanisms, but causes also a permanent DNA damage which cannot be restored by normal repair devices. Such damage results in cell death via induction of apoptosis (Todd and Lippard 2009) mediated by the activation of various signal transduction pathways, including calcium signalling, death receptor signalling and the activation of mitochondrial pathways (Dasari and Tchounwou 2014).

Being DNA the primary Cisplatin target (Roberts and Thomson 1979; Lippard 1982), this drug is unable to distinguish between sick and healthy cells, as most of the antineoplastic agents, causing extensive systemic toxicity. Moreover, owed to platinum high affinity for sulphur and selenium donors present in many proteins and peptides, Cisplatin can also interact with and disrupt the functions of different proteins and enzymes, leading to a series of severe drawbacks, such as nephro-, hepato-, oto- and neurotoxicity, decreased blood cell and platelet production in bone marrow (myelosuppression), decreased response to infections (immunosuppression), hair loss, gastrointestinal disorders, anaemia, etc.

Another serious inconvenient of Cisplatin is that it frequently induces resistance and its efficacy can be lost after some chemotherapy cycles as tumour cells learn how to counteract the drug. The way they orchestrate such a defence is still under discussion: enhancement of DNA repair pathways, detoxification of the drug (e.g. inactivation by glutathione) or changes in uptake and efflux of the drug may be three of the possible mechanisms, which moreover can work synergistically (Stordal and Davey 2007). The result is that also Cisplatin derivatives sharing the same DNA binding pattern and cytotoxicity pathways are able to induce cross-resistance to Cisplatin itself.

The development of different strategies to avoid both toxicity and resistance is highly desirable, and it is based on suitable structural modifications of Cisplatin scaffold or functionalization (Komeda and Casini 2012; Johnstone et al. 2016). For instance, the use of bulky ligands (vide infra): *cis*-Pt(II) compounds with sterically hindered amines (e.g. Picoplatin) are able to form DNA adducts in an analogous way as Cisplatin, but their interaction with thiol-containing molecules is less effective, thus hindering the cell adaptive improvement of the detoxification mechanisms mediated by glutathione and metallothioneins.

Another option could be the employment of *trans*-Pt(II) species (vide infra): once *trans*-diamminedichloroplatinum (Transplatin) were dismissed as therapeutically ineffective compared to its *cis* stereoisomer, *trans* complexes have been long overlooked, but are now raising attention as promising anticancer agents following the experimental evidences slowly emerging. Substitution of the two ammonia ligands with a gamut of amines sided by N-donor heterocyclic ligands gives complexes which platinate DNA with significant toxicity, while those in which the two chlorides have been replaced by acetate groups, and bear bulky aromatic ligands are effective against Cisplatin-resistant cancers.

The third approach to circumvent resistance is the use of polynuclear Pt(II) compounds (vide infra), in which two or more platinum centres are linked by aliphatic polyamine ligands (spermine, spermidine, etc.). The way polynuclear species bind DNA is different with respect to Cisplatin and its derivatives: cationic polynuclear Pt(II) complexes, for instance, are able to bind DNA through non-covalent interactions. Their positive charge can give rise to electrostatic (non-coordinative) pre-association with DNA, which in turn is negatively charged, before the formation of coordinative interactions, so that they produce a more extended damage and hairpin loops that can elude the repairing mechanisms activated by the cell.

While considering the disadvantages of using Cisplatin in cancer treatment, the scarce bioavailability and lack of selectivity of this drug cannot be ignored. In fact, after administration Cisplatin reaches DNA in very low amounts (less than 1% of the administered dose gets to the target, being mostly dispersed within the plasma and the cells via the bonding with a plethora of other coordinating molecules), causing platinum overload of the organism and development of the aforementioned drawbacks. One way to overcome this problem is the use of carriers that can increase the drug availability by a better transport system (nanoparticles, liposomes, micelles, polymers, etc.) or the attachment to specific carriers, such as hormones, that can selectively deliver the platinum drug to the cancer cells, thus saving the healthy ones.

All these problems and disadvantages led to the preparation of numerous novel platinum complexes with a wide range of ligands or ligand combinations both in the attempt of improving Cisplatin performances and also in the search for a completely different alternative to the lead drug, with different mechanisms of action and less prone to resistance.

1.2.1 Polynuclear Pt(II) Complexes

As previously mentioned, polynuclear platinum complexes may adopt different cytotoxic mechanisms with respect to Cisplatin that can enhance their anticancer action. For instance, in the case of the azolato-bridged dinuclear complex $[\{cis\text{-Pt}(NH_3)_2\}_2(\mu\text{-OH})(\mu\text{-pyrazolate})]^{2+}$ (AMPZ), the efficiency against several tumour cell lines was considerably higher than Cisplatin. It was demonstrated, for the first time on this system, that little conformational distortions induced by AMPZ in highly polymeric DNA with a random nucleotide sequence are less efficiently mended by DNA repair systems than those induced by Cisplatin (Mlcouskova et al. 2012). This can improve the antitumour effects of such new compounds, also considering that a tetrazolato-bridged dinuclear platinum(II) complex has markedly high in vivo antitumour activity against pancreatic cancer, indicating this species as potentially active against non-Cisplatin responsive tumours (Komeda et al. 2011).

An analogous disruptive effect on DNA, but driven by a more complex mechanism, was found for a tridentate trinuclear Pt(II) complex, $[Pt_3Cl_3(hptab)]^{3+}$ (hptab = N,N,N′,N′,N″,N″-hexakis(2-pyridylmethyl)-1,3,5-tris(aminomethyl)benzene), which has remarkable cytotoxic effects in human and mouse tumour cells, including some Cisplatin-resistant strains (Olivova et al. 2011). While elucidating the coordination modes of $[Pt_3Cl_3(hptab)]^{3+}$ towards DNA, it was found that, in the absence of other biological targets, this complex is able to form trifunctional intrastrand cross-links with the duplex. Instead, when proteins are present, as it happens in the cellular milieu, the complex is able to cross-link proteins to DNA. Moreover, when a molecular crowding agent is added to mimic environmental conditions in cell nucleus, the trinuclear species cross-links two DNA duplexes in a high yield, a feature here observed for the first time in antitumour trinuclear platinum complexes (Olivova et al. 2011). Other dinuclear complexes with aromatic diamine and picoline derivatives when tested against cancer cells yielded comparable or higher cytotoxicity than Cisplatin, but with different cellular responses with respect to those caused by the lead drug (Bielawska et al. 2010; Lin et al. 2011).

Finally, in the scenery of polynuclear compounds, it is important to report the results achieved with mixed multinuclear Ru(III)/Pt(II) complexes as potential antineoplastic and antimetastatic agents, which are encouraging and open new perspectives on this topic (Pelletier et al. 2010; González-Pantoja et al. 2011; Wenzel et al. 2011; Anderson et al. 2012; Nieto et al. 2012).

1.2.2 Trans-Pt(II) Derivatives

Trans-platinum complexes are not only able to bind DNA (Quiroga 2012), in analogy with their *cis* counterparts, but they can also target different proteins, as reported for *trans*-Pt(II) species bearing aliphatic amines (Cubo et al. 2010a). Transplatin derivatives in which one of the canonical NH_3 ligands is replaced by aromatic N-heterocycles (such as pyridine, thiazole and quinoline) display a cytotoxicity similar to Cisplatin, but almost no cross-resistance. Their design is based on the use of more labile leaving groups (e.g. carboxylates), and their interaction with different kinds of DNA evidences the synergistic effects of different structural modifications, all leading to DNA damage (Musetti et al. 2011). The substitution of NH_3 with pyridine ligands seems to afford more efficient alternatives to Transplatin. For example, when 2-(2-hydroxyethyl)pyridine (2-hepy) is used, the corresponding *trans*-$[PtCl_2(2\text{-hepy})_2]$ species possesses higher anticancer activity compared to Transplatin, Cisplatin, Carboplatin and Oxaliplatin (Icsel et al. 2013). Also oxime-containing *trans*-configured Pt(II) complexes can be rather active, like in the case of *trans*-$[PtCl_2(Me_2C = NOH)_2]$ which is up to 20 times more potent than Cisplatin depending on the cancer cell line tested (Scaffidi-Domianello et al. 2010).

Very promising results have been obtained by introducing sulfonamide ligands into *trans* complexes (Pérez et al. 2014; Agudo-López et al. 2017). Sulfonamides are commonly employed as antibiotics, anticonvulsants and also enzyme inhibitors. A series of *trans*-Pt(II) mono-sulfonamide complexes have been tested for their antiproliferative activity against a panel of representative human tumour cells using Cisplatin as the reference drug. They exhibited a much higher activity depending on the structure of the sulfonamide ligand, the cellular line tested, and interestingly, also on the halide used as the anionic ligand (chloride or iodide). When chiral sulfonamides have been used, one of the two enantiomers was more efficient than the other, showing that chiral conformation matters in these cases (del Solar et al. 2013).

1.2.3 Pt(II) and Pt(IV) Carriers

Scarce bioavailability is one of the major problems concerning platinum drugs, since absorption by the gastrointestinal tract is hardly avoidable and during the travel towards their target, the Pt(II) ions meet a number of possible coordinating species able to sequester and deactivate them. Intravenous administration can help, but again the amount of Pt(II) ions getting to the target is still very low. Poor selectivity is another issue, for platinum drugs attack both healthy and sick cells. One approach to circumvent these troubles may be the derivatization of Pt-drugs with appropriate carriers. In this way, the drug could be transported across the cellular membrane and/or be selectively directed towards cancer cells. Targeting and delivery strategies are based on two kinds of mechanisms: active or passive transport paths. A wide range of nanocarriers (nanoparticles, micelles, liposomes and polymers) can be used as passive transporters (Xiao et al. 2011; Rafi et al. 2012; Kraszewski et al. 2013; Oberoi et al. 2013; Silva et al. 2013a, b; Wang and Guo 2013), based on their physical–chemical properties or by taking advantage of the biological differences between normal and cancerous cells metabolism to increase selectivity. In the latter case, permeability and retention effects can be both exploited: macromolecules have a higher permeability in tumour tissues, where they can accumulate due to a scarce lymphatic clearance and slow venous return (Matsumura and Maeda 1986; Maeda et al. 2009). On the other hand, platinum complexes are relatively small so that they can rapidly cross the membranes of both normal and cancerous tissues and then be cleared, but when they are grafted to liposomes, micelles and polymeric carriers, they selectively concentrate in neoplastic cells (Maeda et al. 2009).

Sensitivity to hormones, like estrogens and progesterone in some breast and ovarian cancers, or testosterone in prostate cancer, can be exploited for active transportation of platinum drugs. In fact, hormones bind to receptors on the tumour cells and induce modifications in the expression of specific genes, leading to an increase in cell growth. When platinum complexes are appended to a hormone or a suitable derivative, they can get inside the cancer cell with higher efficacy and selectivity. Platinum complexes have been derivatized with androgens (Huxley et al. 2010), testosterone derivatives (Fortin et al. 2013), estradiol (Kvasnica et al. 2012; Saha et al. 2012, Brasseur et al. 2013; Zhang et al. 2013) and lipophilic ethisterone (Ruiz et al. 2011a, b), and scored better performances than the reference traditional metallo-drugs both in targeting and efficiency. Also peptides, proteins, carbohydrates and bisphosphonates (the latter used for bone strengthening and prevention of bone mass loss in osteoporosis patients) have been used as carriers with different results (Wang and Guo 2013). Another interesting consideration is that glucose metabolism and glucose dependence are increased in cancer cells; for this reason, polysaccharides too could be used as carriers and a key to penetrate neoplastic tissues (Wild et al. 2012).

Finally, carbon nanoparticles (Biswas and Torchilin 2014; Sakhrani and Padh 2013; Yoong et al. 2014) or properly functionalized peptides (Chen et al. 2013a, b; Wisnovsky et al. 2013) can be designed to carry and deliver platinum complexes to mitochondria, where they can cause apoptosis by binding to mitochondrial DNA (mtDNA). This could diminish the chemotherapy side effects since platinum drugs-mediated mtDNA disruption per se is able to induce cell death without damaging nuclear DNA.

1.2.4 Pt(IV) Complexes

Pt(IV) octahedral complexes (like Iproplatin and Satraplatin) are less reactive towards biomolecules such as proteins and enzymes compared to Pt(II) compounds, resulting in a lower cytotoxicity, and they produce fewer side effects on the organism. Furthermore, Pt(IV) complexes with carboxylate axial ligands (e.g. Satraplatin) are better absorbed by the gastrointestinal tract than their divalent counterparts, show improved toxicity profiles and reduced cross-resistance to Cisplatin, and can be orally administered while all of the currently marketed platinum analogues must be dispensed via intravenous infusion (Bhargava and Vaishampayan 2009).

The strategy behind Pt(IV) complexes design is often to prepare octahedral derivatives of clinically established platinum(II) compounds, such as Oxaliplatin (Göschl et al. 2017) or Carboplatin (Almotairy et al. 2017), with better pharmacokinetics, less side effects and reduced resistance. Pt(IV) species are considered as prodrugs, leading to Pt(II) active species via an 'activation by reduction' mechanism. Reduction can take place anywhere in the body to form reactive metabolites for DNA targeting.

Reduction is not the only mechanism to produce active species (Cubo et al. 2011): light, for instance, is involved in the activation of new Pt(IV) species, which are normally inactive or modestly active in the dark and are selectively activated by UV and/or visible light. Such Pt(IV) complexes generally have *trans* configuration and bind two (not necessarily equal) N-donor ligands, such as amines (Cubo et al. 2010b), imines (Farrer et al. 2010), azido ligands (Farrer et al. 2010; Westendorf et al. 2011, 2012) or mixed diazido-amine systems (Zhao et al. 2013). When one or two ammino ligands are substituted by pyridine, the efficiency of the complex is enhanced, even up to 50–65 times higher than Cisplatin under the same conditions (Farrer et al. 2010). Elucidation of the activation mechanism evidenced that under light of the proper wavelength, one or more ligands are dissociated to give different active Pt(II) photoproducts, seldom Pt(IV) species, able to target DNA and damage it in a way that cannot be recognized by HMGB1 protein, in contrast to

Cisplatin-type lesions (Zhao et al. 2013), or to cause death through non-apoptotic pathways (Westendorf et al. 2012).

1.2.5 Looking for New Anticancer Pt(II) Drugs

The fortuitous recognition of Cisplatin anticancer properties demonstrates that the discovery of an effective metallo-drug is often serendipitous and can be a matter of sheer luck. Thus, the search for an alternative to Cisplatin, with higher selectivity and efficacy, and fewer drawbacks, is mainly carried out towards two directions: making changes on Cisplatin structure in order to tune its characteristics and adjust its properties, or trying something completely new and hope to make a big discovery. Nevertheless, another very common approach is to replace the conventional ligands with drugs or other molecules that possess biological activity per se, expecting a synergistic effect leading to a massive increase in a metal's efficacy.

As previously seen, sulfonamides have been used in *trans*-Pt(II) complexes with interesting results (vide supra). Another example is given by thiosemicarbazones (Fig. 1.2), a class of compounds with relevant biological properties (antiviral, antifungal, antibacterial, antitumour, anticarcinogenic and insulin mimetic). In particular, Triapine (3-aminopyridine-2-carboxaldehyde thiosemicarbazone, Vion Pharmaceuticals, New Haven, CT), a small molecule chelator that blocks a critical step in DNA synthesis by inhibiting ribonuclease reductase, is currently under screening for antitumour activity using the National Cancer Institute panel of 60 tumour cell lines and was successful against cervical cancer in Phase I and II clinical trials (Liu et al. 1992, 1995; Finch et al. 1999, 2000; Alvero et al. 2006), also in association with Cisplatin and radiation. Different thiosemicarbazones have been thus used to develop platinum complexes with high cytotoxicity, low nephrotoxicity and good activity against normal and resistant cancer lines (Gomez et al. 2011; Karakucuk-Iyidogan et al. 2011; Mansouri-Torshizi et al. 2011; Matesanz et al. 2011a, b, 2012; Ibrahim et al. 2014). Other Pt(II) complexes have been prepared using a range of antitumour agents, such as podophyllotoxin (Liu et al. 2013a, b, c), camptothecin (Cincinelli et al. 2013) and endoxifen (Ding et al. 2013), all showing interesting results for their high cytotoxicity and DNA cleavage capabilities.

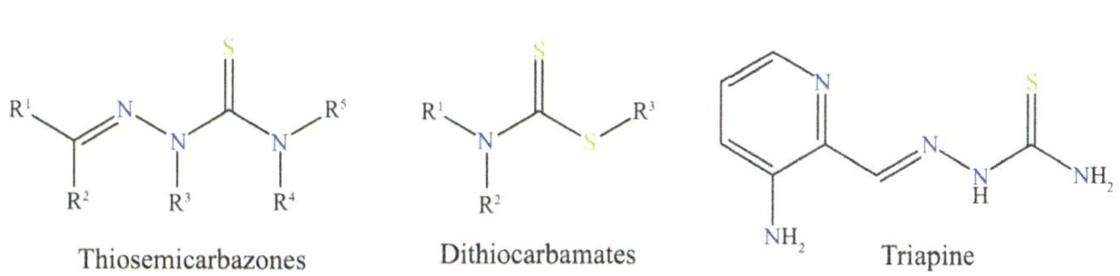

Fig. 1.2 N,S-based drugs used as ligands for Pt(II) complexes

Another approach to obtain efficient anticancer agents is to use intercalating molecules, such as polypyridines and other polycyclic aromatic derivatives, as the ligands. In fact, DNA binding with metallointercalators results in a covalent interaction causing the double helix disentanglement and facilitating π-stacking interactions between the ring cloud of the base pairs and the intercalating planar aromatic systems. Although research on this topic is rather dated (Lippard and co-workers in the late 1970s), platinum complexes with pyridines (Icsel et al. 2013), bipyridines (Coban et al. 2013), terpyridines (Wei et al. 2013), phenanthrolines (Davis et al. 2012; Shahabadi and Nemati 2012; Coban et al. 2013), naphthalene (Duskova et al. 2012), anthraquinones (Ruiz et al. 2011a, b) and their derivatives continue to be synthesized and tested for their possible anticancer activity, effectiveness of DNA binding, DNA cleavage and telomerase inhibition activity.

1.2.6 Other Biological Activities

Pt complexes are mainly designed and prepared for their potential antineoplastic action. Nevertheless, due to the fact that cytotoxicity on cancer cells and bacteria is based almost on the same mechanisms, they often possess also antibacterial properties, and the two activities are frequently evaluated together. For example, Pt(II) complexes with benzothiazoline ligands are effective against fungi (*Fusarium oxysporum* and *Alternaria alternata*) and bacteria (*Pseudomonas aeruginosa* and *Escherichia coli*) (Sharma et al. 2011), while Pt(II) dithiocarbazate species containing triphenylphosphine as the co-ligand are more active against *Trypanosoma cruzi* than the reference drugs for this parasite (Maia et al. 2010).

Finally, an unexpected property for a platinum derivative is the ability to reduce amyloid plaques in the brain tissue of transgenic mouse models affected by Alzheimer's disease as demonstrated by a Pt(II) complex with a quinoline ligand (Kenche et al. 2013).

1.3 Palladium

Pd(II) coordination chemistry is very similar to that of Pt(II) ions; thus, palladium could appear as the perfect alternative to platinum in the design of novel metallo-drugs. Nonetheless, Pd(II) complexes differ from platinum analogues in several features, and perhaps this is the reason why palladium was long overlooked in anticancer research, regaining interest only a decade or two ago. Pd(II) complexes are more labile than their Pt(II) counterparts, as the tendency to exchange their ligands is about 10^5 times higher, leading to a fast hydrolysis of palladium species. Such a rapid dissociation of the complexes produces very active species able to react with any donor they meet in the bloodstream and the cellular milieu, a process that prevents them from getting to their target (DNA) and at the same times produces extended toxic effects. A decrease in the hydrolysis rate can be achieved by the use of bulky chelating ligands, for instance, while the complex could be effectively stabilized by strongly coordinating donors (e.g. N-containing ligands) and an accurate selection of the leaving group(s). In this way, the in vivo structural integrity of the complex could be maintained long enough to accomplish its therapeutic action. Another feature distinguishing palladium from platinum is that the former mainly gives *trans* isomers, so that some *cis*-Pd(II) complexes spontaneously change into their *trans* derivatives, which cannot be considered as a negative aspect at all since, when *cis* and *trans* complexes of both platinum and palladium were compared, most *trans*-palladium species showed higher activity than their *cis*-platinum analogues, even comparable or higher than those of Cisplatin, Carboplatin and Oxaliplatin in vitro (al-Allaf and Rashan 2001). Moreover, Pd-complexes are more soluble compared to platinum, which is an advantage in view of their administration and bioavailability.

Pd(II) complexes evidenced cytotoxic activity against a number of cancers, such as human cervical epitheloid carcinoma, human chronic myelogenous leukaemia, osteogenic sarcoma, malignant melanoma, breast cancer, lung cancer, glioma, human colorectal adenocarcinoma, head and neck squamous cancer, prostate cancer and ovarian cancer (Medici et al. 2015).

In analogy with platinum, the structural variety of Pd(II) compounds for antitumor applications is ruled by sulphur-containing ligands such as thiosemicarbazones and thiocarbamates (Fig. 1.2), nitrogen-based heterocycles (pyridines, bipy, terpy, phenanthrolines and quinolines) or more often a combination of them. Also polyamines forming polynuclear complexes have been employed. Sometimes these Pd(II) complexes exhibit higher activity than their Pt(II) analogues, some other just comparable to Cisplatin and other approved Pt-drugs.

1.3.1 Pd(II) Complexes with Sulphur-Containing Ligands

As previously mentioned thiosemicarbazones show relevant biological properties against viruses, bacteria and cancer. In particular, compounds in which the thiosemicarbazone side chain bears an N-heterocyclic ring in α position, namely, α-N-heterocyclic thiosemicarbazones, have evidenced good antineoplastic action per se and a strong tendency to chelate metals. By introducing them as ligands in transition metal complexes, their activity should improve, as demonstrated by some Pd(II) derivatives which revealed to be more active than thiosemicarbazone alone, with antiproliferative action similar to or higher than Cisplatin, even against resistant tumour cells or in non-Cisplatin responsive cancers (Matesanz et al. 2013).

Effective Pd(II) complexes with thiosemicarbazones can be prepared in the form of both mono- (Jagadeesh et al. 2013) and bis-chelated species, or sided by co-ligands such as planar N-heterocycles (Gomez et al. 2011), phosphines (Matesanz et al. 2011a, b; Kalaivani et al. 2012a, b; Hernandez et al. 2013) and even arsines (Prabhakaran et al. 2013). An interesting modification in thiosemicarbazones design may be a suitable derivatization with N-heterocycles (Afrasiabi et al. 2013; Matesanz et al. 2013) in order to exploit the intercalative properties of the planar aromatic moiety, especially in resistant cancers. Most of these complexes, besides being evaluated as antitumour drugs, exhibit intriguing antimicrobial properties.

Another class of ligands exploited in Pd(II) complexes are dithiocarbamates, a family of biologically active molecules which have been tested for their efficiency at preventing Cisplatin-induced nephrotoxicity, caused by platinum binding and inactivation of thiol-containing enzymes. Dithiocarbamates (Fig. 1.2) have a high propensity to coordinate transition metals, and their Pt(II) and Pd(II) complexes possess both a high antitumour activity and a reduced toxicity, compared to Cisplatin and related compounds. Hence, the strong bonds between platinum (or palladium) and dithiocarbamates may hinder metal interaction with sulphur-containing renal proteins, preventing, or at least reducing, their nephrotoxicity. Finally, Pd(II) mixed ligand dithiocarbamate-amine species not only possess antitumour activity comparable to Cisplatin but are also able to avoid cross-resistance (Buac et al. 2012; Hogarth 2012).

1.3.2 Multinuclear Pd(II) Complexes

Polynuclear Pd(II) complexes with polyamines, as the analogous di- and trinuclear Pt(II) species, were conceived to cause a more extended damage to DNA, by blocking repair mechanisms and development of resistance in cancer cells treated with Cisplatin and its derivatives. They demonstrated to exert high cytotoxic effects both in vitro and in vivo when compared to many platinum-based anticancer drugs; nevertheless, none of these compounds have yet entered the clinical trials. Although Pt(II) and Pd(II) complexes share some aspects in their mode of action as cytotoxic agents, it is improbable that structure–activity relationships attributed to platinum species can be successfully exploited also in Pd(II) systems. Thus, the interactions of the polynuclear Pd(II) complexes with DNA should have completely different bases compared to Pt(II) analogues.

Spermine is the most used diamine ligand in Pd(II) dinuclear complexes with high activity against tumours (Tummala et al. 2010; Fiuza et al. 2011). Their mechanism of interaction with DNA is still under study, but it is clear that such an interaction is very specific, as it induces deformation and local denaturation of B-DNA structures with the release of guanine bases (Corduneanu et al. 2010). The DNA strands partially split to allow palladium intra- and interstrand cross-links, leading to the formation of DNA adducts and aggregates.

Norspermidine is a triamine found in some species of plants, bacteria and algae, but not in humans, and it possesses antineoplastic activity against different types of tumours in mice. Thus, its trinuclear Pd(II) complex has been studied for its anticancer properties, demonstrating that this compound is more active than the Pt(II) analogue, leading to growth inhibition and cell death in different cancer cell lines.

Another interesting aspect is that both norspermidine and its Pd(II) complex are able to abate the number of colonies in breast cancer cell lines, evidencing their potential in reducing such malignancies (Silva et al. 2013a, b).

1.3.3 Other Biological Activities

Palladium complexes with isonicotinamide are more active against *Mycobacterium tuberculosis* than isonicotinamide as such and pyrazinamide (de Souza et al. 2010), and this represents good news in a scenario where the search for new antituberculosis drugs is highly desirable, since Rifampicin, the last class of antibiotics introduced for the first-line treatment, was discovered more than 50 years ago. Moreover, this disease, which seemed vanquished only a couple of decades ago, has regained vitality as a consequence of migration fluxes from the poorest countries. The treatment of tuberculosis is long and costly, based on a 6-month regimen over a mix of antibiotics, but it is ineffective against multidrug and extensive drug-resistant strains and incompatible with many antiretroviral drugs, so that new advances in this field are strongly recommended. Also palladium complexes with antibiotic drugs, such as capreomycin, kanamycin and ofloxacin, have been evaluated for their activity against tuberculosis, both on the *M. tuberculosis* strain and tuberculosis-infected THP-1 (human leukaemia) cell lines. The results indicate that such complexes have extracellular activity comparable to that of their parent drugs and show an improved efficacy against intracellular infection of *M. tuberculosis* (Giovagnoli et al. 2014).

Pd(II) compounds with new steroidal thiosemicarbazones, in turn, possess a remarkable antibacterial activity against *Staphylococcus aureus*, *Streptococcus pyogenes*, *Salmonella typhimurium* and *E. coli* compared to the reference drug, amoxicillin (Asiri and Khan 2010).

A completely different application of palladium in the medical practice involves its ^{103}Pd isotope in the so-called brachytherapy, an internal radiotherapy used in the treatment of cancer (mainly cervical, prostate, breast and skin cancer). ^{103}Pd is the radiation source placed inside or close to the area requiring treatment. Recently, this approach has been also applied to ophthalmology for the treatment of T3- and T4-staged choroidal melanomas (Semenova and Finger 2013, 2014).

1.4 Silver

Silver (Ag) has been used in medicine to heal burns and wounds since very early historical ages, while in recent times, its biological properties have been mainly exploited against bacteria rather than anticancer therapy (although its efficacy has been recognized also in the latter field), contrarily to most of the other noble metals. In fact, silver is not (or almost not highly) toxic to humans, but lethal to lower organisms. Before the introduction of antibiotics, colloidal silver was commonly used in hospitals as a bactericide, and lately is regaining interest as antibiotic resistance is becoming a serious threat to human health. Moreover, silver is currently considered as an 'alternative' drug against a number of pathologies and diseases, especially on the Internet.

During the past century, silver salts were used to treat infections as gonorrhoea, syphilis, conjunctivitis and gastroenteritis. A diluted solution of silver nitrate ($AgNO_3$) was the only therapy for neonatal conjunctivitis (the so-called Credé method, after the physician introduced this practice in 1881), but also found application in the treatment of burns (Bellinger and Conway 1970) and cutaneous warts (Sterling et al. 2001).

Silver proteinates (e.g. Protargol and Argyrol) were used against venereal diseases (Vaupel 2005). Argyrol was also applied against local infections in mucous membrane-lined organs, and to prevent gonorrheal blindness and other ophthalmic infections in infants.

Silver sulfadiazine is an Ag(I) complex with a sulfonamide antibiotic discovered in the 1960s and introduced in the medical practice to prevent burn wounds infection, but also to heal skin wounds in general. Silver sulfadiazine is reported on the World Health Organization's List of Essential Medicines and is still commercially available and recommended, in spite of a long-lasting dispute about its effectiveness and side effects (Storm-Versloot et al. 2010; Wasiak et al. 2013). Nevertheless, and regardless of the lack of controlled comparative studies, silver sulfadiazine is still considered by many clinicians as one of the topical anti-infective agents of choice in burn patients (Monafo and West 1990; Palmieri and Greenlaugh 2002; Atiyeh et al. 2007; Castellano et al. 2007), and there are new studies about its possible advanced applications.

Silver toxic effects against lower organisms (although not recognized) have been acknowledged and exploited for centuries, but only recently, the mechanisms behind such toxicity have slowly been unveiled. They depend on both the nature of the silver compound and its cellular targets; nevertheless, they all share a common aspect: the biologically active species is always the silver cation, Ag^+, whether released by silver salts, complexes or nanoparticles.

The cytotoxic mechanisms of silver ions are based on a series of damages caused by Ag^+ to bacteria, fungi and protozoa, but seem to be also applicable to cancer cells (Ebrahiminezhad et al. 2016; Medici et al. 2016):

- Ion exchange disruption: Ag^+ inhibits phosphate uptake and exchange while increasing the release of K^+ ions, leading to cell death via impairment of proton motive force through the cytoplasmic membrane.
- Complex formation between Ag^+ and DNA or RNA, determining malfunctions in replication processes.
- Enzyme inactivation and protein denaturation by Ag^+ binding with thiol and phosphate moieties, but also with other O- and N-donor groups on proteins and enzymes (Banti et al. 2012, 2014) or selenium in the selenoenzyme thioredoxin reductase (Pellei et al. 2012).

- Disruption of cell and mitochondrial membranes by Ag^+ interaction causes structural modification (Lemire et al. 2013) leading to membrane ruptures and inducing a massive leakage of protons (Dibrov et al. 2002). Moreover, silver can disturb mitochondrial homeostasis leading to its dysregulation and membrane depolarization (Eloy et al. 2012; Li et al. 2014a, b; Saturnino et al. 2016).

The examination of such mechanisms explains why silver seldom causes the development of resistance in bacteria, which is instead rather frequent with classic antibiotics. Actually, bacterial resistance to silver is very rare and often transitory (Silver 2003; Percival et al. 2005). Only a single case is reported about a silver-resistant strain of *Pseudomonas stutzeri* isolated in a silver mine (Slawson et al. 1994), while three silver resistance genes were identified in *E. coli* isolates with extended-spectrum beta-lactamases of the CTX-M type (Sütterlin et al. 2014). The fact that clinical incidence of silver-resistant bacteria is negligible may be due to silver multiple disruptive mechanisms and its different targets within the bacterial cells (Percival et al. 2005) making adaptive countermeasures difficult to build up.

The lethal behaviour of silver on bacteria and other lower organisms seems not to extend to humans. A relevant number of studies assessed silver safety to mammals, but several others reported toxic evidences, and the discussion is still wide open. Nevertheless, the association of low toxicity with high biological activity is attractive and explains the renewed interest in silver-based drugs both as antibacterial and anticancer agents.

1.4.1 Silver Complexes

Research on Ag(I) complexes has evidenced their remarkable biological properties, as they possess antibacterial, antifungal, antiprotozoan, antimalarial (Rai et al. 2017) and anticancer (Medici et al. 2015, 2016) activity. The mechanisms behind silver toxicity have been previously discussed (vide supra).

The therapeutic efficiency of silver complexes depends on several factors: water solubility and stability, lipophilicity, redox behaviour and rate of silver ions release. The nature of the ligands and their steric and electronic properties are the features determining the above characteristics. Still, even the most accurate design of Ag(I) complexes for therapeutic applications can result in a failure under in vivo conditions since a series of drawbacks can affect the performances of the most promising metal species. In fact, although the activity of silver compounds as anticancer agents in vitro and their low cytotoxicity are well documented (Medici et al. 2015, 2016), the information about their in vivo activity is rather scarce or lacking. Nearly nothing is known about possible side effects that could occur after human administration of Ag(I) complexes, although silver per se is still considered to be non-toxic to humans and other mammalians. Moreover, the estimated bioavailability for Ag(I) coordination compounds, albeit low, is considered to be slightly higher than similar Pt(II) or Au(I) species in vitro, but it could be further decreased in vivo by precipitation as AgCl or sequestration as Ag-protein complexes. Encapsulation into biodegradable polymers could help encompass this problem.

However, these considerations do not stop the research, and novel silver complexes for therapeutic uses have been developed with a wide gamut of ligands, although those reporting the highest activities normally contain N-heterocyclic carbenes (NHC), phosphines and N-heterocycles (pyridines and polypyridines, phenanthrolines, etc.) (Medici et al. 2016).

Also in the case of silver coordination compounds, their design often incorporates other biologically active molecules as the ligands, with the aim of enhancing their performances in a synergistic way, although this might not always be the case. Usually, antibiotics (sulfachloropyridazine, sulfamoxole, metronidazole, vancomycin, etc.) and natural drugs or their derivatives (coumarin, salicylic acid, isonicotinic acid, etc.) have been employed for this purpose with discrete success (Medici et al. 2016).

A very interesting property of silver compounds is their activity against biofilms. Biofilms are one of the two growth ways for bacterial cells, so that they can be found either in a planktonic state, i.e. freely suspended as single cells in the aqueous media, or in sessile aggregates, adhering both to living and nonliving surfaces (Donlan 2002; Jamal et al. 2015). Such aggregates can be formed either by a single species or different types of microorganisms enclosed in a self-produced matrix of extracellular polymeric substances (EPS), mainly polysaccharides, but also incorporating proteins (including enzymes), DNA and RNA in an aqueous environment.

The typical example of a biofilm is dental plaque, but recently, it has been found that such bacterial assemblies are involved in most of the common infective processes, and that the EPS matrix is poorly penetrable by antibiotics and human immune system cells, so that bacteria in their sessile forms are 100–1000 times less susceptible to antibiotics than suspended species, thus posing a serious threat to public health. Silver sulfadiazine is one of the complexes showing higher activity against biofilms, especially against mature *P. aeruginosa* biofilms which are commonly diffused conditions in burn wounds (Bjarnsholt et al. 2007). It has been evidenced that the concentration of silver required to eradicate the biofilm is 10–100 times higher than that effective on planktonic forms, due to the resistance of bacterial aggregates to standard treatments. Another efficient class of Ag(I) complexes is based on N-heterocyclic carbenes (NHCs), especially the lipophilic Ag(I) species possessing aromatic groups on the NHC ligand, which have been screened against different bacterial strains (Bernardi et al. 2014).

Finally, a highly promising silver complex against biofilms is the ‘exotic’ silver oxynitrate, $Ag(Ag_3O_4)_2NO_3$, which is a mixed complex where both the Ag(II) and Ag(III) oxidation states stabilized by oxygen atoms coexist steadily at room temperature (Lemire et al. 2017). This complex has been tested against a series of bacterial strains and their antibiotic-resistant counterparts with considerably better results than a wide gamut of silver salts, oxides and complexes (Lemire et al. 2015). It was also demonstrated, via biocompatibility tests, that $Ag(Ag_3O_4)_2NO_3$ is safe for cytotoxicity, acute systemic toxicity, irritation and sensitization, opening the path to its use in the medical practice (Kalan et al. 2017).

Being the toxicological profile of orally administered silver still to be resolved, topical application for the treatment of chronic wounds remains the favoured way of administration, also for the new drugs under trial.

1.5 Ruthenium

Ruthenium is without doubt Cisplatin heir in the present search for therapeutic agents, with impressive efforts devoted to the synthesis of new Ru(II) and Ru(III) complexes as potential anticancer drugs and to the elucidation of their mechanism(s) of action. Ruthenium compounds have also been investigated, such as those containing antibiotics, antiviral and antimalarial agents.

The first ruthenium complexes with biological activity were reported in 1980, when some Cisplatin analogues, i.e. chloro-ammine-Ru(III) compounds, showed anticancer activity in rats. Their action was limited due to low solubility, but 4 years later, a dimethylsulfoxide-Ru(II) species, *cis*-[$RuCl_2(dmso)_4$], although less effective but also less toxic than Cisplatin, was found to be active on both primary and metastatic cancers. Activity on metastatic cancers is an important feature common to other Ruthenium complexes, some of which have recently entered the clinic trials (Fig. 1.3).

Ruthenium species suitable for biomedical applications belong to Ru(II) and Ru(III) oxidation states, the latter appearing to be less reactive. Both states can form hexacoordinate octahedral species, affording a better control on the steric and electronic properties of the complex due to the two 'extra' axial ligands. The rate of ligands exchange in ruthenium complexes (within the range of 10^{-2}–10^{-3} s^{-1}) is comparable to that of platinum and stretches over the span of an average cell's

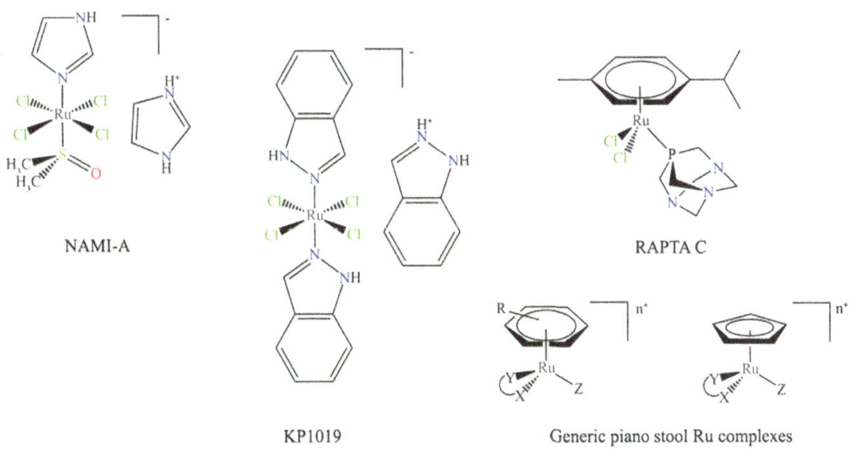

Fig. 1.3 Ruthenium complexes currently in clinical trials and generic 'piano stool' compounds

lifetime, conferring the molecules high kinetic stability and avoiding rapid equilibration processes. The complexes do not decompose during their journey towards the target and remain viable throughout their permanence inside the cell. Higher stability of the complexes can be achieved through a fine-tuning of the ligands so that even the unstable Ru(II) oxidation state can be maintained in oxygen-rich environments and physiological conditions, to give low-reactive species even when organometallic bonds are present.

Ru(III) complexes are considered as prodrugs due to their relative inertness compared to Ru(II) species. As in the case of Pt(IV) derivatives, it is believed that they should undergo 'activation by reduction' to transform into the active drug, although some researchers diverge from this opinion (Bergamo and Sava 2011). Such a mechanism, anyhow, seems to be more likely in solid tumours, where fast-growing cells with insufficient vascularisation lower the pH and induce a hypoxic (reducing) environment. Furthermore, transferrin is often overexpressed in tumour cells: since ruthenium is able to mimic iron while interacting with this protein (but also with albumin), it can exploit this fact to be transported and selectively enter the cancer tissues.

Although the mechanisms behind ruthenium antineoplastic activity are more intricate and less understood than those of platinum, it is clear that also in this case, DNA binding should be the main event, but other different interactions inside and outside the cancer cells are as well slowly being unveiled (Bergamo et al. 2012). Some ruthenium polypyridyl complexes, for instance, are able to induce apoptosis via mitochondrial pathways, due to disruption of mitochondrial membrane potential (Du et al. 2014) followed by release of cytochrome c (Chen et al. 2013a, b), or increase of reactive oxygen species levels (Lin et al. 2013; Qian et al. 2013; Ye et al. 2013). Lipophilic ruthenium complexes, on the other hand, can selectively accumulate in mitochondria (Pisani et al. 2010, 2011) inducing apoptosis via programmed mitochondria death.

Ru complexes possessing biological activity can be divided into three major classes: Ru-dimethylsulfoxide compounds (e.g. NAMI-A), Ru(III) complexes of the [LH]*trans*-$[RuCl_4(L)_2]$ type (e.g. KP1019) and organometallic Ru(II)-arene complexes with general formula $[(\eta^6\text{-arene})Ru(en)Cl][PF_6]$ (e.g. RAPTA-C). The three groups display different chemical and biological properties, which reflect on their in vivo anticancer activity: some compounds are effective against primary tumours, and others against metastases only. Thus, there is not a prevalent indication for the design of new active species (Bergamo et al. 2012).

1.5.1 Ruthenium–Arene Complexes

Arene–ruthenium-based anticancer drugs are characterized by an amphiphilic profile in which a hydrophobic arene ligand is bound to the hydrophilic metal centre; moreover, the synthetic flexibility of the arene moiety provides a versatile backbone on which different side chains for targeted chemotherapy may be appended (Süss-Fink 2010; Smith and Therrien 2011). The foremost cytotoxic ruthenium–arene complex was reported by Tocher et al. (1992), but the first prototypes of this family to be tested for their anticancer activity appeared in 2001: (η^6-p-MeC$_6$H$_4$Pri)Ru(P-pta)Cl$_2$ (pta = 1,3,5-triaza-7-phospha-tricyclo-[3.3.1.1] decane), named RAPTA-C, by Dyson's group, together with some analogues by Sadler. Although RAPTA-C exhibits only a low activity in vitro, it is very active in vivo against metastatic tumours. Following this synthetic indication, new organometallic Ru(II)-arene complexes have been prepared, also bearing phosphines, amines and sulfoxides as co-ligands (Komeda and Casini 2012).

Recently, an improvement in Ru-arene performances was sought through the introduction of intercalating ligands, causing an effective DNA cleavage and reporting activity comparable to Cisplatin (Ganeshpandian et al. 2014). The choice of the proper arene ligand is fundamental for the complex activity. The most exploited one is para-cymene, which has been associated with such an ample gamut of N, S and O donors that a thorough classification and description would go beyond the scopes of this chapter. The co-ligands involved in effective antiproliferative or cytotoxic responses, however, are mainly conjugated biological molecules or biologically active species such as peptides, antibiotic glycosides, flavones, curcumin, steroids, thiosemicarbazones, am(m)ines and heterocycles (Medici et al. 2015).

The employment of heterocyclic arene ligands such as mercaptobenzothiazole and mercaptobenzoxazole in half-sandwich arene-Ru complexes leads to a selective action against several cancer cell lines while sparing the healthy ones, with a mechanism involving a non-intercalative DNA interaction (Mitra et al. 2012). It has also been evidenced that substitution of the aromatic ring of the heterocycle, or addition of a second hydrogen-bond donor on the heterocycle itself, is able to decrease the cytotoxicity of the complex.

When the arene moiety is a cyclopentadienyl ligand, a high antitumour activity is achieved. The $[Ru(II)(\eta^5\text{-}C_5H_5)(bipy)(PPh_3)]^+$ species was indicated as a very promising large spectrum anticancer drug, being more efficient than Cisplatin against several cancer cell lines, and also in Cisplatin-resistant tumours (Tomaz et al. 2012). Comparable results were obtained with analogous Ru(II) complexes where a bipyridine was substituted by N,O or N,N' heteroaromatic ligands, like 2-benzoylpyridine, 2-acetylpyridine, 1-isoquinolinyl phenyl ketone and di(2-pyridyl)ketone (Morais et al. 2012).

1.5.2 Polypyridyl-Ru(II) Complexes

Polypyridine ligands such as bipyridines, o-phenanthrolines and terpyridines are able to induce photoluminescent properties in metal complexes via a metal-to-ligand charge transfer, but also behave as intercalating agents, useful for their anticancer activity. By conjugating these two aspects, Ru(II) polypyridyl complexes have emerged both as promising probes of DNA structure and anticancer agents due to their unique photophysical and cytotoxic properties (Gill and Thomas 2012).

Polypyridines are often associated with other coordinating species to give ruthenium complexes whose mechanism of action most of the times is connected to photo-cleavage reactions (Du et al. 2011; Guo et al. 2012; Sun et al. 2012; Yu et al. 2012; Yadav et al. 2013). Once a Ru(II)-polypyridyl complex is appended to suitable nanoparticles, like mesoporous silica, it can be targeted to cancer cells, cleaved by visible light and released into the cellular environment as an active aquo species, with promising results (Frasconi et al. 2013). The presence of flat heterocyclic compounds suggests that intercalation could be the most probable mechanism of action (Liu et al. 2011; Very et al. 2012; Liu et al. 2013a, b, c) for this kind of complexes, but in some cases, DNA photobinding (Wachter et al. 2012) and photocleavage (Liu et al. 2012) could also be involved, or cancer cell apoptosis achieved through mitochondrial pathways disruption (Chen et al. 2010).

1.5.3 Ruthenium Complexes with Thiosemicarbazones (TSC)

Ruthenium complexes with thiosemicarbazones have been widely synthesized and tested as therapeutic agents, after Beckford et al. (2009) reported the first structurally characterized ruthenium–arene half-sandwich complexes containing both the {(η^6-p-cymene)Ru(II)} moiety and 9-anthracenyl-thiosemicarbazone derivatives as the ligands. Following these results, polycyclic aromatic TSC have been often introduced in Ru(II) compounds (Beckford et al. 2011a, b; Anitha et al. 2013).

TSC-containing species in general possess high cytotoxicity against different human cancer cell lines, and their biological activities are apparently modulated by the TSC moiety. Their electronic, steric and functional properties have thus been tuned by different approaches, also by the accurate choice of the co-ligands, going from arenes (Beckford et al. 2011a, b; Demoro et al. 2013a, b; Su et al. 2013) to phosphines and arsines (Prabhakaran et al. 2011a, b; Selvamurugan et al. 2013), and their results are rather encouraging, although their distinct mechanisms of action and biological targets still need to be clarified.

1.5.4 Other Biological Activities

Ruthenium (Ru) complexes exhibit both antibacterial and antiparasitic activity with high efficacy. Currently, the most studied species are of two kinds: octahedral derivatives with Schiff bases and complexes with planar ligands and an overall flattened geometry, useful for DNA intercalation. To increase water solubility, the presence of the PTA (1,3,5-triaza-7-phospha-tricyclo-[3.3.1.1] decane) ligand is often recommendable.

Ru(II) species bearing polypyridyl ligands mixed with N-phenyl-substituted diazafluorene possess antibacterial activity against methicillin-resistant *S. aureus* with significant improvement in both minimum inhibitory concentration and minimum bactericidal concentration with respect to methicillin (used as the reference drug). These compounds did not evidence cytotoxic effects on normal human skin keratinocytes so that they can find applications in the formulation of topic antibiotics (Lam et al. 2014). Dinuclear Ru(II) 1,10-phenanthroline complexes were tested against *S. aureus*, methicillin-resistant *S. aureus*, *E. coli* and *P. aeruginosa* with remarkable results, being able to kill these bacteria within 2–6 h (Li et al. 2012a, b). Ru(II) polypyridyl complexes in general exhibit antibacterial activity due to DNA binding and intercalation, although molecular docking studies also evidenced DNA interactions with complexes through hydrogen bonding and van der Waal's interactions (Srishailam et al. 2013).

Ru(II) complexes as well have been explored in the search for effective antituberculosis agents, with activity higher than the reference antibiotics, low cytotoxicity and high selectivity (Pavan et al. 2011, 2013). Moreover, Ru(II) species were found highly effective against different protozoa, such as in the case of Leishmania (Pereira et al. 2010), promastigotes and intracellular amastigotes of Leishmania major (Iniguez et al. 2013), alveolar echinococcosis (Kuster et al. 2012) and Trypanosomes (*T. cruzi*, *T. brucei* and *T. vaginalis*) (Adams et al. 2013; Demoro et al. 2013a, b).

1.6 Gold

As other noble metals, like silver and copper, also gold has a very long history in the medicinal field, but found a new application under the form of Au(I) complexes only in the 1930s, against rheumatoid arthritis. The very first gold species used as prototypes were Au(I) thiolates which evolved to give the drug Au(I) thiolate-triethylphosphine, sold under the commercial name of Auranofin, introduced in the medical practice in 1985. Since then, no other gold compound has been admitted in clinical use, for either rheumatoid arthritis or any other disease.

1.6.1 Gold Complexes as Antirheumatic Drugs

The use of gold (chrysotherapy or aurotherapy, from the Greek and Latin words for gold, respectively) to treat rheumatoid arthritis is probably the outcome of a series of erroneous but yet fortunate observations, starting with Robert Koch's report that gold cyanide in dilutions of one in two million inhibited the in vitro growth of *Mycobacterium tuberculosis*. After this observation, gold salts had been employed first in experimental trials and subsequently in humans to treat tuberculosis. Since both discoid lupus erythematosus and rheumatoid arthritis were thought to be caused by tuberculosis, gold salts started to be also used in the standard treatment of these diseases. Forestier tested gold salts injections in 48 patients in 1932 (Forestier 1932) although his first report appeared in 1929. Gold compounds commonly used at that time were sodium aurothiosulphate (Sanochrysin), sodium aurothiomalate (Myochrisine) and aurothioglucose (Solganol). The treatment was indeed effective but several drawbacks were recorded, such as toxicity or hypersensitivity. The adverse reactions most commonly observed (in order of frequency) were rashes, dermatitis, stomatitis, renal irritation, leukopenia, thrombopenia with or without purpura and toxic hepatitis (Hartung 1943). Other gold compounds were applied in chrysotherapy: Allochrisine (sodium aurothiopropanol sulfonate) and Krysolgan (sodium 4-amino-2-aurothiosalicylate), for instance, which in analogy with their aforementioned analogues form chains of general formula $\{Au(SR)\}_n$ containing alternating Au(I) ions and RS ligands, with bridging sulphur atoms between the Au(I) centres. All of these gold compounds should be considered as prodrugs since the Au(I) ion is the active species and they simply work as a source of biologically available gold. The ligands used in these complexes afford both the necessary solubility for the gold complexes to be easily administered and sufficient stability for transportation and storage prior to clinical use. Moreover, the triethylphosphine ligand in the oral drug Auranofin is lipophilic and confers membrane solubility to the complex. After administration, ligands are quickly dissociated, and the Au(I) ion is free to interact with a number of donors present in the organism, although its affinity for sulphur-containing molecules suggests that free thiol groups present on proteins or GSH in the blood would be its first target. Indeed, serum albumin is able to bind and carry 80–95% of gold circulating in the blood, and the process of transferring Au(I) ions to this protein can take place within about 20 minutes.

Gold is a very slow acting agent, needing months to start being effective and attenuate the destructive process in rheumatoid arthritis. The mechanism of gold anti-inflammatory effect is not fully understood, although evidence suggests that this metal is stored in lysosomes whereby it inhibits the processing of antigenic agents and the release of pro-inflammatory cytokines. Moreover, gold is able to decrease levels of COX-2, IL-6 and MMP-3 as a consequence of MAP phosphatase-1 inhibition (Nieminen et al. 2010). Though not commonly in use, and in spite of several side effects, for some patients chrysotherapy is still the most effective mode of treatment. For this reason, the anti-inflammatory properties of new Au(I) complexes are still being evaluated in the treatment of rheumatoid arthritis (Travnicek et al. 2012).

1.6.2 Gold Complexes as Anticancer Agents

As many other metal-based drugs, also Auranofin exhibited cytotoxicity together with an in vitro anticancer activity comparable to that of Cisplatin, but never found applications as a chemotherapeutic against cancer. Following these evidences, a series of Au(I) complexes were prepared and tested against hemolymphatic cancer with high cytotoxicity, especially with diphosphine ligands. Unfortunately, these complexes were also highly cardiotoxic; thus, they never made it to the clinical trials.

Together with Au(I) species, also Au(III) compounds have been prepared for anticancer applications and seemed to be rather promising, since Au(III) is isoelectronic with Pt(II) and similarly forms square planar tetracoordinated complexes with slow exchange kinetics, being slightly faster with respect to Au(I). The weakness of Au(III) complexes, though, resides in their low chemical stability in solution so that no major progress was possible in this field until the use of N-containing stabilizing ligands, introduced in the 1990s, guaranteed a discrete stability under physiological conditions. Although a conspicuous number of square planar Au(III) complexes have been prepared and exhibited anticancer activity, nevertheless, their mechanism of action is far from being understood, since different cytotoxic routes have been evidenced in different complexes. What seems clear, though, is that in spite of their structural similarities, Au(III) compounds do not behave as Cisplatin in inducing cell death. Some complexes, especially those carrying flat polyaromatic ligands, such as terpyridine, interact with DNA, but in the intercalative mode. In other cases, interaction with DNA strands was demonstrated but seemed to be rather weak. On the contrary, a strong bond with serum proteins was ascertained, especially with sulphur-containing proteins such as glutathione and thioredoxin reductase, or with albumin.

What Au(III) complexes have in common with Cisplatin are a number of drawbacks: high toxicity, drug resistance, low cancer cell specificity and limited bioavailability. Nevertheless, several gold complexes have been prepared following a rational design in order to decrease toxicity and increase selectivity, with the aim of site-specific delivery, especially for complexes based on sulphur donors like dithiocarbamates (Nardon et al. 2014a, b).

1.6.2.1 Dithiocarbamate Complexes with Au(I) and Au(III)

As it was previously mentioned, thiocarbamates are used to decrease systemic and renal toxicity induced by metal-based drugs during cancer treatments. Au(III) species bearing dithiocarbamate ligands possess remarkable in vitro and in vivo antitumour properties (Marzano et al. 2011; Nagy et al. 2012; Nardon et al. 2014a, b), while Au(I) phosphino-dithiocarbamate compounds are active against a number of cancers, their efficacy depending on the nature of the phosphine ligand. For instance, triphenylphosphine increases both stability and cytotoxicity, while 1,6-bis (diphenylphosphino)hexane increases the selectivity towards HeLa cancer cells (Jamaludin et al. 2013; Keter et al. 2014). Another approach is to prepare dithiocarbamate Au(III) mixed complexes also containing oligopeptides, in order to take advantage of their peptidomimetic properties for a selective transportation inside the cancer cells: this strategy produced appreciable results against triple negative breast cancer (Nardon et al. 2014a, b) and other cancer cell lines (Kouodom et al. 2012; Nardon et al. 2014a, b).

1.6.2.2 Phosphine and Phosphine-Derivatives Au(I) Complexes

Antiarthritic drug Auranofin as previously remarked also exerts cytotoxic activity which can be exploited in cancer therapy. In fact, several series of Auranofin derivatives such as bis(phosphine)Au(I), phosphine-gold-halides and phosphine-gold-alkynyl complexes have been synthesized with this purpose and possess remarkable activity. Their mechanism of action seems to be mainly related to the inhibition of thioredoxin reductase (Lima and Rodriguez 2011; Jortzik et al. 2014; Ortego et al. 2014), by binding to selenocysteine residue (Wang et al. 2013) without targeting other well-known selenol and thiol groups contained in biomolecules (Vergara et al. 2010), while interaction with DNA was not significant.

Solubility is always a problem with metal complexes for therapeutic applications, especially those bearing phosphines. But associating the phosphine with a suitable co-ligand, as in the case of azolate derivatives, such as pyrazolates and imidazolates substituted with deactivating groups like trifluoromethyl, nitro or chloride, not only results in more active complexes but also improves their solubility in water and other polar media. Such strategy led to the preparation of gold(I) compounds with antiproliferative power up to 70 times higher than Cisplatin (Galassi et al. 2012). A similarly fortunate approach consists in adding a polar moiety directly onto the phosphine ligand, like in 1,3,5-triaza-7-phosphaadamantane, 3,7-diacetyl-1,3,7-triaza-5-phosphabicyclo[3.3.1]nonane, sodium triphenylphosphane monosulfonate and sodium triphenylphosphane trisulfonate which, in association with a thiolate ligand, led to potent antiproliferative complexes even in the case of Cisplatin-resistant cell lines (Vergara et al. 2011). The apoptotic activity of this kind of complexes is often linked to their lipophilicity (Wetzel et al. 2011), as well as to the steric hindrance of the substituents on the phosphorus atom (being the highest for the phenyl and the lowest for the methyl group) together with the length of the linker connecting the two phosphorus atoms in the case of diphosphines (the highest with five or six carbon atoms). These evidences demonstrate that both steric and electronic properties are crucial in the design of effective gold complexes (Horvath et al. 2012).

1.6.2.3 Au(I) and Au(III) Organometallic Complexes

Organogold complexes in both Au(I) and Au(III) oxidation states seem to be rather stable in aqueous solutions, leading to a wide variety of compounds owing anti-cancer activity, such as gold N-heterocyclic carbene (NHC), cyclometalated Au(III) and gold alkynyl complexes (Bertrand and Casini 2014). NHC-gold species in particular have been widely applied, and, together with phosphines-derivatives, they represent the most investigated class of gold-based potential antitumour drugs (Liu et al. 2013a, b, c; Oehninger et al. 2013; Bertrand and Casini 2014).

1.6.3 Other Biological Activities

Gold compounds can be active against several parasites and protozoa, so that they have been tested against leishmaniasis, malaria, tuberculosis and also HIV infection.

Auranofin demonstrated to be effective against Leishmania (Sharlow et al. 2014), together with Au(I) and Au(III) complexes of benzimidazole derivatives (Mota et al. 2014). While free benzimidazoles were completely inert, their gold complexes exhibited a strong activity against Leishmania protozoa and high selectivity, with Au(I) complexes being almost 50 times more toxic to the parasite than to macrophages. The mechanism of action against Leishmania parasites may be connected to the inhibition of the enzyme trypanothione reductase (Colotti et al. 2013): trypanothione is an uncommon form of glutathione in which two molecules of glutathione are linked by a spermidine chain, found in parasitic protozoa such as Leishmania and trypanosomes, as the name suggests. Its principal function is to protect the protozoa from oxidative stress; thus, impairment of its reduction enzyme may cause severe damage to these microorganisms.

Gold complexes possessing antimalarial activity (Khanye et al. 2010; Coetzee et al. 2011; Molter et al. 2011) exert their action via inhibition of the parasite cysteine protease falcipain-2, although studies carried out to ascertain this mechanism were not able to establish any direct correlation between enzyme inhibition and reduction of *Plasmodium falciparum* growth, indicating that falcipain-2 inhibition represents just one of the different mechanisms gold compounds use to prevent *P. falciparum* replication (Micale et al. 2011).

An antiviral action of gold compounds appeared when some of them were tested against HIV infection, with interesting preliminary results which seem to be outstanding when the incredible complexity of this disease is taken into account. The compounds evaluated in these studies are based on Au(III) tetrachlorides complexes (Mphahlele et al. 2012), which are able to inhibit the integrase enzymatic activity, most likely through protein oxidation; bis(thiosemicarbazonate) Au(III) complexes, on the other hand, show to inhibit HIV replication at cytostatic concentrations (Fonteh et al. 2011).

1.7 Copper

Among the noble metals, copper is the only essential one in all organisms living under aerobic conditions, being crucial in a number of biochemical processes; thus, its homeostasis is strictly regulated. Copper is a catalytic cofactor and a structural component for proteins; in fact, it is present in proteins and metallo-enzymes implicated in both antioxidative activity (copper-zinc superoxido dismutases and oxidative phosphorylation) and energy metabolism (cytochrome c oxidases); it takes part in the development and function of bones, heart and brain, sugar and cholesterol metabolism, erythrocytes formation, iron metabolism, connective tissue synthesis, pigment formation, immunity, free radical control, oxygen transport, and cell signalling; and it has a role in the development of diabetes (Denoyer et al. 2015).

The redox properties of copper are crucial for enzymatic processes but represent just one side of the same coin, since due to this activity copper can be potentially toxic. The production of free radicals can be catalyzed by copper ions, leading to damage in DNA, proteins, lipids and other biomolecules. Moreover, copper inhibits the activity of metal-containing proteins by interacting with iron–sulphur clusters or displacing other metals such as zinc from metalloproteins (Denoyer et al. 2015). Finally, copper seems to be involved in cancer mechanisms since aberrant levels of this metal have been found in cancerous tissues of tumour-bearing mice and in cancer patients, suggesting its dysregulation in cancer states, and was indicated as a potential carcinogen and diagnostic/prognostic marker (Denoyer et al. 2015).

Copper compounds have a wide biological activity. They find therapeutic applications mostly as antibacterial and anticancer agents, but also behave as good antimalarial and antifungal drugs. Moreover, copper species seem to be effective on diabetes, inflammatory states (e.g. rheumatoid arthritis), leishmaniasis and skin wounds. They demonstrate to modulate copper homeostasis in the brain, leading to protective effects in several models of neurodegeneration, so that they have been tested in the treatment of Alzheimer's and Parkinson's diseases, and amyotrophic lateral sclerosis. Finally, their ability to increase SOD activity, resulting in relief of oxidative stress, can be exploited in coronary heart disease and other cardiovascular problems (Duncan and White 2012).

1.7.1 Copper as an Antibiotic Agent

Although most of the noble metal compounds are mainly studied for their anticancer activity, copper and silver are the only two being strongly efficient in killing bacteria, viruses, yeasts and fungi, both in their metal state and as coordination complexes or salts. Moreover, copper is also commonly used as an algaecide and pesticide.

The Egyptians used to store water in copper vessels to keep it uncontaminated and fresh for long times, but also modern Indians do the same, following an Ayurvedic practice. Thus, a new interest is rising about the antibacterial properties of copper metal containers or surfaces, which can be exploited in different situations where it is necessary to control bacterial proliferation: the use of copper jars to store drinking water has been proposed as a means to support water disinfection practices in rural areas of undeveloped countries where a potabilisation plant could be unaffordable and water purification is a real problem together with the mortality consequent to the spreading of diseases and infections. In fact, it was proved that 16 h is enough to destroy the bacterial load of important diarrhoeagenic bacteria when contaminated water is kept in copper pots, including *Vibrio cholerae*, *Shigella flexneri*, enterotoxigenic *E. coli*, enteropathogenic *E. coli*, *Salmonella enterica Typhi* and *Salmonella enterica Paratyphi*. The decontamination process is so effective and absolute that any attempt to revitalize these bacteria fails, even after culturing in enrichment broth, followed by plating on selective media (Sudha et al. 2012). Another interesting application is the use of copper nanofilms to cover touch surfaces in hospitals and healthcare settings, where bacterial proliferation and resistance is becoming a serious problem. As a matter of fact, thin layers of copper on objects and surfaces are effective in inhibiting the growth of a number of nosocomial germs and *Enterobacter* species (Codita et al. 2010; Grass et al. 2011) exploiting an effect called 'contact killing'. These remarkable properties led to the approval of metallic copper as the first solid antimicrobial material by the U.S. Environmental Protection Agency. Nevertheless, the feasibility of such practice should be carefully evaluated. In fact, while silver-induced resistance is a rare and mostly transient phenomenon (vide supra), there are evidences that bacteria are able to respond to copper toxicity in several ways, and thus, they are able to develop resistance. Copper has a double role in living organisms: it is necessary to accomplish many biological functions, but at high concentration, it is poisonous, no species excluded. One of the reasons for its toxicity may be found in the fact that copper degrades iron–sulphur clusters in dehydratases through iron displacement, leading to the inactivation of these fundamental enzymes. Once iron is released from the iron–sulphur clusters, it may initiate the Fenton reaction causing oxidative damage inside the cell (Macomber and Imlay 2009). For this reason, both eukaryotic and prokaryotic cells have developed detoxification mechanism to maintain a perfect equilibrium in copper homeostasis. The processes involved in bacterial cells are intra- and extracellular sequestration, enzymatic detoxification and active efflux. Extracellular sequestration is possible due to the production of exopolysaccharides that bind copper ions due to electrostatic interactions and keep them trapped outside the cell (González et al. 2010). Bacteria can enhance and improve these mechanisms in order to get rid of extra copper and build up resistance (Bondarczuk and Piotrowska-Seget 2013). The widespread use of copper-containing products in medicine, agriculture and farming (e.g. copper supplements in animal feed to stimulate growth) has thus led to prolonged exposure of bacterial cells to copper, resulting in the selection of Cu-resistant/tolerant strains, which poses some limits to the application of copper in the above-mentioned fields and demands careful evaluation of either risks and benefits.

Copper complexes show antimicrobial activity both in their Cu(I) and Cu(II) oxidation states, the latter being the most utilized. Normally, Cu(II) complexes bear mixed ligands, among which phenthrolines often associated with amino acids (Li et al. 2011; Tabassum et al. 2012; Liu et al. 2013a, b, c; Starosta et al. 2013), other polypyridyl ligands (Kharadi 2014) and especially antibiotic molecules, in order to enhance the activity of the drug itself. The association of 1,10-phenanthroline with antibiotics increases the stability of the Cu(II)-antibiotic complex, as in the case of lomefloxacin. Studies on the ternary complex against several *E. coli* strains revealed that the free antibiotic and its copper derivative have the same activity, while their cell intake route appeared to be completely different (Fernandes et al. 2014), an aspect common to other Cu(II)-antibiotic compounds (Sousa et al. 2012).

Sparfloxacin (a fluoroquinolone) was used in a series of mononuclear Cu(II) complexes with a terpyridine derivative (Patel et al. 2013) and tested against several bacterial strains. All complexes were more active than the free drug and exhibited DNA intercalative binding and cleavage, together with an SOD-like activity. Cu(II) compounds of sparfloxacin and levofloxacin associated with 1,10-phenanthroline were more effective against protozoan *T. cruzi* than benznidazole, the reference drug for this infectious agent (Martins et al. 2012).

Amphotericin B is an antibiotic extracted from *Streptomyces nodosus* and has been used for more than 50 years in the treatment of acute systemic fungal infections and protozoan pathogens with relatively rare resistance (Chudzik et al. 2013). Its copper(II) complex was successfully tested against *Candida albicans*, evidencing insertion of Cu(II) ions into the fungal cell membranes. The increased antifungal activity of the copper complex was not just the sum of the toxic effects of the antibiotic and Cu(II) ions, but was due to the unique structure of the resulting compound.

Tobramycin and its copper complex exert anti-inflammatory effects on inflammation states related to cystic fibrosis. Moreover, a series of experiments demonstrated that Tobramycin alone is active due to the spontaneous formation of a copper–tobramycin complex inside the cell, suggesting that copper–tobramycin may result in a stronger action. Also, this copper–antibiotic complex exerts an SOD-like activity (Gziut et al. 2013).

Thus, copper complexes with antibiotics commonly have comparable or higher activities with respect to the free drugs and could be used in antimicrobial therapies due to their different paths of cellular intake and mechanisms of action.

1.7.2 Anticancer Activity of Copper Complexes

As all its noble metal congeners, also copper can be active against cancer, albeit the mechanisms behind its activity are not yet fully clarified. One of the most probable pathways is the intracellular formation of reactive oxygen species (ROS) via a thiol-mediated reduction of Cu(II) to Cu(I), as diffusedly proposed by the most recent research (Kowol et al. 2012). DNA cleavage was demonstrated in several cases where the ligands were extended aromatic systems, such as polypyridines and polyphenols (Li et al. 2012a, b).

1.7.2.1 Copper Complexes with Polypyridyl Ligands

As previously mentioned, polypyridyl ligands (bipyridines, terpyridines, phenanthrolines, etc.) have been widely used in the preparation of metal complexes for therapeutic applications, since they are able to interact with DNA in the intercalative way, an aspect that can be highly desirable in cancer treatment. Thus, copper complexes with polypyridyl ligands have been assessed as cytotoxic compounds with remarkable results. 1,10-phenanthrolines derivatives exert the highest anticancer power and gathered conspicuous interest for this, so they will be discussed in a dedicated section.

Instead, the activity of polypyridine Cu(II) complexes depends on the co-ligand. With quinolinato species, the efficacy against human hosteosarcoma and breast carcinoma is evident already at low, micromolar doses: their mechanism is based on a multiple action including DNA cleavage, SOD-mimic activity and binding to sulphur-containing biomolecules, like cysteine and reduced glutathione (Buchtik et al. 2011, 2012). When polypyridines are associated with a phenolate ligand, the resulting copper complexes show cytotoxic activity higher than Cisplatin on breast and cervical cancer, based also in this case on DNA cleavage at micromolar concentrations (Jaividhya et al. 2012). Cu(II) complexes of terpyridine derivatives, instead, exhibit a high cytotoxicity against lung adenocarcinoma (Rajalakshmi et al. 2011; Manikandamathavan et al. 2012) and breast cancer cell lines, with a low toxicity against normal ones (Rajalakshmi et al. 2012), showing a certain degree of selectivity. Nevertheless, the most effective Cu(II) derivative bore an anthracenyl-terpy ligand and exhibited outstanding cytotoxicity against a wide range of cancer lines (Kumar et al. 2011). Also in this case, the mechanism of action is based on DNA intercalation and cleavage. Finally, bipy Cu(II) complexes with the amino acid glycine are active against breast and liver cancer (Mohamed et al. 2012).

1.7.2.2 Copper Complexes with 1,10-Phenanthrolines

Copper–phenanthroline complexes are very important species since they act as nucleases, causing oxidative damage and cleaving nucleic acids (Chen and Sigman 1986; Gallagher et al. 1996). It was recently reported that 1,10-phenanthroline per se is able to promote copper complexes into tumour cells and induce apoptosis by inhibiting the proteasome activity; thus, its ternary complexes are expected to be effective anticancer drugs (Zhang et al. 2012). Normally, 1,10-phenanthroline ternary copper complexes are tested as chemotherapeutics, and different co-ligands are examined in order to improve their activity and reduce toxicity, at the same time aiming at explaining their modes of action. Following these evidences, a combination of ternary Cu(II) mixed complexes bearing different 1,10-phenanthrolines or bipyridines together with an amino acid has been recently patented under the name of Casiopeinas® (Ruiz-Azuara 1992–1999). These complexes exert cytostatic, cytotoxic and antineoplastic activity, with promising applications for their use as clinical antitumour drugs. Studies on their mechanism of action revealed that they induce oxidative stress and mitochondrial dysfunctions together with DNA fragmentation and base oxidation, indicating that reactive oxygen species (ROS) generation after copper reduction may be the cause of their high activity (Kachadourian et al. 2010; Ruiz-Azuara and Bravo-Gomez 2010; Serment-Guerrero et al. 2011). Interesting results have been obtained with oxazolidin-carboxylates against a vast range of cancer lines, with activities higher than Cisplatin and some degree of selectivity (Ng et al. 2013). A dimetallic complex with terephthalate, on the other hand, causes a potent oxidative DNA cleavage with the production of ROS already at nanomolar concentration (Prisecaru et al. 2012a, b) and is effective against Cisplatin-resistant cancer lines. Photocleavage can be a very useful aid in cancer treatment, as previously seen in the case of ruthenium complexes. UV-light induced DNA cleavage is also at the basis of the anticancer activity of several copper complexes containing 1,10-phenanthrolines, as in the case of two tetracycline derivatives, which are some of the most potent DNA cleavers to date (Bortolotto et al. 2011; Silva et al. 2011), a ferrocene-conjugated tryptophan compound (Goswami et al. 2011) or naphthalene sulfonamides (Garcia-Gimenez et al. 2013).

1.7.2.3 Polynuclear Copper Complexes

The cytotoxic activity of Cu(II) di- and trinuclear complexes is well recognized and can be also flanked by the antiangiogenic properties associated with some of these polynuclear compounds (Qin et al. 2013). Their efficacy can be linked to ROS formation pathways, but DNA binding and intercalation may also be the favoured pathways, like in the case of a trimetallic species containing μ-oxamido-bridged ligands (Li et al. 2013). This is not an isolated case since DNA binding and cleavage was also observed in polynuclear complexes containing a disubstituted terpyridine which evidenced that cleavage activity depends on the number of copper atoms present in the complex, decreasing in the order $3 > 2 > 1$. The trimetallic species is very active against leukaemia, with a good propensity to enter the cell and localize in its nucleus (Suntharalingam et al. 2012). This demonstrates that polypyridyl ligands are able to confer high cytotoxicity also to Cu(II) polynuclear species, through different mechanisms of action according to the kind of ligand, going from oxidation of the DNA duplex through ROS formation (Prisecaru et al. 2012) or DNA binding and cleavage, as in the case of salen or salophen Cu(II) dinuclear complexes (Reddy and Shilpa 2011).

In a research dominated by Cu(II) species, it is interesting to note that also polynuclear Cu(I) complexes exert potential anticancer activity. The ligands used in these complexes are of the cyclodiphosphazane and pyridyl types, giving compounds that are more active than Cisplatin on different cancer cell lines and able to damage DNA, block the cells in the G1 phase of their cycle and induce apoptosis via a p53-dependent pathway (Balakrishna et al. 2010).

1.7.2.4 Thiosemicarbazones Cu(II) Complexes

Thiosemicarbazones (TSC) are one of the most versatile families of ligands for metal complexes owning anticancer activity, and copper is not exception (Paterson and Donnelly 2011). Cu(II) complexes with TSC bearing halogen substituents are effective on liver cancer (Jagadeesh et al. 2014), while cytotoxicity is evidenced on different colon cancer lines when TSC are based on the piperonal structure (Beckford et al. 2012) or conjugated to D-proline (the L-enantiomer is less effective) (Milunovic et al. 2012), or formed a bis(thiosemicarbazone) species (Palanimuthu et al. 2013). In all these cases, the mechanism of action does not involve DNA binding and needs to be elucidated.

1.8 Conclusions

The search for an alternative to Cisplatin and its derivatives, with lower toxicity and less side effects, has produced an impressive number of metal-based compounds which have been evaluated for their anticancer activity with remarkable results. Noble metals take the lion's share in the field of biomedical applications, with platinum, palladium, ruthenium, silver, gold and copper as the most widely studied metals for their possible therapeutic uses. Nevertheless, there is a growing interest around other, more 'exotic' transition metals, such as rhodium, iridium, rhenium and osmium, for their notable properties and performances as potential drugs, which will be discussed in Chap. 2.

In spite of the impressive results obtained by non-platinum complexes not only against cancer but also against bacteria, fungi and protozoa, only a very small number of them, namely, three ruthenium compounds, have accessed the clinical trials in the past few years. Some of the possible reasons reside in the differences between the in vitro and in vivo behaviour of the complexes, since their activity can be significantly reduced by many factors, decreasing their bioavailability: low solubility, sequestration by other biomolecules, redox equilibria, complex stability, increased detoxification mechanisms and so on. Moreover, intrinsic toxicity can be a major drawback, but this aspect is rarely evaluated by researchers that mostly focus on the cytotoxic activity of the compounds and seldom concentrate on their toxicity in animal models.

Still, the potentialities of this class of compounds are vast and can be exploited in an extensive way. The possibility to choose between several metals and a virtually infinite range of ligands gives the opportunity to better tune the properties of the resulting complexes, thus regulating their activity and toxicity. Proper functionalization of the complexes can result in better performances in transportation, bioavailability and selectivity. Thus, the noble metals field represents an exciting ground for research exploration with extraordinary potentialities in biomedical applications.

References

Adams M, Li Y, Khot H, De Kock C, Smith PJ, Land K, Chibale K, Smith GS (2013) The synthesis and antiparasitic activity of aryl- and ferrocenyl-derived thiosemicarbazone ruthenium(II)-arene complexes. Dalton Trans 42:4677–4685

Afrasiabi Z, Stovall P, Finley K, Choudhury A, Barnes C, Ahmad A, Sarkar F, Vyas A, Padhye S (2013) Targeting triple negative breast cancer cells by N3-substituted 9,10-phenanthrenequinone thiosemicarbazones and their metal complexes. Spectrochim Acta Part A Mol Biomol Spectrosc 114:114–119

Agudo-López A, Prieto-García E, Alemán J, Pérez C, Díaz-García CV, Parrilla-Rubio L, Cabrera S, Navarro-Ranninger C, Cortés-Funes H, López-Martín JA, Agulló-Ortuño MT (2017) Mechanistic added value of a trans-Sulfonamide-Platinum-Complex in human melanoma cell lines and synergism with cis-Platin. Mol Cancer 16(1):45

al-Allaf TA, Rashan LJ (2001) Cis- and trans-platinum and palladium complexes: a comparative study review as antitumour agents. Boll Chim Farm 140(3):205–210

Almotairy ARZ, Gandin V, Morrison L, Marzano C, Montagner D, Erxleben A (2017) Antitumor platinum(IV) derivatives of carboplatin and the histone deacetylase inhibitor 4-phenylbutyric acid. J Inorg Biochem 177:1–7

Alvero AB, Chen W, Sartorelli AC, Schwartz P, Rutherford T, Mor G (2006) Triapine (3-aminopyridine-2-carboxaldehyde thiosemicarbazone) induces apoptosis in ovarian cancer cells. J Soc Gynecol Invest 3:145–152

Anderson CM, Taylor IR, Tibbetts MF, Philpott J, Hu Y, Tanski JM (2012) Hetero-multinuclear ruthenium(III)/platinum(II) complexes that potentially exhibit both antimetastatic and antineoplastic properties. Inorg Chem 51:12917–12924

Anitha P, Chitrapriya N, Jang YJ, Viswanathamurthi P (2013) Synthesis, characterization, DNA interaction, antioxidant and anticancer activity of new ruthenium(II) complexes of thiosemicarbazone/semicarbazone bearing 9,10-phenanthrenequinone. J Photochem Photobiol, B 129:17–26

Asiri AM, Khan SA (2010) Palladium(II) complexes of NS donor ligands derived from steroidal thiosemicarbazones as antibacterial agents. Molecules 15:4784–4791

Atiyeh BS, Costagliola M, Hayek SN, Dibo SA (2007) Effect of silver on burn wound infection control and healing: review of the literature. Burns 33:139–148

Balakrishna MS, Suresh D, Rai A, Mague JT, Panda D (2010) Dinuclear copper(I) complexes containing cyclodiphosphazane derivatives and pyridyl ligands: Synthesis, structural studies, and antiproliferative activity toward human cervical and breast cancer cells. Inorg Chem 49:8790–8801

Banti CN, Giannoulis AD, Kourkoumelis N, Owczarzak AM, Poyraz M, Kubicki M, Charalabopoulos K, Hadjikakou SK (2012) Mixed ligand-silver(I) complexes with anti-inflammatory agents which can bind to lipoxygenase and calf-thymus DNA, modulating their function and inducing apoptosis. Metallomics 4:545–560

Banti CN, Kyros L, Geromichalos GD, Kourkoumelis N, Kubicki M, Hadjikakou SK (2014) A novel silver iodide metalo-drug: experimental and computational modelling assessment of its interaction with intracellular DNA, lipoxygenase and glutathione. Eur J Med Chem 77:388–399

Beckford F, Dourth D, Shaloski M, Didion J, Thessing J, Woods J, Crowell V, Gerasimchuk N, Gonzalez-Sarrias A, Seeram NP (2011a) Half-sandwich ruthenium-arene complexes with thiosemicarbazones: synthesis and biological evaluation of [(η^6-p-cymene)Ru(piperonal thiosemicarbazones)Cl]Cl complexes. J Inorg Biochem 105:1019–1029

Beckford F, Thessing J, Woods J, Didion J, Gerasimchuk N, Gonzalez-Sarrias A, Seeram NP (2011b) Synthesis and structure of [(η^6–p-cymene)Ru(2-anthracen-9 ylmethylene-N-ethylhydrazinecarbothioamide)Cl]Cl: biological evaluation, topoisomerase-II inhibition and reaction with DNA and human serum albumin. Metallomics 3:491–502

Beckford FA, Thessing J, Stott A, Holder AA, Poluektov OG, Li L, Seeram NP (2012) Anticancer activity and biophysical reactivity of copper complexes of 2-(benzo[d][1,3]dioxol-5-ylmethylene)-N-alkylhydrazinecarbothioamides. Inorg Chem Commun 15:225–229

Bellinger CG, Conway H (1970) Effects of silver nitrate and sulfamylon on epithelial regeneration. Plast Reconstr Surg 45:582–585

Bergamo A, Sava G (2011) Ruthenium anticancer compounds: myths and realities of the emerging metal-based drugs. Dalton Trans 40:7817–7823

Bergamo A, Gaiddon C, Schellens JH, Beijnen JH, Sava G (2012) Approaching tumour therapy beyond platinum drugs: status of the art and perspectives of ruthenium drug candidates. J Inorg Biochem 106:90–99

Bernardi T, Badel S, Mayer P, Groelly J, de Frémont P, Jacques B, Braunstein P, Teyssot ML, Gaulier C, Cisnetti F, Gautier A, Roland S (2014) High-throughput screening of metal-N-heterocyclic carbene complexes against biofilm formation by pathogenic bacteria. ChemMedChem 9(6):1140–1144

Bertrand B, Casini A (2014) A golden future in medicinal inorganic chemistry: the promise of anticancer gold organometallic compounds. Dalton Trans 43:4209–4219

Bhargava A, Vaishampayan UN (2009) Satraplatin: leading the new generation of oral platinum agents. Expert Opin Investig Drugs 18(1). https://doi.org/10.1517/13543780903362437

Bielawska A, Poplawska B, Surazynski A, Czarnomysy R, Bielawski K (2010) Cytotoxic efficacy of a novel dinuclear platinum(II) complex in human breast cancer cells. Eur J Pharmacol 643:34–41

Biswas S, Torchilin VP (2014) Nano-preparations for organelle-specific delivery in cancer. Adv Drug Delivery Rev 66:26–41

Bjarnsholt T, Kirketerp-Moller K, Kristiansen S, Phipps R, Nielsen AK, Jensen PO, Hoiby N, Givskov M (2007) Silver against Pseudomonas aeruginosa biofilms. APMIS 115:921–928

Bondarczuk K, Piotrowska-Seget Z (2013) Molecular basis of active copper resistance mechanisms in Gram-negative bacteria. Cell Biol Toxicol 29(6):397–405

Bortolotto T, Silva PP, Neves A, Pereira-Maia EC, Terenzi H (2011) Photoinduced DNA cleavage promoted by two copper(II) complexes of tetracyclines and 1,10-henanthroline. Inorg Chem 50:10519–10521

Brasseur K, Leblanc V, Fabi F, Parent S, Descoteaux C, Berube G, Asselin E (2013) ERα-targeted therapy in ovarian cancer cells by a novel estradiol-platinum(II) hybrid. Endocrinology 154:2281–2295

Bruijnincx PC, Sadler PJ (2008) New trends for metal complexes with anticancer activity. Curr Opin Chem Biol 12:197–206

Buac D, Schmitt S, Ventro G, Kona FR, Dou QP (2012) Dithiocarbamate-based coordination compounds as potent proteasome inhibitors in human cancer cells. Mini-Rev Med Chem 12:1193–1201

Buchtik R, Travnicek Z, Vanco J, Herchel R, Dvorak Z (2011) Synthesis, characterization, DNA interaction and cleavage, and in vitro cytotoxicity of copper(II) mixed-ligand complexes with 2-phenyl-3-hydroxy-4(1H)-quinolinone. Dalton Trans 40:9404–9412

Buchtik R, Travnicek Z, Vanco J (2012) In vitro cytotoxicity, DNA cleavage and SOD-mimic activity of copper(II) mixed-ligand quinolinonato complexes. J Inorg Biochem 116:163–171

Castellano JJ, Shafii SM, Ko F, Donate G, Wright TE, Mannari RJ, Payne WG, Smith DJ, Robson MC (2007) Comparative evaluation of silver-containing antimicrobial dressings and drugs. Int Wound J 4:114–122

Chen CH, Sigman DS (1986) Nuclease activity of 1,10-phenanthroline-copper: sequence-specific targeting. Proc Nat Acad Sci USA 83:7147–7151

Chen T, Liu Y, Zheng WJ, Liu J, Wong YS (2010) Ruthenium polypyridyl complexes that induce mitochondria-mediated apoptosis in cancer cells. Inorg Chem 49:6366–6368

Chen WH, Xu XD, Luo GF, Jia HZ, Lei Q, Cheng SX, Zhuo RX, Zhang XZ (2013a) Dual-targeting pro-apoptotic peptide for programmed cancer cell death via specific mitochondria damage. Sci Rep 3:3468

Chen Y, Qin MY, Wu JH, Wang L, Chao H, Ji LN, Xu AL (2013b) Synthesis, characterization, and anticancer activity of ruthenium(II)-β-carboline complex. Eur J Med Chem 70:120–129

Chudzik B, Tracz IB, Czernel G, Fiolka MJ, Borsuk G, Gagos M (2013) Amphotericin B-copper(II) complex as a potential agent with higher antifungal activity against *Candida albicans*. Eur J Pharm Sci 49:850–857

Cincinelli R, Musso L, Dallavalle S, Artali R, Tinelli S, Colangelo D, Zunino F, De Cesare M, Beretta GL, Zaffaroni N (2013) Design, modeling, synthesis and biological activity evaluation of camptothecin-linked platinum anticancer agents. Eur J Med Chem 63:387–400

Coban B, Yildiz U, Sengul A (2013) Synthesis, characterization, and DNA binding of complexes [Pt(bpy)(pip)](2 +) and [Pt(bpy)(hpip)] (2 +). J Biol Inorg Chem 18:461–471

Codita I, Caplan DM, Dragulescu EC, Lixandru BE, Coldea IL, Dragomirescu CC, Surdu-Bob C, Badulescu M (2010) Antimicrobial activity of copper and silver nanofilms on nosocomial bacterial species. Rom Arch Microbiol Immunol 69:204–212

Coetzee J, Cronje S, Dobrzanska L, Raubenheimer HG, Joone G, Nell MJ, Hoppe HC (2011) Novel N-heterocyclic ylideneamine gold(I) complexes: synthesis, characterisation and screening for antitumour and antimalarial activity. Dalton Trans 40:1471–1483

Colotti G, Ilari A, Fiorillo A, Baiocco P, Cinellu MA, Maiore L, Scaletti F, Gabbiani C, Messori L (2013) Metal-based compounds as prospective antileishmanial agents: inhibition of trypanothione reductase by selected gold complexes. ChemMedChem 8(10):1634–1637

Corduneanu O, Chiorcea-Paquim AM, Diculescu V, Fiuza SM, Marques MP, Oliveira-Brett AM (2010) DNA interaction with palladium chelates of biogenic polyamines using atomic force microscopy and voltammetric characterization. Anal Chem 82:1245–1252

Cubo L, Groessl M, Dyson PJ, Quiroga AG, Navarro-Ranninger C, Casini A (2010a) Proteins as possible targets for cytotoxic trans-platinum(II) complexes with aliphatic amine ligands: further exceptions to the DNA paradigm. ChemMedChem 5:1335–1343

Cubo L, Pizarro AM, Quiroga AG, Salassa L, Navarro-Ranninger C, Sadler PJ (2010b) Photoactivation of trans diamine platinum complexes in aqueous solution and effect on reactivity towards nucleotides. J Inorg Biochem 104:909–918

Cubo L, Hambley TW, Sanz Miguel PJ, Carnero A, Navarro-Ranninger C, Quiroga AG (2011) The preparation and characterization of trans-platinum(IV) complexes with unusually high cytotoxicity. Dalton Trans 40:344–347

Dasari S, Tchounwou PB (2014) Cisplatin in cancer therapy: molecular mechanisms of action. Eur J Pharmacol 740:364–378

Davis KJ, Carrall JA, Lai B, Aldrich-Wright JR, Ralph SF, Dillon CT (2012) Does cytotoxicity of metallointercalators correlate with cellular uptake or DNA affinity? Dalton Trans 41:9417–9426

de Souza RA, Stevanato A, Treu-Filho O, Netto AV, Mauro AE, Castellano EE, Carlos IZ, Pavan FR, Leite CQ (2010) Antimycobacterial and antitumor activities of palladium(II) complexes containing isonicotinamide (isn): X-ray structure of trans-[Pd(N3)2(isn)(2)]. Eur J Med Chem 45:4863–4868

Del Solar V, Quinones-Lombrana A, Cabrera S, Padron JM, Rios-Luci C, Alvarez-Valdes A, Navarro-Ranninger C, Aleman J (2013) Expanding the synthesis of new trans-sulfonamide platinum complexes: cytotoxicity, SAR, fluorescent cell assays and stability studies. J Inorg Biochem 127:128–140

Demoro B, de Almeida RF, Marques F, Matos CP, Otero L, Costa Pessoa J, Santos I, Rodriguez A, Moreno V, Lorenzo J, Gambino D, Tomaz AI (2013a) Screening organometallic binuclear thiosemicarbazone ruthenium complexes as potential anti-tumour agents: cytotoxic activity and human serum albumin binding mechanism. Dalton Trans 42:7131–7146

Demoro B, Rossi M, Caruso F, Liebowitz D, Olea-Azar C, Kemmerling U, Maya JD, Guiset H, Moreno V, Pizzo C, Mahler G, Otero L, Gambino D (2013b) Potential mechanism of the anti-trypanosomal activity of organoruthenium complexes with bioactive thiosemicarbazones. Biol Trace Element Res 153:371–381

Denoyer D, Masaldan S, La Fontaine S, Cater MA (2015) Targeting copper in cancer therapy: copper that cancer. Metallomics 7(11):1459–1476

Dibrov P, Dzioba J, Gosink KK, Häse CC (2002) Chemiosmotic mechanism of antimicrobial activity of Ag^{+} in *Vibrio cholera*. Antimicrob Agents Chemother 46(8):2668–2670
Ding S, Qiao X, Kucera GL, Bierbach U (2013) Design of a platinum-acridine-endoxifen conjugate targeted at hormone-dependent breast cancer. Chem Commun 49:2415–2417
Donlan RM (2002) Biofilms: microbial life on surfaces. Emerg Infect Dis 8(9):881–890
Du KJ, Wang JQ, Kou JF, Li GY, Wang LL, Chao H, Ji LN (2011) Synthesis, DNA-binding and topoisomerase inhibitory activity of ruthenium(II) polypyridyl complexes. Eur J Med Chem 46:1056–1065
Du Y, Fu X, Li H, Chen B, Guo Y, Su G, Zhang H, Ning F, Lin Y, Mei W, Chen T (2014) Mitochondrial fragmentation is an important cellular event induced by ruthenium(II) polypyridyl complexes in osteosarcoma cells. ChemMedChem 9:714–718
Duncan C, White AR (2012) Copper complexes as therapeutic agents. Metallomics 4:127–138
Duskova K, Sierra S, Fernandez MJ, Gude L, Lorente A (2012) Synthesis and DNA interaction of ethylenediamine platinum(II) complexes linked to DNA intercalants. Bioorg Med Chem 20:7112–7118
Ebrahiminezhad A, Raee MJ, Manafi Z, Jahromi AS, Ghasemi Y (2016) Ancient and novel forms of silver in medicine and biomedicine. J Adv Med Sci Appl Technol 2(1):122–128
Eloy L, Jarrousse AS, Teyssot ML, Gautier A, Morel L, Jolivalt C, Cresteil T, Roland S (2012) Anticancer activity of silver-N-heterocyclic carbene complexes: caspase-independent induction of apoptosis via mitochondrial apoptosis-inducing factor (AIF). ChemMedChem 7(5):805–814
Farrer NJ, Woods JA, Salassa L, Zhao Y, Robinson KS, Clarkson G, Mackay FS, Sadler PJ (2010) A potent trans-diimine platinum anticancer complex photoactivated by visible light. Angew Chem 49:8905–8908 (International edition in English)
Fernandes P, Sousa I, Cunha-Silva L, Ferreira M, de-Castro B, Pereira EF, Feio MJ, Gameiro P (2014) Synthesis, characterization and antibacterial studies of a copper(II) lomefloxacin ternary complex. J Inorg Biochem 131:21–29
Finch RA, Liu M, Grill SP, Rose WC, Loomis R, Vasquez KM, Cheng Y, Sartorelli AC (2000) Triapine (3-aminopyridine-2-carboxaldehyde- thiosemicarbazone): a potent inhibitor of ribonucleotide reductase activity with broad spectrum antitumor activity. Biochem Pharmacol 59:983–991
Finch RA, Liu MC, Cory AH, Cory JG, Sartorelli AC (1999) Triapine (3-aminopyridine-2-carboxaldehyde thiosemicarbazone; 3-AP): an inhibitor of ribonucleotide reductase with antineoplastic activity. Adv Enzyme Regul 39:3–12
Fiuza SM, Holy J, Batista de Carvalho LA, Marques MP (2011) Biologic activity of a dinuclear Pd (II)-spermine complex toward human breast cancer. Chem Biol Drug Des 77:477–488
Fonteh PN, Keter FK, Meyer D (2011) New bis(thiosemicarbazonate) gold(III) complexes inhibit HIV replication at cytostatic concentrations: potential for incorporation into virostatic cocktails. J Inorg Biochem 105:1173–1180
Forestier J (1932) The treatment of rheumatoid arthritis with gold salts injection. Lancet 1:441–444
Fortin S, Brasseur K, Morin N, Asselin E, Berube G (2013) New platinum(II) complexes conjugated at position 7α of 17β-acetyl-testosterone as new combi-molecules against prostate cancer: design, synthesis, structure-activity relationships and biological evaluation. Eur J Med Chem 68:433–443
Frasconi M, Liu Z, LeiJ WuY, Strekalova E, Malin D, Ambrogio MW, Chen X, Botros YY, Cryns VL, Sauvage JP, Stoddart JF (2013) Photoexpulsion of surface-grafted ruthenium complexes and subsequent release of cytotoxic cargos to cancer cells from mesoporous silica nanoparticles. J Am Chem Soc 135:11603–11613
Gabano E, Ravera M, Osella D (2009) The drug targeting and delivery approach applied to pt-antitumour complexes A coordination point of view. CurrMedChem 16:4544–4580
Galassi R, Burini A, Ricci S, Pellei M, Rigobello MP, Citta A, Dolmella A, Gandin V, Marzano C (2012) Synthesis and characterization of azolate gold(I) phosphane complexes as thioredoxin reductase inhibiting antitumor agents. Dalton Trans 41:5307–5318

Gallagher J, Chen CH, Pan CQ, Perrin DM, Cho YM, Sigman DS (1996) Optimizing the targeted chemical nuclease activity of 1,10-phenanthroline-copper by ligand modification. Bioconjug Chem 7:413–420

Ganeshpandian M, Loganathan R, Suresh E, Riyasdeen A, Akbarsha MA, Palaniandavar M (2014) New ruthenium(II) arene complexes of anthracenyl-appended diazacycloalkanes: effect of ligand intercalation and hydrophobicity on DNA and protein binding and cleavage and cytotoxicity. Dalton Trans 43:1203–1219

Garcia-Gimenez JL, Hernandez-Gil J, Martinez-Ruiz A, Castineiras A, Liu-Gonzalez M, Pallardo FV, Borras J, Alzuet-Pina G (2013) DNA binding, nuclease activity, DNA photocleavage and cytotoxic properties of Cu(II) complexes of N-substituted sulfonamides. J Inorg Biochem 121:167–178

Gill MR, Thomas JA (2012) New ruthenium(II) arene complexes of anthracenyl-appended diazacycloalkanes: effect of ligand intercalation and hydrophobicity on DNA and protein binding and cleavage and cytotoxicity. Chem Soc Rev 41:3179–3192

Giovagnoli S, Marenzoni ML, Nocchetti M, Santi C, Blasi P, Schoubben A, Ricci M (2014) Synthesis, characterization and in vitro extracellular and intracellular activity against *Mycobacterium tuberculosis* infection of new second-line antitubercular drug-palladium complexes. J Pharm Pharmacol 66:106–121

Gomez N, Santos D, Vazquez R, Suescun L, Mombru A, Vermeulen M, Finkielsztein L, Shayo C, Moglioni A, Gambino D, Davio C (2011) Synthesis, structural characterization, and pro-apoptotic activity of 1-indanone thiosemicarbazone platinum(II) and palladium(II) complexes: potential as antileukemic agents. ChemMedChem 6:1485–1494

González AG, Shirokova LS, Pokrovsky OS, Emnova EE, Martínez RE, Santana-Casiano JM, González-Dávila M, Pokrovski GS (2010) Adsorption of copper on *Pseudomonas aureofaciens*: protective role of surface exopolysaccharides. J Colloid Interface Sci 350:305–314

González-Pantoja JF, Stern M, Jarzecki AA, Royo E, Robles-Escajeda E, Varela-Ramírez A, Aguilera RJ, Contel M (2011) Titanocene-phosphine derivatives as precursors to cytotoxic heterometallic $TiAu_2$ and TiM (M = Pd, Pt) compounds Studies of their interactions with DNA. Inorg Chem 50:11099–11110

Göschl S, Schreiber-Brynzak E, Pichler V, Cseh K, Heffeter P, Jungwirth U, Jakupec MA, Berger W, Keppler BK (2017) Comparative studies of oxaliplatin-based platinum(iv) complexes in different in vitro and in vivo tumor models. Metallomics 9(3):309–322

Goswami TK, Chakravarthi BV, Roy M, Karande AA, Chakravarty AR (2011) Ferrocene-conjugated L-tryptophan copper(II) complexes of phenanthroline bases showing DNA photocleavage activity and cytotoxicity. Inorg Chem 50:8452–8464

Grass G, Rensing C, Solioz M (2011) Metallic copper as an antimicrobial surface. Appl Environ Microbiol 77:1541–1547

Guo QF, Liu SH, Liu QH, Xu HH, Zhao JH, Wu HF, Li XY, Wang JW (2012) Cytotoxicity, apoptosis, cellular uptake, cell cycle distribution, and DNA-binding investigation of ruthenium complexes. DNA Cell Biol 31:1205–1213

Gziut M, MacGregor HJ, Nevell TG, Mason T, Laight D, Shute JK (2013) Anti-inflammatory effects of tobramycin and a copper-tobramycin complex with superoxide dismutase-like activity. Br J Pharmacol 168:1165–1181

Harper BW, Krause-Heuer AM, Grant MP, Manohar M, Garbutcheon-Singh KB, Aldrich-Wright JR (2010) Advances in platinum chemotherapeutics. Chemistry 16:7064–7077

Hartung EF (1943) The treatment of rheumatoid arthritis including gold salts therapy. Bull NY Acad Med 19(10):693–703

Healy ML, Lim KKT, Travers R (2009) Jacques Forestier (1890–1978) and gold therapy. Int J Rheum Dis 12:145–148

Hernandez W, Paz J, Carrasco F, Vaisberg A, Spodine E, Manzur J, Hennig L, Sieler J, Blaurock S, Beyer L (2013) Synthesis and characterization of new palladium(II) thiosemicarbazone complexes and their cytotoxic activity against various human tumor cell lines. Bioinorg Chem Appl 2013:1

Hill WR, Pillsbury DM (1939) Argyria: the pharmacology of silver. Williams & Wilkins Baltimore

Hogarth G (2012) Metal-dithiocarbamate complexes: chemistry and biological activity. Mini-Rev Med Chem 12:1202–1215

Horvath UE, Dobrzanska L, Strasser CE, Bouwer Nee Potgieter W, Joone G, van Rensburg CE, Cronje S, Raubenheimer HG (2012) Amides of gold(I) diphosphines prepared from N-heterocyclic sources and their in vitro and in vivo screening for anticancer activity. J Inorg Biochem 111:80–90

Huxley M, Sanchez-Cano C, Browning MJ, Navarro-Ranninger C, Quiroga AG, Rodger A, Hannon MJ (2010) An androgenic steroid delivery vector that imparts activity to a non-conventional platinum(II) metallo-drug. Dalton Trans 39:11353–11364

Ibrahim AA, Khaledi H, Hassandarvish P, Mohd Ali H, Karimian H (2014) Indole-7-carbaldehyde thiosemicarbazone as a flexidentate ligand toward ZnII, CdII, PdII and PtII ions: cytotoxic and apoptosis-inducing properties of the PtII complex. Dalton Trans 43:3850–3860

Icsel C, Yilmaz VT, Ari F, Ulukaya E, Harrison WT (2013) Trans-Dichloridopalladium(II) and platinum(II) complexes with 2-(hydroxymethyl)pyridine and 2-(2-hydroxyethyl)pyridine: synthesis, structural characterization, DNA binding and in vitro cytotoxicity studies. Eur J Med Chem 60:386–394

Iniguez E, Sanchez A, Vasquez MA, Martinez A, Olivas J, Sattler A, Sanchez-Delgado RA, Maldonado RA (2013) Metal-drug synergy: new ruthenium(II) complexes of ketoconazole are highly active against Leishmania major and Trypanosoma cruzi and nontoxic to human or murine normal cells. J Biol Inorg Chem 18:779–790

Jagadeesh M, Kalangi SK, Sivarama Krishna L, Reddy AV (2014) Halo-substituted thiosemicarbazones and their copper(II), nickel(II) complexes: detailed spectroscopic characterization and study of antitumour activity against HepG2 human hepatoblastoma cells. Spectrochim Acta Part A Mol Biomol Spectrosc 118:552–556

Jagadeesh M, Rashmi HK, Subba Rao Y, Sreenath Reddy A, Prathima B, Uma Maheswari Devi P, Reddy AV (2013) Synthesis and spectroscopic characterization of 3,4-difluoroacetophenone-thiosemicarbazone and its palladium(II) complex: evaluation of antimicrobial and antitumour activity. Spectrochim Acta Part A Mol Biomol Spectrosc 115:583–587

Jaividhya P, Dhivya R, Akbarsha MA, Palaniandavar M (2012) Efficient DNA cleavage mediated by mononuclear mixed ligand copper(II) phenolate complexes: the role of co-ligand planarity on DNA binding and cleavage and anticancer activity. J Inorg Biochem 114:94–105

Jamal M, Tasneem U, Hussain T, Andleeb S (2015) Bacterial biofilm: its composition, formation and role in human, infections. Res Rev J Microbiol Biotechnol 4(3):1–14

Jamaludin NS, Goh ZJ, Cheah YK, Ang KP, Sim JH, Khoo CH, Fairuz ZA, Halim SN, Ng SW, Seng HL, Tiekink ER (2013) Phosphanegold(I) dithiocarbamates, $R_3PAu[SC(=S)N((i)Pr)CH_2CH_2OH]$ for R = Ph, Cy and Et: role of phosphane-bound R substituents upon in vitro cytotoxicity against MCF-7R breast cancer cells and cell death pathways. Eur J Med Chem 67:127–141

Johnstone TC, Suntharalingam K, Lippard SJ (2016) The next generation of platinum drugs: targeted Pt(II) agents, nanoparticle delivery and Pt(IV) prodrugs. Chem Rev 116(5):3436–3486

Jortzik E, Farhadi M, Ahmadi R, Toth K, Lohr J, Helmke BM, Kehr S, Unterberg A, Ott I, Gust R, Deborde V, Davioud-Charvet E, Reau R, Herold-Mende C, Reau R (2014) Antiglioma activity of GoPI-sugar, a novel gold(I)-phosphole inhibitor: chemical synthesis, mechanistic studies, and effectiveness in vivo. Biochem Biophys Acta 1844(8):1415–1426

Kachadourian R, Brechbuhl HM, Ruiz-Azuara L, Gracia-Mora I, Day BJ (2010) Casiopeína IIgly-induced oxidative stress and mitochondrial dysfunction in human lung cancer A549 and H157 cells. Toxicology 268:176–183

Kalaivani P, Prabhakaran R, Dallemer F, Poornima P, Vaishnavi E, Ramachandran E, Padma VV, Renganathan R, Natarajan K (2012a) DNA, protein binding, cytotoxicity, cellular uptake and antibacterial activities of new palladium(II) complexes of thiosemicarbazone ligands: effects of substitution on biological activity. Metallomics 4:101–113

Kalaivani P, Prabhakaran R, Ramachandran E, Dallemer F, Paramaguru G, Renganathan R Poornima, Poornima P, Vijaya Padma V, Natarajan K (2012b) Influence of terminal substitution on structural, DNA, protein binding, anticancer and antibacterial activities of palladium(II) complexes containing 3-methoxy salicylaldehyde-4(N) substituted thiosemicarbazones. Dalton Trans 41:2486–2499

Kalan LR, Pepin DM, Ul-Haq I, Miller SB, Hay ME, Precht RJ (2017) Targeting biofilms of multidrug-resistant bacteria with silver oxynitrate. Int J Antimicrob Agents 49(6):719–726

Karakucuk-Iyidogan A, Tasdemir D, Oruc-Emre EE, Balzarini J (2011) Novel platinum(II) and palladium(II) complexes of thiosemicarbazones derived from 5-substitutedthiophene-2-carboxaldehydes and their antiviral and cytotoxic activities. Eur J Med Chem 46:5616–5624

Kenche VB, Hung LW, Perez K, Volitakes I, Ciccotosto G, Kwok J, Critch N, Sherratt N, Cortes M, Lal V, Masters CL, Murakami K, Cappai R, Adlard PA, Barnham KJ (2013) Novel platinum(II) and palladium(II) complexes of thiosemicarbazones derived from 5-substitutedthiophene-2-carboxaldehydes and their antiviral and cytotoxic activities. Angew Chem 52:3374–3378 (International Edition in English)

Keter FK, Guzei IA, Nell M, Zyl WE, Darkwa J (2014) Phosphinogold(I) dithiocarbamate complexes: effect of the nature of phosphine ligand on anticancer properties. Inorg Chem 53:2058–2067

Khanye SD, Smith GS, Lategan C, Smith PJ, Gut J, Rosenthal PJ, Chibale K (2010) Synthesis and in vitro evaluation of gold(I) thiosemicarbazone complexes for antimalarial activity. J Inorg Biochem 104:1079–1083

Kharadi GJ (2014) Effect of substituent of terpyridines on the in vitro antioxidant, antitubercular, biocidal and fluorescence studies of copper(II) complexes with clioquinol. Spectrochim Acta Part A Mol Biomol Spectrosc 117:662–668

Komeda S, Casini A (2012) Next-generation anticancer metallodrugs. Curr Top Med Chem 12:219–235

Komeda S, Lin YL, Chikuma M (2011) A tetrazolato-bridged dinuclear platinum(II) complex exhibits markedly high in vivo antitumor activity against pancreatic cancer. ChemMedChem 6:987–990

Kouodom MN, Boscutti G, Celegato M, Crisma M, Sitran S, Aldinucci D, Formaggio F, Ronconi L, Fregona D (2012) Rational design of gold(III)-dithiocarbamato peptidomimetics for the targeted anticancer chemotherapy. J Inorg Biochem 117:248–260

Kowol CR, Heffeter P, Miklos W, Gille L, Trondl R, Cappellacci L, Berger W, Keppler BK (2012) Mechanisms underlying reductant-induced reactive oxygen species formation by anticancer copper(II) compounds. J Biol Inorg Chem 17:409–423

Kraszewski S, Duverger E, Ramseyer C, Picaud F (2013) Theoretical study of amino derivatives and anticancer platinum drug grafted on various carbon nanostructures. J Chem Phys 139:174704

Kumar A, Chinta JP, Ajay AK, Bhat MK, Rao CP (2011) Synthesis, characterization, plasmid cleavage and cytotoxicity of cancer cells by a copper(II) complex of anthracenyl-terpyridine. Dalton Trans 40:10865–10872

Kuster T, Lense N, Barna F, Hemphill A, Kindermann MK, Heinicke JW, Vock CA (2012) A new promising application for highly cytotoxic metal compounds: η^6-areneruthenium(II) phosphite complexes for the treatment of alveolar echinococcosis. J Med Chem 55:4178–4188

Kvasnica M, Rarova L, Oklestkova J, Budesinsky M, Kohout L (2012) Synthesis and cytotoxic activities of estrone and estradiol cis-dichloroplatinum(II) complexes. Bioorg Med Chem 20:6969–6978

Lam PL, Lu GL, Hon KM, Lee KW, Ho CL, Wang X, Tang JC, Lam KH, Wong RS, Kok SH, Bian ZX, Li H, Lee KK, Gambari R, Chui CH, Wong WY (2014) Development of ruthenium (II) complexes as topical antibiotics against methicillin resistant *Staphylococcus aureus*. Dalton Trans 43:3949–3957

Lemire JA, Harrison JJ, Turner RJ (2013) Antimicrobial activity of metals: mechanisms, molecular targets and applications. Nat Rev Microbiol 11:371–384

Lemire JA, Kalan L, Bradu A, Turner RJ (2015) Silver oxynitrate, an unexplored silver compound with antimicrobial and antibiofilm activity. Antimicrob Agents Chemother 59(7):4031–4039
Lemire JA, Kalan L, Gugala N, Bradu A, Turner RJ (2017) Silver oxynitrate—an efficacious compound for the prevention and eradication of dual-species biofilms. Biofouling 33(6):460–469
Li X, Zhang Z, Wang C, Zhang T, He K, Deng F (2011) Synthesis, crystal structure and action on *Escherichia coli* by microcalorimetry of copper complexes with 1,10-phenanthroline and amino acid. J Inorg Biochem 105:23–30
Li XW, Li XJ, Li YT, Wu ZY, Yan CW (2013) Syntheses and structures of new trimetallic complexes bridged by N-(5-chloro-2-hydroxyphenyl)-N'-[3-(dimethylamino)propyl]oxamide: cytotoxic activities, and reactivities towards DNA and protein. J Photochem Photobiol B Biol 118:22–32
Li F, Feterl M, Mulyana Y, Warner JM, Collins JG, Keene FR (2012a) In vitro susceptibility and cellular uptake for a new class of antimicrobial agents: dinuclear ruthenium(II) complexes. Antimicrob Agents Chemother 67:2686–2695
Li Z, Yang X, Dong S, Li X (2012b) DNA breakage induced by piceatannol and copper(II): mechanism and anticancer properties. Oncol Lett 3:1087–1094
Li S, Zhang S, Jin X, Tan X, Lou J, Zhang X, Zhao Y (2014a) Singly protonated dehydronorcantharidin silver coordination polymer induces apoptosis of lung cancer cells via reactive oxygen species-mediated mitochondrial pathway. Eur J Med Chem 86:1–11
Li Y, Liu GF, Tan CP, Ji LN, Mao ZW (2014b) Antitumor properties and mechanisms of mitochondria-targeted Ag(I) and Au(I) complexes containing N-heterocyclic carbenes derived from cyclophanes. Metallomics 6(8):1460–1468
Lima JC, Rodriguez L (2011) Phosphine-gold(I) compounds as anticancer agents: general description and mechanisms of action. Anti-Cancer Agents Med Chem 11:921–928
Lin GJ, Jiang GB, Xie YY, Huang HL, Liang ZH, Liu YJ (2013) Cytotoxicity, apoptosis, cell cycle arrest, reactive oxygen species, mitochondrial membrane potential, and Western blotting analysis of ruthenium(II) complexes. J Biol Inorg Chem 18:873–882
Lin M, Wang X, Zhu J, Fan D, Zhang Y, Zhang J, Guo Z (2011) Cellular and biomolecular responses of human ovarian cancer cells to cytostatic dinuclear platinum(II) complexes. Apoptosis 16:288–300
Lippard SJ (1982) New chemistry of an old molecule: cis-[Pt(NH3)2Cl2]. Science 218:1075–1082
Liu MC, Lin TS, Sartorelli AC (1992) Synthesis and antitumor activity of amino derivatives of pyridine-2-carboxaldehyde thiosemicarbazone. J Med Chem 35:3672–3677
Liu MC, Lin TS, Sartorelli AC (1995) Chemical and biological properties of cytotoxic alpha-(N)-heterocyclic carboxaldehyde thiosemicarbazones. Prog Med Chem 32:1–35
Liu W, Gust R (2013) Metal N-heterocyclic carbene complexes as potential antitumor metallodrugs. Chem Soc Rev 42:755–773
Liu X, Li X, Zhang Z, Dong Y, Liu P, Zhang C (2013a) Studies on antibacterial mechanisms of copper complexes with 1,10-phenanthroline and amino acid on *Escherichia coli*. Biol Trace Elem Res 154:150–155
Liu X, Zhang LL, Xu XH, Hui L, Zhang JB, Chen SW (2013b) Synthesis and anticancer activity of dichloroplatinum(II) complexes of podophyllotoxin. Bioorg Med Chem Lett 23:3780–3784
Liu XW, Chem ZG, Li L, Chen YD, Lu JL, Zhang DS (2013c) DNA-binding, photocleavage studies of ruthenium(II) complexes with 2-(2-quinolinyl) imidazo[4,5-f][1,10]phenanthroline. Spectrochim Acta Part A Mol Biomol Spectrosc 102:142–149
Liu XW, Chen YD, Li L, Lu JL, Zhang DS (2012) DNA-binding and photocleavage studies of ruthenium(II) complexes containing asymmetric intercalative ligand. Spectrochim Acta Part A Mol Biomol Spectrosc 86:554–561
Liu YJ, Li ZZ, Liang ZH, Yao JH, Huang HL (2011) Cytotoxicity, apoptosis, cellular uptake, cell cycle arrest, photocleavage, and antioxidant activity of 1, 10-henanthroline ruthenium(II) complexes. DNA Cell Biol 30:839–848
Lovejoy KS, Lippard SJ (2009) Non-traditional platinum compounds for improved accumulation, oral bioavailability, and tumor targeting. Dalton Trans 48:10651–10659

Macomber L, Imlay JA (2009) The iron-sulfur clusters of dehydratases are primary intracellular targets of copper toxicity. PNAS 106:8344–8349

Maeda H, Bharate GY, Daruwalla J (2009) Polymeric drugs for efficient tumor-targeted drug delivery based on EPR-effect. Eur J Pharm Biopharm 71:409–419

Maia PI, Fernandes AG, Silva JJ, Andricopulo AD, Lemos SS, Lang ES, Abram U, Deflon VM (2010) Dithiocarbazate complexes with the $[M(PPh_3)]^{2+}$ (M = Pd or Pt) moiety: synthesis, characterization and anti-*Trypanosoma cruzi* activity. J Inorg Biochem 104:1276–1282

Manikandamathavan VM, Rajapandian V, Freddy AJ, Weyhermuller T, Subramanian V, Nair BU (2012) Effect of coordinated ligands on antiproliferative activity and DNA cleavage property of three mononuclear Cu(II)-terpyridine complexes. Eur J Med Chem 57:449–458

Mansouri-Torshizi H, Eslami-Moghadam M, Divsalar A, Saboury AA (2011) DNA-binding studies of some potential antitumor 2,2'-bipyridine Pt(II)/Pd(II) complexes of piperidinedithiocarbamate their synthesis, spectroscopy and cytotoxicity. Acta Chim Slov 58:811–822

Martins DA, Gouvea LR, da Gama Jean Batista D, da Silva PB, Louro SR, de Nazare CSM, Teixeira LR (2012) Copper(II)-fluoroquinolone complexes with anti-*Trypanosoma cruzi* activity and DNA binding ability. Biometals 25:951–960

Marzano C, Ronconi L, Chiara F, Giron MC, Faustinelli I, Cristofori P, Trevisan A, Fregona D (2011) Gold(III)-dithiocarbamato anticancer agents: activity, toxicology and histopathological studies in rodents. Int J Cancer 129:487–496

Matesanz AI, Hernandez C, Rodriguez A, Souza P (2011a) 3,5-diacetyl-1,2,4-triazol bis (4N-substituted thiosemicarbazone) palladium(II) complexes: synthesis, structure, antiproliferative activity and low toxicity on normal kidney cells. J Inorg Biochem 105:1613–1622

Matesanz AI, Hernandez C, Rodriguez A, Souza P (2011b) Novel bis(thiosemicarbazones) of the 3,5-diacetyl-1,2,4-triazol series and their platinum(II) complexes: chemistry, antiproliferative activity and preliminary nephrotoxicity studies. Dalton Trans 40:5738–5745

Matesanz AI, Leitao I, Souza P (2013) Palladium(II) and platinum(II) bis(thiosemicarbazone) complexes of the 2,6-diacetylpyridine series with high cytotoxic activity in cisplatin resistant A2780cisR tumor cells and reduced toxicity. J Inorg Biochem 125:26–31

Matesanz AI, Perles J, Souza P (2012) New palladium and platinum complexes with bioactive 3,5-diacetyl-1,2,4-triazol bis(4-cyclohexyl thiosemicarbazone) ligand: chemistry, antiproliferative activity and preliminary toxicity studies. Dalton Trans 41:12538–12547

Matsumura Y, Maeda H (1986) A new concept for macromolecular therapeutics in cancer chemotherapy: mechanism of tumoritropic accumulation of proteins and the antitumor agent smancs. Cancer Res 46:6387–6392

Medici S, Peana MF, Crisponi G, Nurchi VM, Lachowicz JI, Remelli M, Zoroddu MA (2016) Silver coordination compounds: a new horizon in medicine. Coord Chem Rev 327–328:349–359

Medici S, Peana MF, Nurchi VM, Lachowicz JI, Crisponi G, Zoroddu MA (2015) Noble metals in medicine: latest advances. Coord Chem Rev 284:329–350

Micale N, Cinellu MA, Maiore L, Sannella AR, Severini C, Schirmeister T, Gabbiani C, Messori L (2011) Selected gold compounds cause pronounced inhibition of Falcipain 2 and effectively block *P. falciparum* growth in vitro. J Inorg Biochem 105:1576–1579

Milunovic MN, Enyedy E, Nagy NV, Kiss T, Trondl R, Jakupec MA, Keppler BK, Krachler R, Novitchi G, Arion VB (2012) L- and D-proline thiosemicarbazone conjugates: coordination behavior in solution and the effect of copper(II) coordination on their antiproliferative activity. Inorg Chem 51:9309–9321

Mitra R, Das S, Shinde SV, Sinha S, Somasundaram K, Samuelson AG (2012) Anticancer activity of hydrogen-bond-stabilized half-sandwich Ru(II) complexes with heterocycles. Chemistry 18:12278–12291

Mlcouskova J, Kasparkova J, Suchankova T, Komeda S, Brabec V (2012) DNA conformation and repair of polymeric natural DNA damaged by antitumor azolato-bridged dinuclear Pt(II) complex. J Inorg Biochem 114:15–23

Mohamed MS, Shoukry AA, Ali AG (2012) Synthesis and structural characterization of ternary Cu (II) complexes of glycine with 2,2'-bipyridine and 2,2'-dipyridylamine The DNA-binding studies and biological activity. Spectrochim Acta Part A Mol Biomol Spectrosc 86:562–570

Molter A, Rust J, Lehmann CW, Deepa G, Chiba P, Mohr F (2011) Synthesis, structures and anti-malaria activity of some gold(I) phosphine complexes containing seleno- and thiosemicarbazonato ligands. Dalton Trans 40:9810–9820

Monafo WW, West MA (1990) Current treatment recommendations for topical burn therapy. Drugs 40:364–373

Morais TS, Silva TJ, Marques F, Robalo MP, Avecilla F, Amorim Madeira PJ, Mendes PJ, Santos I, Garcia MH (2012) Synthesis of organometallic ruthenium(II) complexes with strong activity against several human cancer cell lines. J Inorg Biochem 114:65–74

Mota VZ, de Carvalho GS, da Silva AD, Costa LA, de Almeida Machado P, Coimbra ES, Ferreira CV, Shishido SM, Cuin A (2014) Gold complexes with benzimidazole derivatives: synthesis, characterization and biological studies. Biometals 27:183–194

Mphahlele M, Papathanasopoulos M, Cinellu MA, Coyanis M, Mosebi S, Traut T, Modise R, Coates J, Hewer R (2012) Modification of HIV-1 reverse transcriptase and integrase activity by gold(III) complexes in direct biochemical assays. Bioorg Med Chem 20:401–407

Musetti C, Nazarov AA, Farrell NP, Sissi C (2011) DNA reactivity profile of trans-platinum planar amine derivatives. ChemMedChem 6:1283–1290

Nagy EM, Ronconi L, Nardon C, Fregona D (2012) Noble metal-dithiocarbamates precious allies in the fight against cancer. Mini Rev Med Chem 12:1216–1229

Nardon C, Boscutti G, Fregona D (2014a) Beyond platinums: gold complexes as anticancer agents. Anticancer Res 34:487–492

Nardon C, Schmitt SM, Yang H, Zuo J, Fregona D, Dou QP (2014b) Gold(III) dithiocarbamato peptidomimetics in the forefront of the targeted anticancer therapy: preclinical studies against human breast neoplasia. PLoS ONE 9:e84248

Ng CH, Wang WS, Chong KV, Win YF, Neo KE, Lee HB, San SL, Raja Abd Rahman RN, Leong WK (2013) Ternary copper(II)-polypyridyl enantiomers: aldol-type condensation, characterization, DNA-binding recognition, BSA-binding and anticancer property. Dalton Trans 42:10233–10243

Nieminen R, Korhonen R, Moilanen T, Clark AR, Moilanen E (2010) Aurothiomalate inhibits cyclooxygenase 2, matrix metalloproteinase 3, and interleukin-6 expression in chondrocytes by increasing MAPK phosphatase 1 expression and decreasing p38 phosphorylation: MAPK phosphatase 1 as a novel target for antirheumatic drugs. Arthritis Rheumatol 62:1650–1659

Nieto D, Gonzalez-Vadillo AM, Bruna S, Pastor CJ, Rios-Luci C, Leon LG, Padron JM, Navarro-Ranninger C, Cuadrado I (2012) Heterometallic platinum(II) compounds with β-aminoethylferrocenes: synthesis, electrochemical behaviour and anticancer activity. Dalton Trans 41:432–441

Oberoi HS, Nukolova NV, Kabanov AV, Bronich TK (2013) Nanocarriers for delivery of platinum anticancer drugs. Adv Drug Delivery Rev 65:1667–1685

Oehninger L, Rubbiani R, Ott I (2013) N-Heterocyclic carbene metal complexes in medicinal chemistry. Dalton Trans 42:3269–3284

Olivova R, Kasparkova J, Vrana O, Vojtiskova M, Suchankova T, Novakova O, He W, Guo Z, Brabec V (2011) Unique DNA binding mode of antitumor trinuclear tridentate platinum(II) compound. Mol Pharm 8:2368–2378

Ortego L, Cardoso F, Martins S, Fillat MF, Laguna A, Meireles M, Villacampa MD, Gimeno MC (2014) Strong inhibition of thioredoxin reductase by highly cytotoxic gold(I) complexes DNA binding studies. J Inorg Biochem 130:32–37

Palanimuthu D, Shinde SV, Somasundaram K, Samuelson AG (2013) In vitro and in vivo anticancer activity of copper bis(thiosemicarbazone) complexes. J Med Chem 56:722–734

Palmieri TL, Greenlaugh DG (2002) Topical treatment of pediatric patients with burns: a practical guide. Am J Clin Dermatol 3:529–534

Patel MN, Joshi HN, Patel CR (2013) Cytotoxic, antibacterial, DNA interaction and superoxide dismutase like activities of sparfloxacin drug based copper(II) complexes with nitrogen donor ligands. Spectrochim Acta Part A Mol Biomol Spectrosc 104:48–55

Paterson BM, Donnelly PS (2011) Copper complexes of bis(thiosemicarbazones): from chemotherapeutics to diagnostic and therapeutic radiopharmaceuticals. Chem Soc Rev 40:3005–3018

Pavan FR, Poelhsitz GV, Barbosa MI, Leite SR, Batista AA, Ellena J, Sato LS, Franzblau SG, Moreno V, Gambino D, Leite CQ (2011) Ruthenium(II) phosphine/diimine/picolinate complexes: inorganic compounds as agents against tuberculosis. Eur J Med Chem 46:5099–5107

Pavan FR, Poelhsitz GV, da Cunha LV, Barbosa MI, Leite SR, Batista AA, Cho SH, Franzblau SG, de Camargo MS, Resende FA, Varanda EA, Leite CQ (2013) In vitro and in vivo activities of ruthenium(II) phosphine/diimine/picolinate complexes (SCAR) against *Mycobacterium tuberculosis*. PLoS ONE 8:e64242

Pellei M, Gandin V, Marinelli M, Marzano C, Yousufuddin M, Dias HV, Santini C (2012) Synthesis and biological activity of ester- and amide-functionalized imidazolium salts and related water-soluble coinage metal N-heterocyclic carbene complexes. Inorg Chem 51:9873–9882

Pelletier FDR, Comte V, Massard A, Wenzel M, Toulot SP, Richard P, Picquet M, Le-Gendre P, Zava O, Edafe F, Casini A, Dyson PJ (2010) Development of bimetallic titanocene-ruthenium-arene complexes as anticancer agents: relationships between structural and biological properties. J Med Chem 53:6923–6933

Percival SL, Bowler PG, Russell D (2005) Bacterial resistance to silver in wound care. J Hosp Infect 60:1–7

Pereira JC, Carregaro V, Costa DL, da Silva JS, Cunha FQ, Franco DW (2010) Antileishmanial activity of ruthenium(II)tetraammine nitrosyl complexes. Eur J Med Chem 45:4180–4187

Pérez C, Díaz-García CV, Agudo-López A, del Solar V, Cabrera S, Agulló-Ortuño MT, Navarro-Ranninger C, Alemán J, López-Martín JA (2014) Evaluation of novel trans-sulfonamide platinum complexes against tumor cell lines. Eur J Med Chem 76:360–368

Pisani MJ, Fromm PD, Mulyana Y, Clarke RJ, Korner H, Heimann K, Collins JG, Keene FR (2011) Mechanism of cytotoxicity and cellular uptake of lipophilic inert dinuclear polypyridylruthenium(II) complexes. ChemMedChem 6:848–858

Pisani MJ, Weber DK, Heimann K, Collins JG, Keene FR (2010) Selective mitochondrial accumulation of cytotoxic dinuclear polypyridyl ruthenium(II) complexes. Metallomics 2:393–396

Prabhakaran R, Anantharaman S, Thilagavathi M, Kaveri MV, Kalaivani P, Karvembu R, Dharmaraj N, Bertagnolli H, Dallemer F, Natarajan K (2011a) Preparation, spectroscopy, EXAFS, electrochemistry and pharmacology of new ruthenium(II) carbonyl complexes containing ferrocenylthiosemicarbazone and triphenylphosphine/arsine. Spectrochim Acta Part A Mol Biomol Spectrosc 78:844–853

Prabhakaran R, Kalaivani P, Jayakumar R, Zeller M, Hunter AD, Renukadevi SV, Ramachandran E, Natarajan K (2011b) Synthesis, structure and biological evaluation of bis salicylaldehyde-4(N)-ethylthiosemicarbazone ruthenium(iii) triphenylphosphine. Metallomics 3:42–48

Prabhakaran R, Kalaivani P, Poornima P, Dallemer F, Huang R, Vijaya Padma V, Natarajan K (2013) Synthesis, DNA/protein binding and in vitro cytotoxic studies of new palladium metallothiosemicarbazones. Bioorg Med Chem 21:6742–6752

Prisecaru A, Devereux M, Barron N, McCann M, Colleran J, Casey A, McKee V, Kellett A (2012a) Potent oxidative DNA cleavage by the di-copper cytotoxin: $[Cu_2(\mu\text{-terephthalate})(1,10\text{-phen})_4]^{2+}$. Chem Commun (Camb) 48:6906–6908

Prisecaru A, Devereux M, Barron N, McCann M, Colleran J, Casey A, McKee V, Kellett A (2012b) Potent oxidative DNA cleavage by the di-copper cytotoxin: $[Cu2(\mu\text{-terephthalate})(1,10\text{-phen})4]^{2+}$. Chem Commun (Camb) 48:6906–6908

Qian C, Wang JQ, Song CL, Wang LL, Ji LN, Chao H (2013) The induction of mitochondria-mediated apoptosis in cancer cells by ruthenium(II) asymmetric complexes. Metallomics 5:844–854

Qin XY, Yang LC, Le FL, Yu QQ, Sun DD, Liu YN, Liu J (2013) Structures and anti-cancer properties of two binuclear copper complexes. Dalton Trans 42:14681–14684

Quiroga AG (2012) Understanding trans platinum complexes as potential antitumor drugs beyond targeting DNA. J Inorg Biochem 114:106–112

Rafi M, Cabral H, Kano MR, Mi P, Iwata C, Yashiro M, Hirakawa K, Miyazono K, Nishiyama N, Kataoka K (2012) Polymeric micelles incorporating (1,2-diaminocyclohexane) platinum (II) suppress the growth of orthotopic scirrhous gastric tumors and their lymph node metastasis. J Control Release 159:189–196

Rai M, Ingle AP, Paralikar P, Gupta I, Medici S, Santos CA (2017) Recent advances in use of silver nanoparticles as antimalarial agents. Int J Pharm 526(1–2):254–270

Rajalakshmi S, Weyhermuller T, Dinesh M, Nair BU (2012) Copper(II) complexes of terpyridine derivatives: a footstep towards development of antiproliferative agent for breast cancer. J Inorg Biochem 117:48–59

Rajalakshmi S, Weyhermuller T, Freddy AJ, Vasanthi HR, Nair BU (2011) Anomalous behavior of pentacoordinate copper complexes of dimethylphenanthroline and derivatives of terpyridine ligands: studies on DNA binding, cleavage and apoptotic activity. Eur J Med Chem 46:608–617

Reddy PR, Shilpa A (2011) Synthesis, characterization, and DNA-binding and cleavage properties of dinuclear Cu(II)-salophen/salen complexes. Chem Biodivers 8:1245–1265

Roberts JJ, Thomson AJ (1979) The mechanism of action of antitumor platinum compounds. Prog Nucleic Acid Res Mol Biol 22:71–133

Rosenberg B, Vancamp L, Krigas T (1965) Inhibition of cell division in *Escherichia Coli* by electrolysis products from a platinum electrode. Nature 205:698–699

Rosenberg B, VanCamp L, Trosko JE, Mansour VH (1969) Platinum compounds: a new class of potent antitumour agents. Nature 222:385–386

Ruiz J, Rodriguez V, Cutillas N, Espinosa A, Hannon MJ (2011a) Novel C, N-chelate platinum(II) antitumor complexes bearing a lipophilic ethisterone pendant. J Inorg Biochem 105:525–531

Ruiz J, Vicente C, de Haro C, Espinosa A (2011b) Synthesis and antiproliferative activity of a C, N-cycloplatinated(II) complex with a potentially intercalative anthraquinone pendant. Inorg Chem 50:2151–2158

Ruiz-Azuara L (1992) México Trade Mark: Casiopeína SECOFI 407543; US Patent 5,107,005

Ruiz-Azuara L (1993) México Patent 172248

Ruiz-Azuara L (1994) México Patent 172967

Ruiz-Azuara L (1996) US Patent 5, 576,326

Ruiz-Azuara L (1997) EP 434444; US Patent Re 35,458

Ruiz-Azuara L (1999) EP 314073

Ruiz-Azuara L, Bravo-Gomez ME (2010) Copper compounds in cancer chemotherapy. Curr Med Chem 17:3606–3615

Saha P, Descoteaux C, Brasseur K, Fortin S, Leblanc V, Parent S, Asselin E, Berube G (2012) Synthesis, antiproliferative activity and estrogen receptor α affinity of novel estradiol-linked platinum(II) complex analogs to carboplatin and oxaliplatin potential vector complexes to target estrogen-dependent tissues. Eur J Med Chem 48:385–390

Sakhrani NM, Padh H (2013) Organelle targeting: third level of drug targeting. Drug Des Dev Ther 7:585–599

Saturnino C, Barone I, Iacopetta D, Mariconda A, Sinicropi MS, Rosano C, Campana A, Catalano S, Longo P, Andò S (2016) N-heterocyclic carbene complexes of silver and gold as novel tools against breast cancer progression. Future Med Chem 8(18):2213–2229

Scaffidi-Domianello YY, Meelich K, Jakupec MA, Arion VB, Kukushkin VY, Galanski M, Keppler BK (2010) Novel cis- and trans-configured bis(oxime)platinum(II) complexes: synthesis, characterization, and cytotoxic activity. Inorg Chem 49:5669–5678

Selvamurugan S, Ramachandran R, Viswanathamurthi P (2013) Ruthenium(II) carbonyl complexes containing S-methylisothiosemicarbazone based tetradentate ligand: synthesis, characterization and biological applications. Biometals 26:741–753

Semenova E, Finger PT (2013) Palladium-103 radiation therapy for small choroidal melanoma. Ophthalmology 120:2353–2357

Semenova E, Finger PT (2014) Palladium-103 plaque radiation therapy for American Joint Committee on cancer T3- and T4-staged choroidal melanomas. JAMA Ophthalmol 132:205–213

Serment-Guerrero J, Cano-Sanchez P, Reyes-Perez E, Velazquez-Garcia F, Bravo-Gomez ME, Ruiz-Azuara L (2011) Genotoxicity of the copper antineoplastic coordination complexes casiopeinas. Toxicol In Vitro 25:1376–1384

Shahabadi N, Nemati L (2012) DNA interaction studies of a platinum(II) complex containing L-histidine and 1,10-phenanthroline ligands. DNA Cell Biol 31:883–890

Sharlow ER, Leimgruber S, Murray S, Lira A, Sciotti RJ, Hickman M, Hudson T, Leed S, Caridha D, Barrios AM, Close D, Grogl M, Lazo JS (2014) Auranofin is an apoptosis-simulating agent with in vitro and in vivo anti-leishmanial activity. ACS Chem Biol 9:663–672

Sharma K, Singh RV, Fahmi N (2011) Palladium(II) and platinum(II) derivatives of benzothiazoline ligands: synthesis, characterization, antimicrobial and antispermatogenic activity. Spectrochim Acta A Mol Biomol Spectrosc 78:80–87

Silva PP, Guerra W, Silveira JN, Ferreira AM, Bortolotto T, Fischer FL, Terenzi H, Neves A, Pereira-Maia EC (2011) Two new ternary complexes of copper(II) with tetracycline or doxycycline and 1,10-phenanthroline and their potential as antitumoral: cytotoxicity and DNA cleavage. Inorg Chem 50:6414–6424

Silva H, Silva AC, Lemos FO, Monte-Neto RL, Fontes AP, Lopes MT, Frezard F (2013a) Improved pharmacological profile of the lipophilic antitumor dichloro-(N-dodecyl)-propanediamine-platinum(II) complex after incorporation into pegylated liposomes. Anticancer Drugs 24:131–139

Silva TM, Andersson S, Sukumaran SK, Marques MP, Persson L, Oredsson S (2013b) Improved pharmacological profile of the lipophilic antitumor dichloro-(N-dodecyl)-propanediamine-platinum(II) complex after incorporation into pegylated liposomes. PLoS ONE 8:13

Silver S (2003) Bacterial silver resistance: molecular biology and uses and misuses of silver compounds. FEMS Microbiol Rev 27:341–353

Slawson RM, Lohmeier-Vogel EM, Lee H, Trevors JT (1994) Silver resistance in *Pseudomonas stutzeri*. Biometals 7:30–40

Smith GS, Therrien B (2011) Targeted and multifunctional arene ruthenium chemotherapeutics. Dalton Trans 40:10793–10800

Sousa I, Claro V, Pereira JL, Amaral AL, Cunha-Silva L, de Castro B, Feio MJ, Pereira E, Gameiro P (2012) Synthesis, characterization and antibacterial studies of a copper(II) levofloxacin ternary complex. J Inorg Biochem 110:64–71

Srishailam A, Kumar YP, Gabra NM, Reddy PV, Deepika N, Veerababu N, Satyanarayana S (2013) Synthesis, DNA-binding, cytotoxicity, photo cleavage, antimicrobial and docking studies of Ru(II) polypyridyl complexes. J Fluoresc 23:897–908

Starosta R, Bykowska A, Kyziol A, Plotek M, Florek M, Krol J, Jezowska-Bojczuk M (2013) Copper(I) (pseudo)halide complexes with neocuproine and aminomethylphosphines derived from morpholine and thiomorpholine -in vitro cytotoxic and antimicrobial activity and the interactions with DNA and serum albumins. Chem Biol Drug Des 82:579–586

Sterling JC, Handfield-Jones S, Hudson PM (2001) Guidelines for the management of cutaneous warts. Br J Dermatol 144(1):4–11

Stordal B, Davey M (2007) Understanding cisplatin resistance using cellular models. IUBMB Life 59:696–699

Storm-Versloot MN, Vos CG, Ubbink DT, Vermeulen H (2010) Topical silver for preventing wound infection. Cochrane Database Syst Rev (Online) 3:CD006478; https://doi.org/10.1002/14651858.cd006478.pub2

Su W, Qian Q, Li P, Lei X, Xiao Q, Huang S, Huang C, Cui J (2013) Synthesis, characterization and anticancer activity of a series of ketone-N(4)-substituted thiosemicarbazones and their ruthenium(II) arene complexes. Inorg Chem 52:12440–12449

Sudha VB, Ganesan S, Pazhani GP, Ramamurthy T, Nair GB, Venkatasubramanian P (2012) Storing drinking-water in copper pots kills contaminating diarrhoeagenic bacteria. J Health Population Nutr 30:17–21

Sun D, Liu Y, Liu D, Zhang R, Yang X, Liu J (2012) Stabilization of G-quadruplex DNA, inhibition of telomerase activity and live cell imaging studies of chiral ruthenium(II) complexes. Chemistry 18:4285–4295

Suntharalingam K, Hunt DJ, Duarte AA, White AJ, Mann DJ, Vilar R (2012) A tri-copper(II) complex displaying DNA-cleaving properties and antiproliferative activity against cancer cells. Chemistry 18:15133–15141

Süss-Fink G (2010) Arene ruthenium complexes as anticancer agents. Dalton Trans 39:1673–1688

Sütterlin S, Edquist P, Sandegren L, Adler M, Tängdén T, Drobni M, Olsen B, Melhus Å (2014) Silver resistance genes are overrepresented among *Escherichia coli* isolates with CTX-M production. Appl Environ Microbiol 80(22):6863–6869

Tabassum S, Asim A, Arjmand F, Afzal M, Bagchi V (2012) Synthesis and characterization of copper(II) and zinc(II)-based potential chemotherapeutic compounds: their biological evaluation viz DNA binding profile, cleavage and antimicrobial activity. Eur J Med Chem 58:308–316

Todd RC, Lippard S (2009) Inhibition of transcription by platinum antitumor compounds. Metallomics 1:280–291

Tomaz AI, Jakusch T, Morais TS, Marques F, de Almeida RF, Mendes F, Enyedy EA, Santos I, Pessoa JC, Kiss T, Garcia MH (2012) $[RuII(\eta^5\text{-}C_5H_5)(bipy)(PPh_3)]^+$, a promising large spectrum antitumor agent: cytotoxic activity and interaction with human serum albumin. J Inorg Biochem 117:261–269

Travnicek Z, Starha P, Vanco J, Silha T, Hosek J, Suchy P Jr, Prazanova G (2012) Anti-inflammatory active gold(I) complexes involving 6-substituted-purine derivatives. J Med Chem 55:4568–4579

Tummala R, Diegelman P, Fiuza SM, Batista de Carvalho LA, Marques MP, Kramer DL, Clark K, Vujcic S, Porter CW, Pendyala L (2010) Characterization of Pt-, Pd-spermine complexes for their effect on polyamine pathway and cisplatin resistance in A2780 ovarian carcinoma cells. Oncol Rep 24:15–24

Vaupel E (2005) Arthur Eichengrün - Tribute to a Forgotten Chemist, Entrepreneur, and German Jew. Angew Chem Int Ed 44:3344–3355

Vergara E, Casini A, Sorrentino F, Zava O, Cerrada E, Rigobello MP, Bindoli A, Laguna M, Dyson PJ (2010) Anticancer therapeutics that target selenoenzymes: synthesis, characterization, in vitro cytotoxicity, and thioredoxin reductase inhibition of a series of gold(I) complexes containing hydrophilic phosphine ligands. ChemMedChem 5:96–102

Vergara E, Cerrada E, Clavel C, Casini A, Laguna M (2011) Thiolato gold(I) complexes containing water-soluble phosphane ligands: a characterization of their chemical and biological properties. Dalton Trans 40:10927–10935

Very T, Despax S, Hebraud P, Monari A, Assfeld X (2012) Spectral properties of polypyridyl ruthenium complexes intercalated in DNA: theoretical insights into the surrounding effects of $[Ru(dppz)(bpy)_2]^{2+}$. Phys Chem Chem Phys 14:12496–12504

Wachter E, Heidary DK, Howerton BS, Parkin S, Glazer EC (2012) Light-activated ruthenium complexes photobind DNA and are cytotoxic in the photodynamic therapy window. Chem Commun (Camb) 48:9649–9651

Wang X (2010) Light-activated ruthenium complexes photobind DNA and are cytotoxic in the photodynamic therapy window. Anticancer Agents Med Chem 10:396–411

Wang X, Guo Z (2013) Targeting and delivery of platinum-based anticancer drugs. Chem Soc Rev 42:202–224

Wang Y, Liu M, Cao R, Zhang W, Yin M, Xiao X, Liu Q, Huang N (2013) A soluble bis-chelated gold(I) diphosphine compound with strong anticancer activity and low toxicity. J Med Chem 56:1455–1466

Wasiak J, Cleland H, Campbell F and Spinks A (2013) Dressings for superficial and partial thickness burns. The Cochrane database of systematic reviews 3: CD002106 PMID 23543513

Wei C, Ren L, Gao N (2013) Interactions of terpyridines and their Pt(II) complexes with G-quadruplex DNAs and telomerase inhibition. Int J Biol Macromol 57:1–8

Wenzel M, Bertrand B, Eymin MJ, Comte V, Harvey JA, Richard P, Groessl M, Zava O, Amrouche H, Harvey PD, Le Gendre P, Picquet M, Casini A (2011) Multinuclear cytotoxic metallodrugs: physicochemical characterization and biological properties of novel heteronuclear gold-titanium complexes. Inorg Chem 50:9472–9480

Westendorf AF, Bodtke A, Bednarski PJ (2011) Studies on the photoactivation of two cytotoxic trans, trans, trans-diazidodiaminodihydroxo-Pt(IV) complexes. Dalton Trans 40:5342–5351

Westendorf AF, Woods JA, Korpis K, Farrer NJ, Salassa L, Robinson K, Appleyard V, Murray K, Grunert R, Thompson AM, Sadler PJ, Bednarski PJ (2012) Trans, trans, trans-[PtIV(N3)2(OH) 2(py)(NH3)]: a light-activated antitumor platinum complex that kills human cancer cells by an apoptosis-independent mechanism. Mol Cancer Ther 11:1894–1904

Wetzel C, Kunz PC, Kassack MU, Hamacher A, Bohler P, Watjen W, Ott I, Rubbiani R, Spingler B (2011) Gold(I) complexes of water-soluble diphos-type ligands: synthesis, anticancer activity, apoptosis and thioredoxin reductase inhibition. Dalton Trans 40:9212–9220

Wild A, Babiuch K, Konig M, Winter A, Hager MD, Gottschaldt M, Prokop A, Schubert US (2012) Synthesis of a glycopolymeric Pt(II) carrier and its induction of apoptosis in resistant cancer cells. Chem Commun (Camb) 48:6357–6359

Wisnovsky SP, Wilson JJ, Radford RJ, Pereira MP, Chan MR, Laposa RR, Lippard SJ, Kelley SO (2013) Targeting mitochondrial DNA with a platinum-based anticancer agent. Chem Biol 20:1323–1328

Xiao H, Qi R, Liu S, Hu X, Duan T, Zheng Y, Huang Y, Jing X (2011) Biodegradable polymer - cisplatin(IV) conjugate as a pro-drug of cisplatin(II). Biomaterials 32:7732–7739

Yadav A, Janaratne T, Krishnan A, Singhal SS, Yadav S, Dayoub AS, Hawkins DL, Awasthi S, MacDonnell FM (2013) Regression of lung cancer by hypoxia-sensitizing ruthenium polypyridyl complexes. Mol Cancer Ther 12:643–653

Ye RR, Ke ZF, Tan CP, He L, Ji LN, Mao ZW (2013) Histone-deacetylase-targeted fluorescent ruthenium(II) polypyridyl complexes as potent anticancer agents. Chemistry 19:10160–10169

Yoong SL, Wong BS, Zhou QL, Chin CF, Li J, Venkatesan T, Ho HK, Yu V, Ang WH, Pastorin G (2014) Enhanced cytotoxicity to cancer cells by mitochondria-targeting MWCNTs containing platinum(IV) prodrug of Cisplatin. Biomaterials 35:748–759

Yu Q, Liu Y, Wang C, Sun D, Yang X, Liu J (2012) Chiral ruthenium(II) polypyridyl complexes: stabilization of g-quadruplex DNA, inhibition of telomerase activity and cellular uptake. PLoS ONE 7:e50902

Zhang P, Yang YW, Shen ZR (2013) Progress in synthesis and antitumor activities of estradiol-linked platinum complex. Mini Rev Med Chem 13:265–272

Zhang Z, Bi C, Schmitt SM, Fan Y, Dong L, Zuo J, Dou QP (2012) 1,10-Phenanthroline promotes copper complexes into tumor cells and induces apoptosis by inhibiting the proteasome activity. J Biol Inorg Chem 17:1257–1267

Zhao Y, Woods JA, Farrer NJ, Robinson KS, Pracharova J, Kasparkova J, Novakova O, Li H, Salassa L, Pizarro AM, Clarkson GJ, Song L, Brabec V, Sadler PJ (2013) Diazido mixed-amine platinum(IV) anticancer complexes activatable by visible-light form novel DNA adducts. Chemistry 19:9578–9591

Chapter 2
The Intriguing Potential of "Minor" Noble Metals: Emerging Trends and New Applications

Massimiliano Francesco Peana, Serenella Medici and Maria Antonietta Zoroddu

Abstract The chemistry of metallodrugs is dominated by a few transition elements belonging to the so-called "noble metals" group, which have considerably drawn the attention as potential pharmaceuticals after the discovery of cisplatin antitumor activity. Platinum compounds have obviously been the most studied derivatives due to the acknowledged biological properties of this element. In addition, palladium, ruthenium, gold, silver, and copper species, under the form of salts, complexes, or nanoparticles formulations, found interesting applications in the biomedical fields as anticancer, antibacterial, antiparasitic, and antifungal agents. Still, there is an emerging trend involving the research on the next generation of non-platinum metal complexes, especially those based on rhodium, iridium, and osmium, which offer intriguing results and new perspectives about the biomedical applications of such compounds.

Keywords Rhodium · Iridium · Biological catalyst · Sensors · Tracking Imaging

2.1 Introduction

Heavy metals can be rather toxic to humans; for this reason, the pharmaceutical industry has ever tried to avoid their use in the design of drugs. Nevertheless, the discovery of cisplatin anticancer properties led to a frenetic search of more potent, second and third generation of platinum derivatives by the development of increasingly cytotoxic compounds, that ended up in the FDA approval of two cisplatin analogs, carboplatin and oxaliplatin, and the introduction of other platinum derivatives in the medical practice all around the world (i.e., lobaplatin, nedaplatin, satraplatin, etc.) (Medici et al. 2015). The rationale behind such research was to prepare novel metal complexes able to coordinate DNA in the same way as

M. F. Peana (✉) · S. Medici · M. A. Zoroddu
Department of Chemistry and Pharmacy, University of Sassari, 07100 Sassari, Italy
e-mail: peana@uniss.it

M. Rai et al. (eds.), *Biomedical Applications of Metals*,
https://doi.org/10.1007/978-3-319-74814-6_2

cisplatin, but with higher efficacy, either by optimizing their uptake or causing DNA lesions less easy to detect and repair. Such "classical" chemotherapeutics were meant to interfere with the replication and/or the mitotic processes of tumor cells, but by doing so they were also harmful to healthy cells and caused severe side effects (e.g., neurotoxicity, nephrotoxicity, leukopenia, thrombocytopenia, nausea, vomiting, and hair loss) and drug resistance (Barabas et al. 2008).

For this reason, the research trend has changed in the recent years and the attention has turned to the development of a new generation of non-platinum drugs with completely different characteristics from cisplatin, able to selectively target cancer cells or to induce cell death via alternative pathways (Medici et al. 2015). The next generation of chemotherapeutics, based on less prominent noble metals, as rhodium and iridium, has thus focused on targeting biomolecules, including proteins, organelles (e.g., mitochondria) and specific DNA lesions, so that a number of interesting compounds have emerged with outstanding properties and activity. The wide photophysical and photochemical features of noble metal complexes provide the opportunity of monitoring their fate within the cancer cell through a series of spectroscopies, which can be exploited in tracking and imaging applications, or to use photoactivation for a more selective therapeutic treatment. Finally, the relatively easy synthetic routes, together with the unique reactivity and coordination geometry of such complexes, make them the ideal candidates for a new tailor-made design of targeted therapeutics.

Having an anticancer activity is indeed the most desirable characteristic of metal complexes and this concept is thus leading the research in the medical field. Nevertheless, in the most recent years, a novel trend has emerged, focusing on different features belonging to coordination compounds, such as their ability to work as catalytic drugs, probes, or sensors for small biological molecules, or as agents for live cell imaging. Iridium complexes, for instance, are experiencing a growing interest for these applications, and other metals are following the same tendency. In this chapter, the new trends in biomedical research will be also examined, in order to give a full account of the remarkable possibilities offered by these incredibly versatile compounds.

2.2 Rhodium

After cisplatin breakthrough in cancer therapy, several other transition metals have been investigated as potential drugs for their antitumor activity. Among them, group 9 elements (i.e., rhodium and iridium) and their relative complexes have raised considerable interest in the therapeutic and bioanalytical fields due to their tunable properties and reactivity (ranging from kinetic susceptibility to substitutional inertness), elevated water solubility, air and moisture stability, and facile synthetic routes. Furthermore, kinetically inert rhodium and iridium complexes have been indicated as alternative options to small organic molecules in enzyme targeting and direct inhibition of protein–protein interfaces, or as luminescent probes for the construction of oligonucleotide-based assays for a wide gamut of analytes.

Rhodium(II) carboxylates were the first compounds of this metal to show cytotoxic properties, back in the early 1970s, after the synthesis of several dirhodium(II) complexes with bridging equatorial ligands, such as the typical dirhodium carboxylate $[Rh_2(RCOO)_4(solvent)_2]$ complexes (Erck et al. 1974; Bear et al. 1975). Such dinuclear species contain a Rh(II)–Rh(II) bond, four equatorial ligands in a lantern arrangement around the metal center, and an axial ligand on either end (Fig. 2.1).

Rh(II) ions have a d^7 configuration and are paramagnetic: the pairing of the two spare electrons in the Rh(II)–Rh(II) system originates a diamagnetic complex. About a decade later, similar compounds were found to be effective against Ehrlich ascites sarcoma and P 388 leukemia (Bear 1986), but too toxic for therapeutic uses, while a Rh(II) butyrate species showed cell cycle phase-specific effects in HeLa cells with high anticancer activity (Rao et al. 1980). More recently, Rh(II) citrate was reported to extend survival and reduce the size of breast carcinoma in mice when administered via maghemite nanoparticles (Peixoto et al. 2015), while Rh(II) acetate found a completely new application in a "turn-on" fluorescent microbead sensor for detecting nitric oxide (Yang et al. 2014). In fact, the dimer can form an adduct with a fluorophore, dansyl-piperazine, which is loaded onto copolymer microbeads. Dansyl-piperazine is fluorescent in its unbound state, while the Rh(II) adduct is not. Reaction of the adduct with nitric oxide (NO) releases dansyl-piperazine in an exchange reaction, resulting in the emission of fluorescent light by the microbeads upon contact with NO. This is an important application since NO is a ubiquitous messenger in the cardiovascular, nervous, and immune systems, and is also related to tumor progression; thus detection and control of the NO concentration are critical in the treatment of cardiovascular, neurological, and cancer-related conditions. Moreover, NO, with its unpaired electron, is an extremely reactive molecule, so it is rapidly and easily converted into other species and its detection in vivo otherwise very complicated.

Also, Rh(I) and Rh(III) mononuclear species have been evaluated for their cytotoxicity against tumor cells. Rh(I), being a d^8 ion, is isoelectronic with Pt(II), and its square planar complexes seem to have some analogies in common with cisplatin, such as the tendency to bind DNA. Although rhodium complexes initially appeared to be less attractive in cancer research due to their kinetic inertness, even

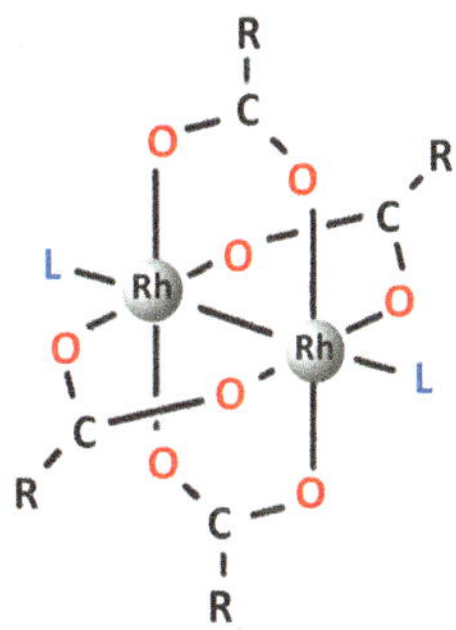

Fig. 2.1 Dirhodium(II) carboxylate $[Rh_2(RCOO)_4(solvent)_2]$ complexes

"unreactive" compounds possess some activity against tumors. In fact, a number of kinetically inert rhodium(III) complexes (together with analogous ruthenium(II) and iridium(III) derivatives) have been developed as inhibitors of protein kinases or protein–protein interactions. However, a careful choice of the ligands, especially cyclometalating molecules, is sufficient to increase the reactivity of inert compounds.

Another interesting application of rhodium complexes in the medical field is their use as catalysts in the synthesis of biologically active molecules, such as succinimide-containing chromones, naphthoquinones, and xanthones (Han et al. 2016), indolines (Jeon et al. 2016), or quinonoid compounds (Jardim et al. 2017).

Finally, rhodium in its metallic form, together with molybdenum, is used in anodes and filters for mammography equipments (Lawaczeck et al. 2005). Rhodium emits its principal characteristic radiation at an energy of 20.3 keV with a less intense emission at 22.7 keV, thus producing a more penetrating X-ray beam than the more conventional molybdenum anode (17.6 and 19.7 keV, respectively). In some mammography systems, a dual-track (molybdenum and rhodium) X-ray tube anode is used. The operator can select the one that is optimum for a specific patient based on breast characteristics, especially density.

Thus, rhodium demonstrates to be a very versatile element in the biomedical field, although its applications as an antineoplastic agent are obviously the most common and thoroughly investigated.

2.2.1 Organorhodium(III) Compounds

Organometallic Rh(III) complexes are the most successful compounds of this element in anticancer studies. In fact, a carbon–metal bond is always rather reactive and this can help overcoming the relative inertness of Rh(III) species, especially when they coordinate neutral arene or, even better, anionic cyclopentadienyl ligands, in the so-called "half-sandwich" or "piano stool" complexes. Also cyclometalating pyridine or phenanthroline derivatives are able to form reactive compounds.

Anionic cyclopentadienyl ligands have been employed in the synthesis of active Rh(III) species, following the idea that the chemistry of cyclopentadienyl Rh(III) complexes could be similar to that of analogous arene ruthenium(II) species, which demonstrated to be powerful anticancer agents (Fig. 2.2).

Like other arene ligands, cyclopentadienyl derivatives provide a lipophilic protecting shield to the metal by occupying three coordination sites at the octahedral center, while the remaining three positions can host ligands with hydrophilic character. Such a strategic expedient, providing an accurate tuning of both the lipophilic/hydrophilic properties of the cyclopentadienyl derivative and the other coordinated ligands, intervenes in modulating the solubility, stability, and ligand exchange kinetics of the complexes (Geldmacher et al. 2012a, b). As a result, pentamethylcyclopentadienyl-based rhodium complexes containing hydroxypyrone

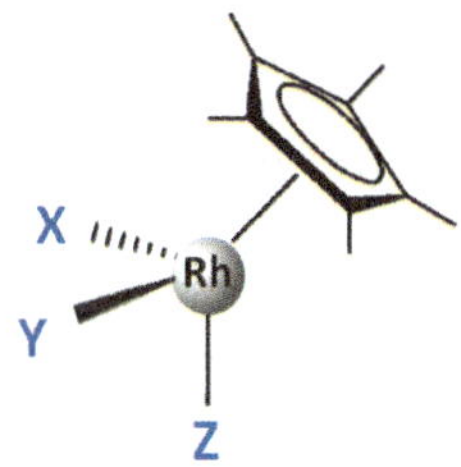

Fig. 2.2 Cyclopentadienyl Rh(III) complexes

(maltol and allomaltol) or piroxicamato ligands exhibit moderate to low cytotoxicity in different human cancer cell lines (Dömötör et al. 2014; Raja et al. 2014).

The mechanisms behind the action of organorhodium(III) complexes have been investigated and seem to be mainly associated with DNA interaction via insertion. Barton and his group (Ernst et al. 2009, 2011; Komor et al. 2012) showed that Rh(III) metalloinsertors can be exploited for their ability in targeting DNA mismatches, since they are capable of recognizing mismatches with high selectivity and bind them with elevated affinity and specificity. For this reason, they accumulate in cells where the mismatch repair (MMR) system is inefficient. In fact, Rh(III) metalloinsertors can selectively aim at MMR-deficient cells, which host 1000-fold more mismatches than MMR-proficient cells. In case the complexes can be subject to photoactivation, such activation is also able to promote single-strand cleavage. Rhodium metalloinsertors are thus preferentially cytotoxic to MMR-deficient cell lines, and it was demonstrated that they cause cell death via a necrotic rather than apoptotic path (Ernst et al. 2011).

A novel rhodium(III) complex with mixed ligands, containing a cyclometalated functionalized pyridine and a derivative of 1,10-phenanthroline, has been reported as the first metal-based inhibitor of autotoxin (ATX) activity in melanoma skin cancer, by binding to this protein (Kang et al. 2017). ATX is a prometastatic enzyme that functions as a motility stimulating factor in melanoma cells, so its inhibition represents a potential target in skin cancer therapy. Additionally, the same complex is cytotoxic and dose-dependently inhibited cell proliferation in three cancer cell lines tested.

It has been determined that the charge of a complex is able to exert important effects on its activity on tumor cells. For instance, the antiproliferative activity of dinuclear di- (neutral) and tri- (cationic) thiolato-bridged pentamethylcyclopentadienyl Rh(III) complexes was tested against cisplatin-sensitive and cisplatin-resistive cancerous human ovarian cell lines, and also on noncancerous human embryonic kidney cells (Gupta et al. 2013). The cationic complexes were especially cytotoxic respect to the neutral ones, perhaps due to an increased intracellular uptake. The nature of the substituent on the thiolato-bridges was determinant for the cytotoxicity of the complexes, and activity was achieved already in the nanomolar range: such an elevated toxicity, in particular on cisplatin-resistant cell lines, supports the hypothesis of a different mechanism of action for this class of rhodium complexes respect to cisplatin.

Rhodium compounds have been extensively used in catalytic reactions, both in the laboratory practice and industrial plants, to favor a wide variety of processes, such as hydrogenation, reduction by hydrogen transfer, C–C bond formation, C–H activation, and allylic substitution, just to quote some. Similarly, organometallic compounds can behave as catalytic drugs, intervening in biochemical transformations like deprotection and functional group modification, degradation of biomolecules, and redox modulation (in photosensitizers, superoxide dismutase mimics, thiol oxidants, and transfer hydrogenation). In this way, catalytic metallodrugs are very interesting since they can lead to low-dose therapy and offer a new design strategy for future medical applications.

Also, rhodium(III) "piano stool" complexes can act as catalytic drugs, as demonstrated by a study conducted on a series of Rh(III) cyclometalated species with general formula [(Cp)Rh(N-N)(Cl)], where N-N can be ethylenediamine (en), 2,2′-bipyridine (bpy), or phenanthroline (phen) and Cp can be pentamethylcyclopentadienyl (Cp) or one of its bulkier derivatives. These complexes were active in the reduction by hydrogen transfer of NAD^+ to NADH, using sodium formate as the hydride source under biologically relevant conditions. Furthermore, they were able to exert antiproliferative activity toward A2780 human ovarian cancer cells, which was increased by up to 50% when administered in combination with non-toxic doses of formate, suggesting that transfer hydrogenation can induce reductive stress in cancer cells (Soldevila-Barreda et al. 2015).

2.2.2 *Polypyridyl Rh(III) Complexes*

As previously reminded, Rh(III) complexes were initially considered as improbable candidates for anticancer therapy due to the typical kinetic inertness of this metal center. However, systematic studies on the cellular response of a wide range of octahedral Rh(III) complexes containing polypyridyl and other aromatic chelating ligands have demonstrated high cytotoxicity in cancer cells and in some cases also a relative tolerance by healthy cells, provided a careful choice of the ancillary ligands was made. Polypyridyl-containing Rh(III) complexes, as in the case of most noble metals, owe their activity to their behavior as DNA intercalators. A number of rhodium polypyridyl complexes can bind DNA, both covalently and non-covalently. Moreover, the cellular uptake of the metal compound can be improved by increasing the surface area and hydrophobicity of the polypyridyl ligand, with a corresponding enhancement in cytotoxicity. Most of these rhodium complexes seem to exert anti-topoisomerase II activity and act as photo-inducible agents (Hackenberg et al. 2011; Geldmacher et al. 2012a, b).

2.2.3 *Rh(I) Carbene Complexes*

Rh(I) compounds are less common than Rh(III) species in biological activity studies. Nevertheless, Rh(I) complexes containing 1,5-cyclooctadiene (COD) or carbonyl (CO) ligands have been effective against Ehrlich ascites (Giraldi et al. 1978; Sartori et al. 1996), leukemia L1210 (Giraldi et al. 1978; Sartori et al. 1996), sarcoma 180 (Craciunescu et al. 1991), and metastatic lung cancer (Sava et al. 1983). Recent studies focused on Rh(I) carbene species and reported novel organorhodium(I) complexes containing both COD and N-heterocyclic carbene (NHC) ligands as cytotoxic to colon cancer cells by targeting DNA, inhibiting metastasis, preventing cell division, and reducing DNA condensation (McConnell et al. 2013) (Fig. 2.3).

In an analogous way, NHC Rh(I) coordination compounds with COD or CO as the co-ligands induced antiproliferative activity, moderate inhibitory action of thioredoxin reductase (TrxR), efficient binding to biomolecules (DNA, albumin), changes in the mitochondrial membrane potential (MMP), and DNA cleavage in wild-type and daunorubicin- or vincristine-resistant Nalm-6 leukemia cells, evidencing a rather intricate mechanism of action within this kind of compounds (Oehninger et al. 2013).

2.3 Iridium

Iridium complexes have been introduced in research studies as anticancer agents only recently (Sava et al. 1983), but iridium's early applications in cancer treatment date back to 1961, when one of its radioactive isotopes, ^{192}Ir, was used for the first time against brain tumors in radiation therapy (Chase et al. 1961). Nowadays, radioisotope ^{192}Ir is commonly employed as a source of gamma radiation for the treatment of cancer in what is called brachytherapy, a form of radiotherapy where a sealed radioactive source (often in the form of "seeds") is placed inside or next to the area requiring treatment. High-dose-rate brachytherapy is a powerful tool in radiation oncology (Milickovic et al. 2017) and represents a specific treatment for

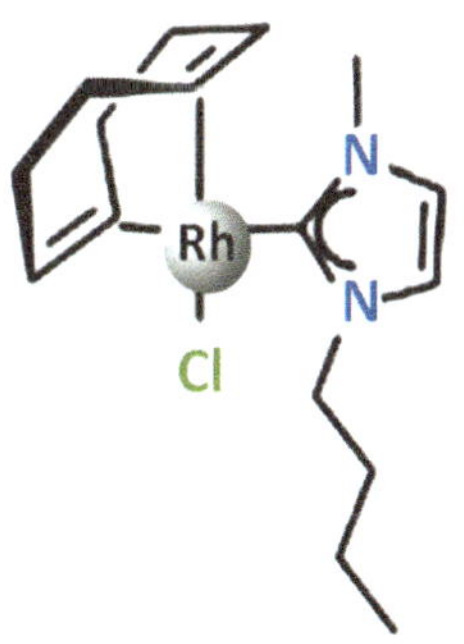

Fig. 2.3 Organorhodium(I) complexes containing 1,5-cyclooctadiene (COD) and N-heterocyclic carbene (NHC) ligands

prostate (Strouthos et al. 2017), bilary duct (Dvorák et al. 2002), and intracavitary cervix tumors (Huang et al. 2013), but can also be used against several other cancer forms localized in breast, skin, brain, eye, head and neck region (Mazeron et al. 2009), respiratory tract, digestive tract, urinary tract, and soft tissues (Gerbaulet et al. 2002).

Iridium complexes are novel theranostic agents in the biomedical field and are emerging at an amazing rate in a series of applications, going from protein staining (Jia et al. 2012; Connell et al. 2015; Zhou et al. 2016) to cellular and mitochondrial imaging, intracellular sensors and probes, peptide labeling, and chemotherapeutic drugs (*vide infra*). Iridium compounds have long been overlooked by the biomedical research, and only very recently they have emerged as interesting compounds for therapeutic uses. A probable reason for this, as it also happened for rhodium species, could be found in iridium inertness: the exchange lifetime for an aqua ligand on $[Ir(H_2O)_6]^{3+}$, for instance, is about 300 years. Similarly to rhodium, also iridium kinetic inertness may be avoided, and the reactivity and biological activity of iridium increased by a suitable choice of auxiliary ligands. In fact, it is known that the reactivity of low-spin d^6 Ir(III) centers, for instance, is highly dependent on the kind of the associated ancillary ligands. The introduction of a cyclopentadienyl substituent, for example, can increase the ligand exchange rate by 14 orders of magnitude.

The first attempts to assess iridium as an anticancer agent immediately followed the discovery of cisplatin. For almost 30 years thereafter, the efforts of reproducing platinum drugs' efficacy had been mainly focused on d^8 Ir(I) compounds with square planar geometry similar to cisplatin, such as [Ir(acac)(COD)] (Giraldi et al. 1978) and its dinuclear analog $[IrCl(COD)]_2$ (Sava et al. 1987). Both the complexes possess high activity: the former against either mice Ehrlich ascites (100% cures) and Lewis lung carcinoma, while the latter showed antimetastatic activity only in the Lewis lung cancer model, but no inhibition of primary tumors. However, not earlier than two decades ago the interest shifted to organoiridium(III) compounds, which are able to exert antiproliferative activity against cancer cells, together with other Ir(III) compounds.

The scheme applied to the design and development of biologically active iridium complexes as anticancer agents is very similar to that reported for rhodium (Leung et al. 2013). Initially, the main strategy was to use a stabilizing ligand, such as the pentamethylcyclopentadienyl anion, to increase the lability of its *trans*-halide ligands and make the complex more reactive; next, a new trend emerged based on the use of appropriate ligands possessing cytotoxic activity per se through specific interactions with biological targets (Leung et al. 2013); finally, modulation of Ir complexes redox activity became one of the most explored approaches in the search of effective therapeutic agents (Romero-Canelon and Sadler 2013).

The most frequently used ligands in the design of iridium complexes for potential therapeutic applications are those forming organoiridium species (arenes, cyclopentadienyl anion derivatives, and 2-phenylpyrydine derivatives), polypyridyl compounds, or a combination of the two.

2.3.1 Half-sandwich Organoiridium(III) Complexes

In the family of organoiridium compounds, "half-sandwich" organometallic Ir (III) cyclopentadienyl complexes are probably the most important (Liu and Sadler 2014), especially those of the pseudo-octahedral pentamethylcyclopentadienyl type, which are indeed the most studied anticancer agents for this metal. Their general formula is $[(\eta^5\text{-Cp})\text{Ir}(\text{L-L}')\text{Z}]^{0/n+}$, where Cp is the cyclopentadienyl anion or its polysubstituted derivatives (phenyltetramethylcyclopentadienyl or biphenyltetramethylcyclopentadienyl), L-L′ is a bidentate ligand with nitrogen, oxygen, and/or carbon donor atoms, and Z is a monodentate ligand (a chloride or a pyridine) (Fig. 2.4).

The role of the Cp ligand, which occupies one face of the octahedron (three coordination sites), is to stabilize the complex and determine its interactions with the target, for example, by intercalation into DNA base pairs, while its hydrophobic character increases the cellular uptake of the complex. The chelating ligand L-L′ provides extra stability for the complex and contributes to tuning the electronic properties of the iridium center. The monodentate ligand Z generally provides a labile site for substitution reactions with target sites. The mechanisms through which such complexes exert their action depend on the ligands on the iridium center: some complexes are able to bind DNA, while others can perturb the redox balance in cells (Liu et al. 2014). Mitochondrial targeting is another possible pathway, leading to cell death via a process that starts with primary redox mediation processes (ROS generation), followed by DNA damage and impairment of protein synthesis due to oxidative stress. For instance, a novel "half-sandwich" organoiridium(III) complex containing also a pyridine ligand was evaluated by the National Cancer Institute NCI-60 Human Tumor Cell Lines Screen and found to be more potent than cisplatin against a wide range of cancer cells. The pyridine ligand protects the iridium complex from rapid reactions with glutathione, while the mechanism behind its anticancer action was demonstrated to be connected to an unprecedented ability of the iridium complexes to generate H_2O_2 by catalytic hydride transfer from the coenzyme NADH to the O_2 molecule, thus substantially increasing the amount of reactive oxygen species (ROS) inside the cancer cells,

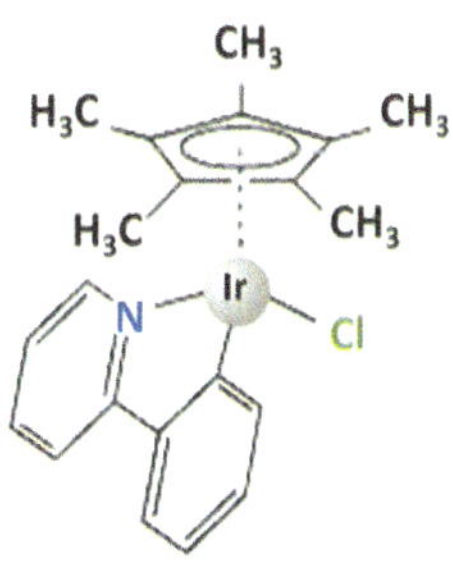

Fig. 2.4 Example of Ir(III) complexes of the general formula is $[(\eta^5\text{-Cp})\text{Ir}(\text{L-L}')\text{Z}]^{0/n+}$, Chloro (pentamethylcyclopentadienyl)[(2-pyridinyl-kN)phenyl-kC]iridium(III)

even in the presence of a ROS scavenger such as a thiol-containing molecule (i.e., N-acetyl-cysteine). The induced oxidative stress subsequently causes cell death via extended damage to various cellular components (Liu et al. 2014).

"Half-sandwich" complexes can also suppress tumor necrosis factor α, promote DNA oxidation, and generate singlet oxygen when photoactivated. Finally, the mechanisms involved in their cellular internalization have been clarified (Novohradsky et al. 2014), evidencing that the action of antitumour agents is a complex, multistep process that involves cell entry or accumulation, drug activation, binding to cellular targets, and responses to the cellular target damage. Thus, an efficient accumulation of iridium complexes in cancer cells is the first and crucial stage determining the success or failure of any iridium compound designed to be a metal–drug.

2.3.2 Cyclometallated Ir(III) Complexes

Organoiridium complexes bearing cyclometallated ligands have raised considerable interest as candidates for the use as luminescent probes in cellular imaging because of their remarkable photophysical properties (*vide infra*). The second aspect of such compounds is that they also exert high cytotoxic activities. An example is given by the case of 2-(2,4-difluorophenyl)pyridine, whose Ir(III) complex was rather effective against SP2 myeloma and Chinese hamster ovary cells, causing blebbing and vacuole formation in living cells (indicative of apoptosis) within 30 min of exposure to the probe, but cell death was markedly faster under irradiation (Dolan et al. 2013). With 2-phenylquinoline as the cyclometalating ligand, the corresponding Ir(III) complex is able to accumulate in mitochondria and causes mitochondrial shortening by conjugation to specific protein targets (Wang et al. 2012). When a derivative of 2-(5′-amino-4′-tolyl)pyridine bearing three amino groups at the 5′-position is used, on the other hand, the corresponding Ir(III) compound photoactivation at 377 or 470 nm causes HeLa-S3 cell death by generating singlet oxygen in a pH-dependent manner. The reactivity of this complex is evidently dependent on the pH; for this reason, it is also able to stain acidic organelles, such as the lysosomes (Moromizato et al. 2012).

Also, a series of valproic acid-containing cyclometalated Ir(III) complexes showed to target and accumulate in mitochondria, causing cell death via a series of mitochondria-mediated events. Such complexes were highly effective in circumventing cisplatin resistance being about 50–90 times more cytotoxic than cisplatin against cisplatin-resistant human lung carcinoma (Ye et al. 2017).

A peculiar cell death pathway has been recognized for some cationic amphiphilic tris-cyclometalated iridium(III) complexes, which have been able to induce cancer cell death via interaction with Ca^{2+}–calmodulin complex accompanied by membrane disruption in Jurkat cells (Hisamatsu et al. 2017). A similar membrane disrupting mechanism was also evidenced for oligoarginine peptide derivatives containing cyclometallated Ir(III) complexes, which were also remarkably cytotoxic

(Salvadó et al. 2016). Other cyclometalated iridium(III) complexes, instead, demonstrated to effectively inhibit tumor necrosis factor-α (Kang et al. 2016).

Iridium hydrides are attractive catalysts for several organic and bioorganic reactions, but have also been tested for their biological properties, among which they exhibit excellent anticancer activity. Song et al. (2013) described the synthesis and properties of novel cyclometalated iridium hydrides prepared by C–H bond activation of aromatic nitrones (based on the antioxidant α-phenyl-N-tert-butylnitrone scaffold) which had a high antiproliferative effect on human hepatocellular liver carcinoma. The most interesting iridium complexes of this series demonstrated to actively interact with DNA and thus cause conformational changes on the helix structure; it was also effective in vivo and possessed reduced toxicity compared to cisplatin.

When a cyclometalating ligand like 2-phenyl-pyridine was combined with polypyridyl species with extended conjugation (i.e., bipyridine, phenanthroline, and diphenylphenanthroline) to form compounds based on a simple model structure, $[Ir(ppy)_2(N\text{-}N)]^+$, where ppy is 2-phenyl-pyridine and N-N the polypyridyl ligand, it was possible to finely tune the lipophilic *versus* hydrophobic properties of the complexes (Cao et al. 2013). All the three complexes exerted anticancer action, but the one carrying the diphenylphenanthroline ligand had the highest cellular uptake efficiency and the highest cytotoxic activity in different cancer cell lines at lower doses than cisplatin. The remarkable cytotoxicity of this complex is connected to its ability to accumulate on the cellular membrane, due to its strong hydrophobic character, thus causing endoplasmic reticulum stress and mitochondria-mediated apoptosis. The conspicuous advantage in using these complexes comes from the fact that they own tunable luminescent properties, and this permits more direct and accurate optical observations of their intracellular location. Their target is the cytoplasm, where the cell death process seems to start.

Lastly, bis-C,N-cyclometalated Ir(III) thiosemicarbazide complexes prepared by Ruiz and his group (Ruiz et al. 2013) are up to fivefold more active than cisplatin on breast cancer cells. Especially remarkable is the very low Resistance Factor (RF in the range 0.9–1.1) for two of the characterized compounds against cancer cells resistant to cisplatin, indicating they can efficiently circumvent one of the most important drawbacks of this drug. These complexes are also able to inhibit cathepsin B, an enzyme overexpressed in several cancer cell lines, and to bind the human serum albumin protein (HAS), which is a transport agent for drugs. More recently, the same research group has successfully synthesized a series of novel iridium benzimidazole cyclometalated complexes containing polyvalent ligands, which can play different and simultaneous functions (Yellol et al. 2013) (Fig. 2.5).

These compounds exhibited good anticancer activity against several cancer cell lines by inducing early and severe apoptotic mechanism; they also demonstrated good accumulation and S-phase cell arrest, together with an efficient binding to HSA protein, while DNA binding at the minor groove was weaker.

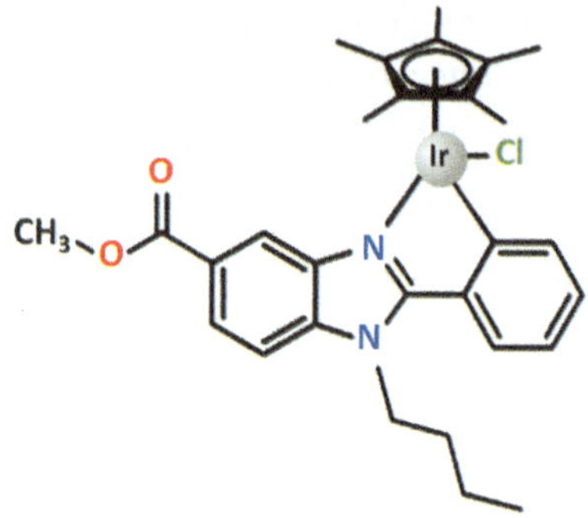

Fig. 2.5 Cyclometalated benzimidazole Ir complexes

2.3.3 *Emerging Trends for Ir(III) Complexes as Theranostics*

During the very latest years, the interest around Ir(III) compounds have been mainly focused on their unique photophysical and photochemical properties, which allow them to be applied in the most recent areas of theranostics: photodynamic therapy, live cell or hypoxia imaging, biosensors and bioprobes, etc. Often, the same complex can find application in two or more of these fields at the same time, since the integration of chemotherapy and photodynamic therapy in a single delivery system is highly desirable for enhancing anticancer therapeutic efficacy (Xiang et al. 2017), as well as the integration of imaging capabilities and anticancer properties (Chen et al. 2017).

Photodynamic therapy (PDT) (also called photochemotherapy) is a treatment in which tumor cells are killed by light-induced generation of the singlet oxygen ($^1O_2$) through the interactions of a photosensitizer, light, and ground-state molecular oxygen ($^3O_2$) in tissue (Schmidt 2006). Singlet oxygen is a very reactive and cytotoxic species so that PDT has been considered as one of the most promising candidates in cancer treatment due to its high efficiency, controllable and high selectivity for the lesion area, and low damage to healthy tissues, especially in image-guided PDT (Tian et al. 2013; Wang et al. 2013; Tang et al. 2016; Li et al. 2017a, b, c).

To guide the treatment, Magnetic Resonance Imaging (MRI) and time-resolved luminescence imaging techniques, for instance, can be applied. However, many efforts have been dedicated to the design and synthesis of agents suitable for a highly efficient image-guided PDT, since agents based on small molecules are often rather cytotoxic, possess low molar absorption coefficient in the visible region, and are poorly soluble in water. Due to the remarkable consumption and subsequent decrease of O_2 in tumor tissues, hypoxia imaging has also been proposed, although the majority of O_2 probes can lead to inaccurate measurement due to external influences. Other techniques for hypoxia imaging are Electron Paramagnetic Resonance (EPR), Magnetic Resonance Imaging (MRI), pulse oximetry, and Positron Emission Tomography (PET), but also optical imaging techniques have received much attention in the detection of intracellular O_2. Phosphorescent transition metal complexes are amongst the most responsive dyes suitable for hypoxia imaging, thanks to their easy phosphorescence quenching by efficient and reversible energy transfer from their excited triplet states to the ground states of O_2, at the same time producing $^1O_2$. Moreover, such complexes show excellent photostability, large Stokes shifts, and relatively long emission lifetimes which are desirable qualities for biosensing and bioimaging agents. In this perspective, iridium(III) complexes are emerging as efficient compounds for this kind of applications, as demonstrated by the outstanding research carried out in the very recent years (Liu et al. 2015, 2017c, d; Sun et al. 2015, 2016; Tobita and Yoshihara 2016; Feng et al. 2017; Li et al. 2017a, b, c).

The photophysical and photochemical properties of Ir(III) complexes have been exploited in tracking, sensing, and detecting biologically relevant molecules, especially those linked to pathological conditions, but also in the imaging of living cells. The two-photon excitation and emission processes of luminescent and phosphorescent iridium compounds have been widely employed in a vast range of applications: intracellular tracking of transcription factor NF-κB in living cells (Wang et al. 2017a, b); and sensors for biothiols, including glutathione (GSH) and hydrogen sulfide (Tso et al. 2017), hydrogen peroxide (Liu et al. 2017d), sialic acids (Liu et al. 2017b), COX-2 enzyme (Liu et al. 2017a), methylglyoxal (Zhang et al. 2017a, b), hypochlorous acid in liver injuries (Zhang et al. 2017a, b) and hypochlorite ions in mitochondria (Li et al. 2015a, b), glutamine (Jiang et al. 2016), sulfur dioxide derivatives (Li et al. 2015a, b), phosphorylated peptides (Kang et al. 2014), a malarial protein biomarker (Davis et al. 2015), intracellular oxygen (Yoshihara et al. 2015), nitric oxide in mitochondria (Chen et al. 2015), hydrogen sulfide (Yu et al. 2015), and heparin (Jiang et al. 2015).

Another important application is the tracking of cell organelles and live cell and lifetime imaging (Rood et al. 2015; Wang et al. 2017a, b). Mitochondria are the preferred targets for many Ir(III) compounds (Zhang et al. 2014; Jin et al. 2015a, b, 2017) but also lysosomes (Qiu et al. 2016) and nuclei as well can be evidenced by such techniques (Li et al. 2011; Liu et al. 2015). Mitochondrial polarity (Li et al. 2017a, b, c) and dynamics (Jin et al. 2015a, b; Huang et al. 2016a, b) have also been monitored via phosphorescent Ir(III) complexes.

Finally, the photophysical properties of a family of neutral cyclometalated iridium(III) tetrazolato complexes and their methylated cationic analogs have been exploited to investigate their intracellular localization, showing that the neutral species accumulated mostly in the endoplasmic reticulum and lipid droplets, whereas the majority of the cationic complexes could be found in the mitochondria, indicating a different behavior linked to the charge of the complex (Caporale et al. 2017). The impressive work done on this kind of iridium complexes shows their growing importance in the theranostic field with a wide range of applications.

2.4 Osmium

Osmium is the heavier relative of ruthenium, and only recently it attracted the attention of several researchers, being practically neglected until 2006. From that year on, osmium complexes have experienced a growing importance in the field of tumor-inhibiting metal species, and can be interesting alternatives to their ruthenium analogs because of their relative inertness and sufficient stability under physiological conditions.

Osmium compounds can be either highly toxic (OsO_4) or relatively inert (Os(II) and Os(III) complexes), so that they were not particularly attractive for therapeutic applications, until the first Os(II) arene complexes exhibited cytotoxicity comparable to cisplatin (Peacock et al. 2008; van Rijt et al. 2009) and researchers started considering them for biomedical employment. Also for osmium compounds, the development of organometallic species containing arene or cyclometallated ligands is the common practice in the search of biologically interesting species. Other strategies include, of course, the synthesis of osmium analogs of ruthenium complexes (Büchel et al. 2011), clusters (Lee et al. 2014), or higher oxidation states for the metal center.

2.4.1 Osmium–Arene Complexes

Organometallic osmium complexes have been prepared and tested against cancer cell lines with discrete success. Nevertheless, the weakness of arene complexes as well as all metallodrugs in general is linked to their instability in water or air. A proper design of osmium complexes for biological activity cannot leave aside a precise control of their chemical reactivity (rate of hydrolysis, acidity of the aqua adducts, dynamic chelate ring opening, and interactions with nucleobases) which are strictly connected to cancer cytotoxicity and this is possible only by a careful tuning of the characteristics of the chelating ligands. This has been achieved by modulating the steric and electronic properties of the substituents, which in turn are able to determine the kinetics and thermodynamics of osmium drugs in the aqueous medium (Peacock et al. 2006, 2007).

Both the in vitro and in vivo anticancer activities for a series of osmium arene complexes were evaluated (Hanif et al. 2014), evidencing that no cross-resistance with platinum-based drugs was observed, as for example with the "piano stool" Os(II) arene complexes (Fu et al. 2011). Such kind of derivatives are very interesting for drug design, since slight changes in the arene ligand can modulate cellular uptake and DNA intercalation, while the other ligands forming the "legs" of the "stool" are devoted to the control of both reactivity and stability. Even the finest modification on the structure of the metal complex can produce a major effect on its biological activity, as, for example, the surprising advantages in the cellular metabolic pathways induced by the substitution of a coordinated chloride by a iodide group in both iminopyridine and azopyridine organometallic Os(II) arene complexes (Romero-Canelon et al. 2013). In this way, the problem of intrinsic or acquired resistance in chemotherapy can be adequately addressed and overcome.

2.4.2 Osmium Complexes in High Oxidation States

A vast gamut of osmium complexes in low oxidation states +2, +3, and +4 (Hanif et al. 2014) demonstrated to exert anticancer activity by inducing cell death through DNA targeting, but also osmium species in high oxidation states have been prepared and tested with higher cytotoxicity respect to the common platinum-based chemotherapeutic drugs: Os(VI) nitrido compounds with tridendate Schiff bases (Ni et al. 2011), monodentate azole heterocycle ligands (Ni et al. 2012) or azopyridine complex (Shnyder et al. 2011), or carrying the 8-quinolinolato ligand and its derivatives (Tang et al. 2013). Recently, the first osmium complex inducing cell death via endoplasmic reticulum stress was prepared by Lippard's group (Suntharalingam et al. 2013) (Fig. 2.6).

While working with Os(VI) nitrido compounds carrying bidentate ligands, they demonstrated that small changes to the ligand periphery are able to induce a series of entirely different cellular responses, ranging from genomic DNA damage (which leads to G2/M phase arrest and apoptosis) to ER stress, and finally to p53-independent, caspase-directed apoptosis (Suntharalingam et al. 2013).

2.5 Rhenium

The preparation of rhenium complexes in order to evaluate their anticancer action started only recently, at the beginning of the 2000s. They are usually derivatives of Re(I) mono- or dinuclear hexacoordinated carbonyl species, in which one or more heteroligands are bound in a mono- or polydentate fashion (Leonidova et al. 2014). Their mechanism of action is still under scrutiny, but it seems it can be linked to DNA interaction.

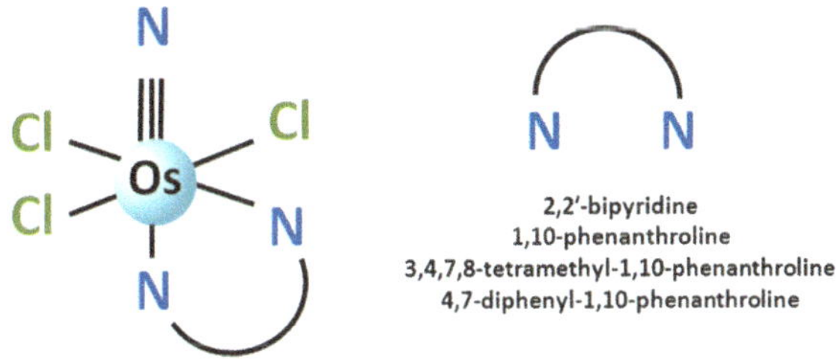

Fig. 2.6 Scheme of Os(VI) nitrido compounds carrying bidentate ligands

The most commonly used ligands in Re(I) compounds are diphosphines and polypyridyl species (Gasser et al. 2011), which can be suitably selected or derivatized to be directed toward both cancer cells or mitochondria (Ferri et al. 2010; Balasingham et al. 2011; Moura et al. 2013; Leonidova and Gasser 2014), since rhenium complexes normally lack in selectivity. The latest trends also include the synthesis of fluorescent (Choi et al. 2012) or photo-activatable (Kastl et al. 2013) Re(I) complexes.

Sometimes, rhenium derivative can be more potent than cisplatinum, as in the case of a tricarbonyl Re(I) complex with thymidine as the co-ligand (Bartholoma et al. 2010, 2011). It was supposed that its mechanism of action could be exerted by inhibition of the thymidine kinase 1 enzyme, but studies demonstrated that this could not be the only process involved.

Re(IV) compounds for therapeutic applications are not very common and normally do not exert high cytotoxic activity in vitro apart from those reported by De Munno and co-workers (Martinez-Lillo et al. 2011). All complexes had the general formula $ReCl_4L$, where L was 2,2′-bipyridine, 2,2′-bipyrimidine; 4,4′-dimethyl-2,2′-bipyridine; and 1,10-phenanthroline: they all demonstrated potent in vitro antiproliferative activity against a number of cancer cell lines (Fig. 2.7).

Rhenium(V) oxo complexes of general formula $[ReO(OMe)(N\text{-}N)Cl_2]$, where N-N is a derivative of 1,10-phenanthroline, can effectively kill cancer cells by triggering necroptosis pathway, a non-apoptotic kind of cell death. These complexes are also able to induce mitochondrial membrane potential depletion as a possible downstream effect of ROS production (Suntharalingam et al. 2015).

A completely different application of rhenium is through its radioactive isotope, ^{188}Re, which was used to prepare complexes with hydroxyethylidenediphosphonate, a bone growth regulator applicable in radiotherapeutic palliative treatment of bone cancer and metastasis (Biersack et al. 2011; van Dodewaard-de Jong et al. 2011; Cheng et al. 2011). Improvement of survival and quality of life have been demonstrated when radiopharmaceuticals were given repeatedly or in combination with chemotherapy, with a considerable reduction of pain.

Fig. 2.7 Scheme of Re(IV) Cl_4L complexes

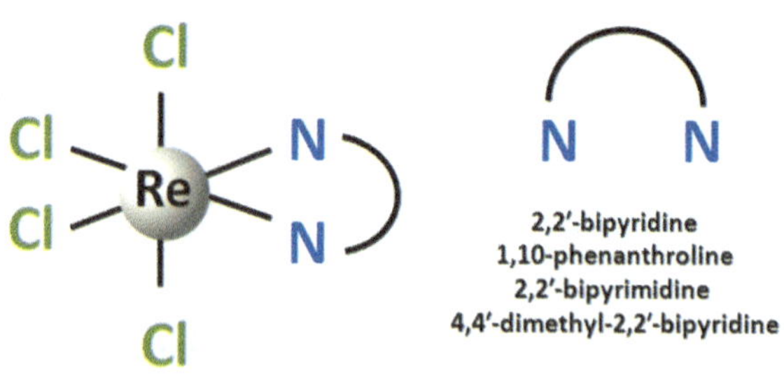

2.6 Conclusions

Although the leading compounds in biomedical applications are those based on relevant noble metals such as platinum, ruthenium, gold, silver, copper, and palladium (Medici et al. 2015; Medici et al. 2016), there is an emerging research trend focused on less common transition elements. Rhodium, iridium, and other minor metals are offering a series of complexes exerting their biological activities by mechanisms which are completely different respect to those of the most common metallodrugs. Such alternative pathways can decrease the toxicity of these compounds, which could soon become new options to the classic chemotherapeuticals. Moreover, the ability of rhodium and iridium compounds to work as catalytic drugs, probes or sensors for small biological molecules, or agents for live cell imaging, opens the scenery for new applications as theranostics which seems not to be feasible for classical noble metal complexes.

References

Balasingham RG, Coogan MP, Thorp-Greenwood FL (2011) Complexes in context: attempting to control the cellular uptake and localisation of rhenium fac-tricarbonyl polypyridyl complexes. Dalton Trans 40:11663–11674

Barabas K, Milner R, Lurie D, Adin C (2008) Cisplatin: a review of toxicities and therapeutic applications. Vet Comp Oncol 6(1):1–18

Bartholoma MD, Vortherms AR, Hillier S, Ploier B, Joyal J, Babich J, Doyle RP, Zubieta J (2010) Synthesis, cytotoxicity, and insight into the mode of action of $Re(CO)_3$ thymidine complexes. Chem Med Chem 5:1513–1529

Bartholoma MD, Vortherms AR, Hillier S, Joyal J, Babich J, Doyle RP, Zubieta J (2011) Synthesis, cytotoxicity and cellular uptake studies of N_3 functionalized $Re(CO)_3$ thymidine complexes. Dalton Trans 40:6216–6225

Bear JL, Gray HB Jr, Rainen L, Chang IM, Howard R, Serio G, Kimball AP (1975) Interaction of rhodium(II) carboxylates with molecules of biologic importance. Cancer Chemother Rep Part I 59(3):611–620

Bear JL (1986) Rhodium compounds for antitumor use. In: Proceedings of 9th International Precious Metals Institute Conference, pp. 337–344

Biersack HJ, Palmedo H, Andris A, Rogenhofer S, Knapp FF, Guhlke S, Ezziddin S, Bucerius J, von Mallek D (2011) Palliation and survival after repeated (188) Re-HEDP therapy of hormone-refractory bone metastases of prostate cancer: a retrospective analysis. J Nucl Med 52:1721–1726

Büchel GE, Stepanenko IN, Hejl M, Jakupec MA, Keppler BK, Arion VB (2011) En route to osmium analogues of KP1019: Synthesis, structure, spectroscopic properties and antiproliferative activity of trans-$[Os(IV)Cl_4(Hazole)_2]$. Inorg Chem 50:7690–7697

Cao R, Jia J, Ma X, Zhou M, Fei H (2013) Membrane localized iridium(III) complex induces endoplasmic reticulum stress and mitochondria-mediated apoptosis in human cancer cells. J Med Chem 56:3636–3644

Caporale C, Bader CA, Sorvina A, MaGee KDM, Skelton BW, Gillam TA, Wright PJ, Raiteri P, Stagni S, Morrison JL, Plush SE, Brooks DA, Massi M (2017) Investigating intracellular localisation and cytotoxicity trends for neutral and cationic iridium tetrazolato complexes in live cells. Chemistry 23(62):15666–15679

Chase NE, Atkins HL, Correll JW (1961) Interstitial irradiation of brain tumors with iridium 192. Radiology 77:842–843

Chen X, Sun L, Chen Y, Cheng X, Wu W, Ji L, Chao H (2015) A fast and selective two- photon phosphorescent probe for the imaging of nitric oxide in mitochondria. Biomaterials 58:72–81

Chen MH, Wang FX, Cao JJ, Tan CP, Ji LN, Mao ZW (2017) Light-up mitophagy in live cells with dual-functional theranostic phosphorescent iridium(III) complexes. ACS Appl Mater Interfaces 9(15):13304–13314

Cheng A, Chen S, Zhang Y, Yin D, Dong M (2011) The tolerance and therapeutic efficacy of rhenium-188 hydroxyethylidene diphosphonate in advanced cancer patients with painful osseous metastases. Cancer Biother Radiopharm 26:237–244

Choi AW, Louie MW, Li SP, Liu HW, Chan BT, Lam TC, Lin AC, Cheng SH, Lo KK (2012) Emissive behavior, cytotoxic activity, cellular uptake, and PEGylation properties of new luminescent rhenium(I) polypyridine poly(ethylene glycol) complexes. Inorg Chem 51:13289–13302

Connell TU, James JL, White AR, Donnelly PS (2015) Protein labelling with versatile phosphorescent metal complexes for live cell luminescence imaging. Chemistry 21(40):14146–14155

Craciunescu DG, Scarcia V, Furlani A, Papaioannou A, Parrondo-Iglesias E, Alonso MP (1991) Pharmacological and toxicological studies on new Rh(I) organometallic complexes. Vivo 5 (4):329–332

Davis KM, Bitting AL, Markwalter CF, Bauer WS, Wright DW (2015) Iridium(III) luminescent probe for detection of the malarial protein biomarker histidine rich protein-II. J Vis Exp 101: e52856

Dolan C, Moriarty RD, Lestini E, Devocelle M, Forster RJ, Keyes TE (2013) Cell uptake and cytotoxicity of a novel cyclometalated iridium(III) complex and its octaarginine peptide conjugate. J Inorg Biochem 119:65–74

Dömötör O, Aicher S, Schmidlehner M, Novak MS, Roller A, Jakupec MA, Kandioller W, Hartinger CG, Keppler BK, Enyedy EA (2014) Antitumor pentamethylcyclopentadienyl rhodium complexes of maltol and allomaltol: Synthesis, solution speciation and bioactivity. J Inorg Biochem 134:57–65

Dvorák J, Jandík P, Melichar B, Jon B, Mergancová J, Zoul Z, Vacek Z, Petera J (2002) Intraluminal high dose rate brachytherapy in the treatment of bile duct and gallbladder carcinomas. Hepatogastroenterology 49(46):916–917

Erck A, Rainen L, Whileyman J, Chang IM, Kimball AP, Bear J (1974) Studies of rhodium (II) carboxylates as potential antitumor agents. Proceed Soc Exp Biol Med 145:1278–1283

Ernst RJ, Song H, Barton JK (2009) DNA mismatch binding and antiproliferative activity of rhodium metalloinsertors. J Am Chem Soc 131:2359–2366

Ernst RJ, Komor AC, Barton JK (2011) Selective cytotoxicity of rhodium metalloinsertors in mismatch repair-deficient cells. Biochemistry 50:10919–10928

Feng Z, Tao P, Zou L, Gao P, Liu Y, Liu X, Wang H, Liu S, Dong Q, Li J, Xu B, Huang W, Wong WY, Zhao Q (2017) Hyperbranched phosphorescent conjugated polymer dots with iridium(III) complex as the core for hypoxia imaging and photodynamic therapy. ACS Appl Mater Interfaces 9(34):28319–28330

Ferri E, Donghi D, Panigati M, Prencipe G, D'Alfonso L, Zanoni I, Baldoli C, Maiorana S, D'Alfonso G, Licandro E (2010) Luminescent conjugates between dinuclear rhenium(I) complexes and peptide nucleic acids (PNA) for cell imaging and DNA targeting. Chem Commun (Camb) 46:6255–6257

Fu Y, Habtemariam A, Basri AMBH, Braddick D, Clarkson GJ, Sadler PJ (2011) Structure-activity relationships for organometallic osmium arene phenylazopyridine complexes with potent anticancer activity. Dalton Trans 40:10553–10562

Gasser G, Ott I, Metzler-Nolte N (2011) Organometallic anticancer compounds. J Med Chem 54:3–25

Geldmacher Y, Oleszak M, Sheldrick WS (2012a) Rhodium(III) and Iridium(III) complexes as anticancer agents. Inorg Chim Acta 393:84–102

Geldmacher Y, Splith K, Kitanovic I, Alborzinia H, Can S, Rubbiani R, Nazif MA, Wefelmeier P, Prokop A, Ott I, Wölfl S, Neundorf I, Sheldrick WS (2012b) Cellular impact and selectivity of half-sandwich organorhodium(III) anticancer complexes and their organoiridium(III) and trichloridorhodium(III) counterparts. J Biol Inorg Chem 17:631–646

Gerbaulet A, Pötter R, Mazeron JJ, Meertens H, van Limbergen E (eds) (2002) The GEC ESTRO handbook of brachytherapy Leuven. European Society for Therapeutic Radiology and Oncology, Belgium

Giraldi T, Sava G, Mestroni G, Zassinovich G, Stolfa D (1978) Antitumor action of rhodium (I) and iridium (I) complexes. Chem Biol Interact 22(2–3):231–238

Gupta G, Garci A, Murray BS, Dyson PJ, Fabre G, Trouillas P, Giannini F, Furrer J, Süss-Fink G, Therrien B (2013) Synthesis, molecular structure, computational study and in vitro anticancer activity of dinuclear thiolato-bridged pentamethylcyclopentadienyl Rh(III) and Ir(III) complexes. Dalton Trans 42(43):15457–15463

Hackenberg F, Oehninger L, Alborzinia H, Can S, Kitanovic I, Geldmacher Y, Kokoschka M, Wölfl S, Ott I, Sheldrick WS (2011) Highly cytotoxic substitutionally inert rhodium(III) tris (chelate) complexes: DNA binding modes and biological impact on human cancer cells. J Inorg Biochem 105:991–999

Han SH, Kim S, De U, Mishra NK, Park J, Sharma S, Kwak JH, Han S, Kim HS, Kim IS (2016) Synthesis of succinimide-containing chromones, naphthoquinones, and xanthones under Rh (III) catalysis: Evaluation of anticancer activity. J Org Chem 81(24):12416–12425

Hanif M, Babak MV, Hartinger CG (2014) Development of anticancer agents: wizardry with osmium. Drug Discov Today 19(10):1640–1648

Hisamatsu Y, Suzuki N, Masum AA, Shibuya A, Abe R, Sato A, Tanuma SI, Aoki S (2017) Cationic amphiphilic tris-cyclometalated iridium(III) complexes induce cancer cell death via interaction with Ca^{2+}-calmodulin complex. Bioconjug Chem 28(2):507–523

Huang EY, Sun LM, Lin H, Lan JH, Chanchien CC, Huang YJ, Wang CY, Wang CJ (2013) A prospective cohort study to compare treatment results between 2 fractionation schedules of high-dose-rate intracavitary brachytherapy (HDR-ICBT) in patients with cervical cancer. Int J Radiat Oncol Biol Phys 85(1):123–128

Huang H, Zhang P, Qiu K, Huang J, Chen Y, Ji L, Chao H (2016a) Mitochondrial dynamics tracking with two-photon phosphorescent terpyridyl iridium(III) complexes. Sci Rep 6:20887

Huang H, Yang L, Zhang P, Qiu K, Huang J, Chen Y, Diao J, Liu J, Ji L, Long J, Chao H (2016b) Real-time tracking mitochondrial dynamic remodeling with two-photon phosphorescent iridium (III) complexes. Biomaterials 83:321–331

Jardim GAM, Silva TL, Goulart MOF, de Simone CA, Barbosa JMC, Salomão K, de Castro SL, Bower JF, da Silva Júnior EN (2017) Rhodium-catalyzed C-H bond activation for the synthesis of quinonoid compounds: Significant Anti-Trypanosoma cruzi activities and electrochemical studies of functionalized quinines. Eur J Med Chem 18(136):406–419

Jeon M, Mishra NK, De U, Sharma S, Oh Y, Choi M, Jo H, Sachan R, Kim HS, Kim IS (2016) Rh (III)-Catalyzed C-H functionalization of indolines with readily accessible amidating reagent: synthesis and anticancer evaluation. J Org Chem 81(20):9878–9885

Jia J, Fei H, Zhou M (2012) Luminescent iridium(III) complexes as novel protein staining agents. Electrophoresis 33(9–10):1397–1401

Jiang J, Zhang C, Lin W, Liu Y, Liu S, Xu Y, Zhao Q, Huang W (2015) Long-lived phosphorescent iridium(III) complexes conjugated with cationic polyfluorenes for heparin sensing and cellular imaging. Macromol Rapid Commun 36(7):640–646

Jiang Q, Wang M, Yang L, Chen H, Mao L (2016) Synergistic coordination and hydrogen bonding interaction modulate the emission of iridium complex for highly sensitive glutamine imaging in live cells. Anal Chem 88(20):10322–10327

Jin C, Liu J, Chen Y, Li G, Guan R, Zhang P, Ji L, Chao H (2015a) Cyclometalated iridium(III) complexes with imidazo[4,5-f][1,10]phenanthroline derivatives for mitochondrial imaging in living cells. Dalton Trans 44(16):7538–7547

Jin C, Liu J, Chen Y, Zeng L, Guan R, Ouyang C, Ji L, Chao H (2015b) Cyclometalated iridium (III) complexes as two-photon phosphorescent probes for specific mitochondrial dynamics tracking in living cells. Chemistry 21(34):12000–12010

Jin C, Guan R, Wu J, Yuan B, Wang L, Huang J, Wang H, Ji L, Chao H (2017) Rational design of NIR-emitting iridium(III) complexes for multimodal phosphorescence imaging of mitochondria under two-photon excitation. Chem Commun (Camb) 53(75):10374–10377

Kang JH, Kim HJ, Kwon TH, Hong JI (2014) Phosphorescent sensor for phosphorylated peptides based on an iridium complex. J Org Chem 79(13):6000–6005

Kang TS, Mao Z, Ng CT, Wang M, Wang W, Wang C, Lee SM, Wang Y, Leung CH, Ma DL (2016) Identification of an Iridium(III)-Based Inhibitor of Tumor Necrosis Factor- α. J Med Chem 59(8):4026–4031

Kang TS, Wang W, Zhong HJ, Liang JX, Ko CN, Lu JJ, Chen XP, Ma DL, Leung CH (2017) A rhodium(III)-based inhibitor of autotaxin with antiproliferative activity. Biochimica Biophysica Acta 1861(2):256–263

Kastl A, Dieckmann S, Wahler K, Volker T, Kastl L, Merkel AL, Vultur A, Shannan B, Harms K, Ocker M, Parak WJ, Herlyn M, Meggers E (2013) Rhenium complexes with visible-light-induced anticancer activity. Chem Med Chem 8:924–927

Komor AC, Schneider CJ, Weidmann AG, Barton JK (2012) Cell-selective biological activity of rhodium metalloinsertors correlates with subcellular localization. J Am Chem Soc 134:19223–19233

Lawaczeck R, Arkadiev V, Diekmann F, Krumrey M (2005) Monochromatic x-rays in digital mammography. Invest Radiol 40(1):33–39

Lee HZ, Leong WK, Top S, Vessieres A (2014) Cytotoxic triosmium carbonyl clusters: a structure-activity relationship study. Chem Med Chem 9(7):1453–1457

Leonidova A, Gasser G (2014) Underestimated potential of organometallic rhenium complexes as anticancer agents. ACS Chem Biol 9(10):2180–2193

Leonidova A, Pierroz V, Rubbiani R, Heier J, Ferrari S, Gasser G (2014) Towards cancer cell-specific phototoxic organometallic rhenium(I) complexes. Dalton Trans 43:4287–4294

Leung CH, Zhong HJ, Chan DSH, Ma DL (2013) bioactive iridium and rhodium complexes as therapeutic agents. Coord Chem Rev 257:1764–1776

Li C, Yu M, Sun Y, Wu Y, Huang C, Li F (2011) A nonemissive iridium(III) complex that specifically lights-up the nuclei of living cells. J Am Chem Soc 133(29):11231–11239

Li G, Lin Q, Sun L, Feng C, Zhang P, Yu B, Chen Y, Wen Y, Wang H, Ji L, Chao H (2015a) A mitochondrial targeted two-photon iridium(III) phosphorescent probe for selective detection of hypochlorite in live cells and in vivo. Biomaterials 53:285–295

Li G, Chen Y, Wang J, Wu J, Gasser G, Ji L, Chao H (2015b) Direct imaging of biological sulfur dioxide derivatives in vivo using a two-photon phosphorescent probe. Biomaterials 63:128–136

Li X, Yin Y, Gao P, Li W, Yan H, Lu C, Zhao Q (2017a) A novel phosphorescent iridium(III) complex bearing a donor-acceptor-type o-carboranylated ligand for endocellular hypoxia imaging. Dalton Trans 46(40):13802–13810

Li X, Kolemen S, Yoon J, Akkaya EU (2017b) Activatable photosensitizers: Agents for selective photodynamic therapy. Adv Func Mater 27:1604053

Li X, Tong X, Yin Y, Yan H, Lu C, Huang W, Zhao Q (2017c) Using highly emissive and environmentally sensitive o-carborane-functionalized metallophosphors to monitor mitochondrial polarity. Chem Sci 8(9):5930–5940

Liu Z, Sadler PJ (2014) Organoiridium complexes: Anticancer agents and catalysts. Acc Chem Res 47:1174–1185

Liu Z, Romero-Canelon I, Qamar B, Hearn JM, Habtemariam A, Barry NP, Pizarro AM, Clarkson GJ and Sadler PJ (2014) The potent oxidant anticancer activity of organoiridium catalysts. Angewandte Chemie [International Edition (English)] 53:3941–3946

Liu S, Liang H, Zhang KY, Zhao Q, Zhou X, Xu W, Huang W (2015) A multifunctional phosphorescent iridium(III) complex for specific nucleus staining and hypoxia monitoring. Chem Commun (Camb) 51(37):7943–7946

Liu C, Yang C, Lu L, Wang W, Tan W, Leung CH, Ma DL (2017a) Luminescent iridium(III) complexes as COX-2-specific imaging agents in cancer cells. Chem Commun (Camb) 53 (19):2822–2825
Liu HW, Law WH, Lee LC, Lau JC and Lo KK (2017b) Cyclometalated iridium(III) bipyridine-phenylboronic acid complexes as bioimaging reagents and luminescent probes for sialic acids. Chem An Asian J 12(13):1545–1556
Liu J, Wu Y, Yu Y, Li K, Ji Y, Wu D (2017c) Quantitative ratiometric phosphorescence hypoxia-sensing nanoprobes based on quantum dots/Ir(III) glycerol monoolein cubic-phase nanoparticles. Biosens Bioelectron 98:119–125
Liu J, Dong ZZ, Yang C, Li G, Wu C, Lee FW, Leung CH, Ma DL (2017d) Turn-on luminescent probe for hydrogen peroxide sensing and imaging in living cells based on an iridium(III) complex-silver nanoparticle platform. Sci Rep 7(1):8980
Martinez-Lillo J, Mastropietro TF, Lappano R, Madeo A, Alberto ME, Russo N, Maggiolini M, De Munno G (2011) Rhenium(IV) compounds inducing apoptosis in cancer cells. Chem Commun (Camb) 47:5283–5285
Mazeron JJ, Ardiet JM, Haie-Méder C, Kovács G, Levendag P, Peiffert D, Polo A, Rovirosa A, Strnad V (2009) GEC-ESTRO recommendations for brachytherapy for head and neck squamous cell carcinomas. Radiother Oncol 91(2):150–156
McConnell JR, Rananaware DP, Ramsey DM, Buys KN, Cole ML, McAlpine SR (2013) A potential rhodium cancer therapy: Studies of a cytotoxic organorhodium (I) complex that binds DNA. Bioorg Med Chem Lett 23:2527–2531
Medici S, Peana M, Nurchi VM, Lachowicz JI, Crisponi G, Zoroddu MA (2015) Noble metals in medicine: latest advances. Coordin Chem Rev 284:329–350
Medici S, Peana M, Crisponi G, Nurchi VM, Lachowicz JI, Remelli M, Zoroddu MA (2016) Silver coordination compounds: a new horizon in medicine. Coordin Chem Rev 327–328: 349–359
Milickovic N, Tselis N, Karagiannis E, Ferentinos K, Zamboglou N (2017) Iridium-knife: Another knife in radiation oncology. Brachytherapy 16(4):884–892
Moromizato S, Hisamatsu Y, Suzuki T, Matsuo Y, Abe R, Aoki S (2012) Design and synthesis of a luminescent cyclometalated iridium(III) complex having N, N-diethylamino group that stains acidic intracellular organelles and induces cell death by photoirradiation. Inorg Chem 51:12697–12706
Moura C, Mendes F, Gano L, Santos I, Paulo A (2013) Mono- and dicationic Re(I)/(99 m)Tc(I) tricarbonyl complexes for the targeting of energized mitochondria. J Inorg Biochem 123:34–45
Ni WX, Man WL, Cheung MT, Sun RW, Shu YL, Lam YW, Che CM, Lau TC (2011) Osmium (VI) complexes as a new class of potential anti-cancer agents. Chem Commun (Camb) 47:2140–2142
Ni WX, Man WL, Yiu SM, Ho M, Cheung MTW, Ko CC, Che CM, Lam YW, Lau TC (2012) Osmium(VI) nitrido complexes bearing azole heterocycles: a new class of antitumor agents. Chem Sci 3:1582–1588
Novohradsky V, Liu Z, Vojtiskova M, Sadler PJ, Brabec V, Kasparkova J (2014) Mechanism of cellular accumulation of an iridium(III) pentamethylcyclopentadienyl anticancer complex containing a C, N-chelating ligand. Metallomics 6:682–690
Oehninger L, Kuster LN, Schmidt C, Munoz-Castro A, Prokop A, Ott I (2013) A chemical-biological evaluation of rhodium(I) N-heterocyclic carbene complexes as prospective anticancer drugs. Chem A Eur J 19:17871–17880
Peacock AF, Habtemariam A, Fernandez R, Walland V, Fabbiani FP, Parsons S, Aird RE, Jodrell DI, Sadler PJ (2006) Tuning the reactivity of osmium(II) and ruthenium(II) arene complexes under physiological conditions. J Am Chem Soc 128:1739–1748
Peacock AF, Parsons S, Sadler PJ (2007) Tuning the hydrolytic aqueous chemistry of osmium arene complexes with N, O-chelating ligands to achieve cancer cell cytotoxicity. J Am Chem Soc 129:3348–3357
Peacock AF and Sadler PJ (2008) Medicinal organometallic chemistry: designing metal arene complexes as anticancer agents. Chemistry – An Asian Journal 3: 1890-1899

Peixoto RC, Miranda-Vilela AL, de Souza Filho J, Carneiro ML, Oliveira RG, da Silva MO, de Souza AR, Báo SN (2015) Antitumor effect of free rhodium (II) citrate and rhodium (II) citrate-loaded maghemite nanoparticles on mice bearing breast cancer: a systemic toxicity assay. Tumour Biol 36(5):3325–3336

Qiu K, Huang H, Liu B, Liu Y, Huang Z, Chen Y, Ji L, Chao H (2016) Long-Term Lysosomes Tracking with a Water-Soluble Two-Photon Phosphorescent Iridium(III) Complex. ACS Appl Mater Interfaces 8(20):12702–12710

Raja MU, Tauchman J, Therrien B, Suss-Fink G, Riedel T, Dyson PJ (2014) Arene ruthenium and pentamethylcyclopentadienyl rhodium and iridium complexes containing N, O-chelating ligands derived from piroxicam: Synthesis, molecular structure and cytotoxicity. Inorg Chim Acta 409:479–483

Rao PN, Smith ML, Pathak S, Howard RA, Bear LJ (1980) Rhodium (II) butyrate: a potential anticancer drug with cell cycle phase-specific effects in HeLa cells. J Nat Cancer Inst 64 (4):905–912

Romero-Canelon I, Sadler PJ (2013) Next-generation metal anticancer complexes: Multitargeting via redox modulation. Inorg Chem 52:12276–12291

Romero-Canelon I, Salassa L, Sadler PJ (2013) The contrasting activity of iodido versus chlorido ruthenium and osmium arene azo- and imino-pyridine anticancer complexes: Control of cell selectivity, cross-resistance, p53 dependence, and apoptosis pathway. J Med Chem 56:1291–1300

Rood MT, Raspe M, ten Hove JB, Jalink K, Velders AH, van Leeuwen FW (2015) MMP- 2/ 9-Specific Activatable Lifetime Imaging Agent. Sensors (Basel) 15(5):11076–11091

Ruiz J, Vicente C, de Haro C, Bautista D (2013) Novel bis-C, N-cyclometalated iridium(III) thiosemicarbazide antitumor complexes: interactions with human serum albumin and DNA, and inhibition of cathepsin B. Inorg Chem 52:974–982

Salvadó I, Gamba I, Montenegro J, Martínez-Costas J, Brea JM, Loza MI, Vázquez López M, Vázquez ME (2016) Membrane-disrupting iridium(III) oligocationic organometallopeptides. Chem Commun (Camb) 52(73):11008–11011

Sartori R, Rencoret G, Mora A, Perez C, Pastene R, Sariego R, Moya SA (1996) The novel use of Rh(I) complexes with naphthyridine ligands and poly(oxyethylene) as antitumorals. Anticancer Drugs 7(1):87–92

Sava G, Giraldi T, Mestroni G, Zassinovich G (1983) Antitumor effects of rhodium(I), iridium(I) and ruthenium(II) complexes in comparison with cis-dichlorodiammino platinum(II) in mice bearing Lewis lung carcinoma. Chem Biol Interact 45(1):1–6

Sava G, Zorzet S, Perissin L, Mestroni G, Zassinovich G, Bontempi A (1987) Coordination metal complexes of Rh(I), Ir(I) and Ru(II): Recent advances on antimetastatic activity on solid mouse tumors. Inorg Chim Acta 137:69–71

Schmidt R (2006) Photosensitized generation of singlet oxygen. Photochem Photobiol 82:1161–1177

Shnyder SD, Fu Y, Habtemariam A, van Rijt SH, Cooper PA, Loadman PM, Sadler PJ (2011) Anti-colorectal cancer activity of an organometallic osmium arene azopyridine complex. Med Chem Comm 2:666–668

Soldevila-Barreda JJ, Habtemariam A, Romero-Canelón I, Sadler PJ (2015) Half-sandwich rhodium(III) transfer hydrogenation catalysts: Reduction of NAD(+) and pyruvate, and antiproliferative activity. J Inorg Biochem 153:322–333

Song X, Qian Y, Ben R, Lu X, Zhu HL, Chao H, Zhao J (2013) Activation of C-H bonds in nitrones leads to iridium hydrides with antitumor activity. J Med Chem 56:6531–6535

Strouthos I, Tselis N, Chatzikonstantinou G, Butt S, Baltas D, Bon D, Milickovic N, Zamboglou N (2017) High dose rate brachytherapy as monotherapy for localised prostate cancer. Radiother Oncology pii S0167–8140(17):32624–32625

Sun L, Li G, Chen X, Chen Y, Jin C, Ji L, Chao H (2015) Azo-based iridium(III) complexes as multicolor phosphorescent probes to detect hypoxia in 3D multicellular tumor spheroids. Sci Rep 5:14837

Sun L, Chen Y, Kuang S, Li G, Guan R, Liu J, Ji L, Chao H (2016) Iridium(III) Anthraquinone complexes as two-photon phosphorescence probes for mitochondria imaging and tracking under hypoxia. Chemistry 22(26):8955–8965

Suntharalingam K, Johnstone TC, Bruno PM, Lin W, Hemann MT, Lippard SJ (2013) Bidentate ligands on osmium(VI) nitrido complexes control intracellular targeting and cell death pathways. J Am Chem Soc 135:14060–14063

Suntharalingam K, Awuah SG, Bruno PM, Johnstone TC, Wang F, Lin W, Zheng Y-R, Page JE, Hemann MT, Lippard SJ (2015) Necroptosis-inducing rhenium(V) oxo complexes. J Am Chem Soc 137(8):2967–2974

Tang Q, Ni WX, Leung CF, Man WL, Lau KK, Liang Y, Lam YW, Wong WY, Peng SM, Liu GJ, Lau TC (2013) Synthesis and antitumor activity of a series of osmium(VI) nitride complexes bearing quinolinolato ligands. Chem Commun (Camb) 49:9980–9982

Tang W, Zhen Z, Wang M, Wang H, Chuang Y-J, Zhang W, Wang GD, Todd T, Cowger T, Chen H, Liu L, Li Z, Xie J (2016) Red blood cell-facilitated photodynamic therapy for cancer treatment. Adv Func Mater 26:1757–1768

Tian J, Ding L, Xu HJ, Shen Z, Ju H, Jia L, Bao L, Yu JS (2013) Cell-specific and pH-activatable rubyrin-loaded nanoparticles for highly selective near-infrared photodynamic therapy against cancer. J Am Chem Soc 135:18850–18858

Tobita S, Yoshihara T (2016) Intracellular and in vivo oxygen sensing using phosphorescent iridium(III) complexes. Curr Opin Chem Biol 33:39–45

Tso KK, Liu HW, Lo KK (2017) Phosphorogenic sensors for biothiols derived from cyclometalated iridium(III) polypyridine complexes containing a dinitrophenyl ether moiety. J Inorg Biochem pii S0162–0134(17):30275–30281

van Dodewaard-de Jong JM, de Klerk JM, Bloemendal HJ, van Bezooijen BP, de Haas MJ, Wilson RH, O'Sullivan JM (2011) A phase I study of combined docetaxel and repeated high activity 186Re-HEDP in castration-resistant prostate cancer (CRPC) metastatic to bone (the TAXIUM trial). Eur J Nucl Med Mol Imaging 38:1990–1998

van Rijt SH, Peacock AFA, Johnstone RDL, Parsons S, Sadler PJ (2009) Organometallic osmium (II) arene anticancer complexes containing picolinate derivatives. Inorg Chem 48:1753–1762

Wang B, Liang Y, Dong H, Tan T, Zhan B, Cheng J, Lo KK, Lam YW, Cheng SH (2012) A luminescent cyclometalated iridium(III) complex accumulates in mitochondria and induces mitochondrial shortening by conjugation to specific protein targets. Chem Bio Chem 13:2729–2737

Wang C, Cheng L, Liu Y, Wang X, Ma X, Deng Z, Li Y, Liu Z (2013) Imaging-guided pH-sensitive photodynamic therapy using charge reversible upconversion nanoparticles under near-infrared light. Adv Func Mater 23:3077–3086

Wang J, Xue J, Yan Z, Zhang S, Qiao J, Zhang X (2017a) Photoluminescence lifetime imaging of synthesized proteins in living cells using an iridium-alkyne probe. Angew Chem, Int Ed Engl 56(47):14928–14932

Wang W, Yang C, Lin S, Vellaisamy K, Li G, Tan W, Leung CH, Ma DL (2017b) First Synthesis of an Oridonin-Conjugated Iridium(III) Complex for the Intracellular Tracking of NF-κB in Living Cells. Chemistry 23(20):4929–4935

Xiang H, Chen H, Tham HP, Phua SZF, Liu JG, Zhao Y (2017) Cyclometalated iridium(III)-complex-based micelles for glutathione-responsive targeted chemotherapy and photodynamic therapy. ACS Appl Mater Interfaces 9(33):27553–27562

Yang LH, Ahn DJ, Koo E (2014) A "turn-on" fluorescent microbead sensor for detecting nitric oxide. Int J Nanomed 10:115–123

Ye RR, Cao JJ, Tan CP, Ji LN, Mao ZW (2017) Valproic acid-functionalized cyclometalated iridium(III) complexes as mitochondria-targeting anticancer agents. Chemistry 23(60):15166–15176

Yellol GS, Donaire A, Yellol JG, Vasylyeva V, Janiak C, Ruiz J (2013) On the antitumor properties of novel cyclometalated benzimidazole Ru(II), Ir(III) and Rh(III) complexes. Chem Commun (Camb) 49:11533–11535

Yoshihara T, Murayama S, Tobita S (2015) Ratiometric molecular probes based on dual emission of a blue fluorescent coumarin and a red phosphorescent cationic iridium(III) complex for intracellular oxygen sensing. Sens (Basel) 15(6):13503–13521

Yu Q, Zhang KY, Liang H, Zhao Q, Yang T, Liu S, Zhang C, Shi Z, Xu W, Huang W (2015) Dual-emissive nanohybrid for ratiometric luminescence and lifetime imaging of intracellular hydrogen sulfide. ACS Appl Mater Interfaces 7(9):5462–5470

Zhang Q, Cao R, Fei H, Zhou M (2014) Mitochondria-targeting phosphorescent iridium(III) complexes for living cell imaging. Dalton Trans 43(44):16872–16879

Zhang F, Liang X, Zhang W, Wang YL, Wang H, Mohammed YH, Song B, Zhang R, Yuan J (2017a) A unique iridium(III) complex-based chemosensor for multi-signal detection and multi-channel imaging of hypochlorous acid in liver injury. Biosens Bioelectron 87:1005–1011

Zhang W, Zhang F, Wang YL, Song B, Zhang R, Yuan J (2017b) Red-emitting ruthenium(II) and iridium(III) complexes as phosphorescent probes for methylglyoxal in vitro and in vivo. Inorg Chem 56(3):1309–1318

Zhou Y, Jia J, Wang X, Guo W, Wu Z, Xu N (2016) Protein staining agents from cationic and neutral luminescent iridium(III) complexes. Chemistry 22(47):16796–16800

Chapter 3
Metal-on-Metal Hip Implants: Progress and Problems

Alexander L. Neuwirth, Blair S. Ashley, William M. Hardaker and Neil P. Sheth

Abstract Once perceived as the future of hip arthroplasty, metal-on-metal (MoM) prostheses have since infamously fallen out of favor. The in vitro advantages of MoM implants, which included improved wear properties, reduced osteolysis, and allowed for the use of larger femoral heads to improve stability, have since been far outweighed by the local and systemic reactions associated with metal-on-metal implants. These adverse reactions stem from local release of chromium and cobalt ions, which result in immune responses locally and the formation of effusions and large solid masses known as pseudotumors or systemic effects on various organ systems. With over 1 million MoM prostheses in circulation worldwide, the revision burden of these devices is expected to increase, and a thorough understanding of the clinical manifestations of adverse reactions and revision strategies is essential for revision arthroplasty surgeons.

Keywords Arthroplasty · Metal-on-metal implants · Pseudotumors
Acetabular component

3.1 Introduction

Metal-on-metal (MoM) hip prostheses have been in use since the 1966 McKee-Farrar prosthesis. With advantages in volumetric wear reduction, and the ability to utilize larger femoral heads to reduce the incidence of dislocations, MoM implants were thought to be a significant step forward from conventional metal on polyethylene designs. As national registry data on MoM implants began to surface demonstrating significantly increased revision rates compared to conventional implants, increased efforts focused on identifying causes of failure, which revealed systemic effects of serum metal ions levels as well as local tissue reactions known as

A. L. Neuwirth · B. S. Ashley · W. M. Hardaker · N. P. Sheth (✉)
Department of Orthopaedic Surgery, University of Pennsylvania,
Philadelphia, PA, USA
e-mail: Neil.Sheth@uphs.upenn.edu

M. Rai et al. (eds.), *Biomedical Applications of Metals*,
https://doi.org/10.1007/978-3-319-74814-6_3

aseptic lymphocyte-dominant vasculitis-associated lesion (ALVAL). The spectrum of conditions associated with MoM implants is referred to as adverse reaction to metal debris (ARMD).

In response to the alarming data, the FDA issued black box warnings in 2011 on MoM implants, ultimately resulting in recalls from three separate implant companies: Depuy's ASR Acetabular system, Smith and Nephew's R3 Acetabular system, and Zimmer's Durom Acetabular system. With increased professional and public awareness, the use of MoM implants has rapidly declined since the recalls, and current use of these devices is rare almost exclusive to hip resurfacing options.

This chapter will review the history of MoM implants as well as the pathophysiology of local and systemic adverse reactions, the biomechanical effects of implant positioning on ion release, prevention and the workup of the patient with these devices.

3.2 History of MoM Hip Implants

Total joint replacement has been a goal pursued by surgeons for over 150 years. The earliest attempt at hip replacement occurred in Germany in 1891 using ivory to replace the femoral heads of patients who had suffered from tuberculosis septic arthritis (Learmonth et al. 2007). In 1925, Marius Smith-Pet created the first mold arthroplasty out of glass which consisted of a hollow hemisphere that fits over the existing femoral head, providing a smooth surface for articulation (Smith-Peterson 1948). Glass, although a biocompatible material, failed to withstand the joint reaction forces acting through the hip and often shattered. Smith-Peterson later joined Philip Wiles in introducing the first metal-on-metal bearing in what is regarded as the first total hip arthroplasty (THA) in 1938 (Wiles 1957). The Wiles prosthesis, made of stainless steel, relieved pain but was prone to loosening and early failure. The introduction of polymethylmethacrylate bone cement in 1960 helped address this issue, leading in part to the McKee-Farrar hip replacement. This method used a modified Thompson stem (a cemented hemiarthroplasty used to treat femoral neck fractures) in combination with a novel one-piece cobalt-chrome socket, which functioned as the acetabulum (McKee and Watson-Farrar 1966).

The poor results seen with this method were superseded by the Charnley low friction arthroplasty. This new system, introduced by Sir John Charnley, incorporated a cemented metal femoral stem and an all-polyethylene acetabular component. Charnley advocated for the use of a small femoral head with smaller surface area in order to reduce polyethylene wear (Charnley 1961). Backed by consistent early positive results, metal-on-polyethylene (MoPE) systems predominated until concern began to emerge about polyethylene wear debris. Polyethylene debris has been shown to lead to periprosthetic osteolysis predominately through inducing a macrophage-based response and the release of cytokines and proteolytic enzymes, ultimately resulting in bone resorption and eventual implant failure (Bizot et al. 2001) (Fig. 3.1). Polyethylene wear debris is cited as the ultimate cause of most

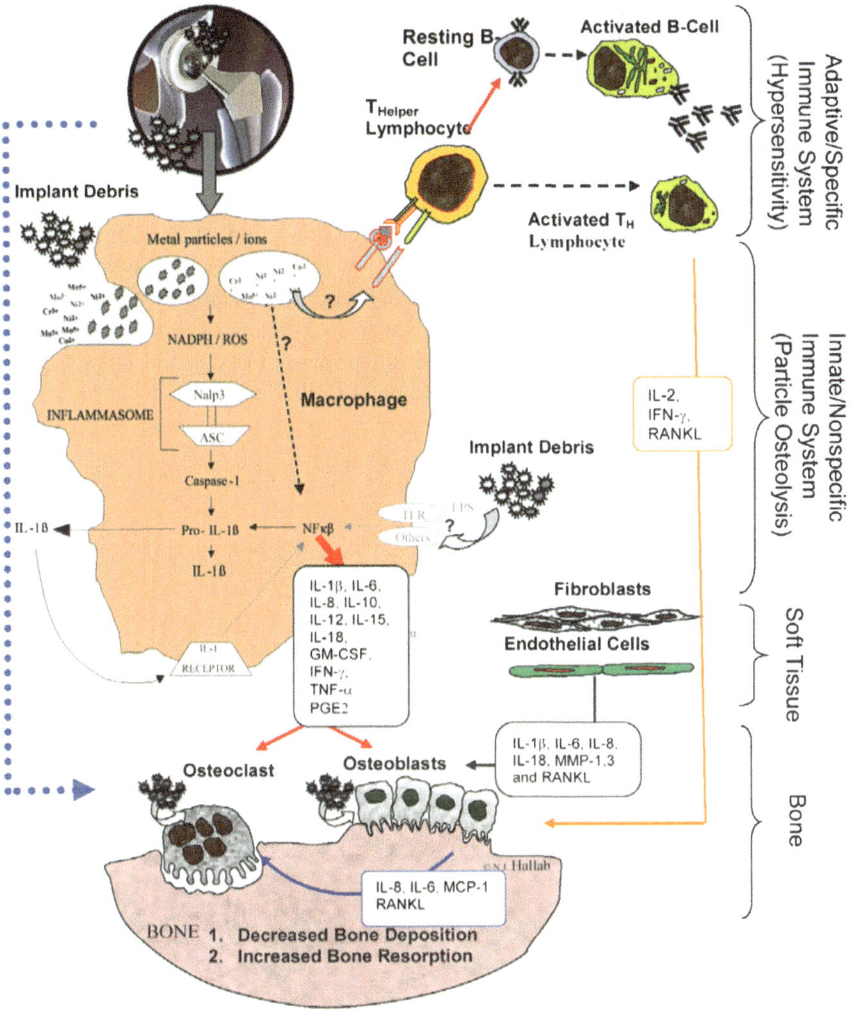

Fig. 3.1 Schematic representation of osteolysis pathway

THA failures today leading to decreased implant longevity and an increased requirement for revision surgery secondary to aseptic loosening (Amstutz 1996).

In the late 1980s and early 1990s, the issue of polyethylene wear debris led to the reintroduction of MoM articulations, which provided two theoretical advantages over metal-on-polyethylene (MoPE) articulations. First, MoM articulations produce significantly less volumetric wear than MoPE articulations, and therefore had the potential to substantially reduce failure rates secondary to wear-induced osteolysis (MacDonald et al. 2003). Second, metal acetabular components can be made thinner than their MoPE counterparts, allowing for larger diameter femoral heads, maximization of the head to neck ratio, and greater range of motion prior to neck impingement on the acetabular shell. These perceived advantages led to the dramatic increase in popularity of the MoM hip implant. It is estimated that since 1996, more than 1 million MoM articulations have been implanted worldwide (Bozic et al. 2009).

The peak of MoM popularity was reached in 2008, when over 40% of all primary THA procedures performed in the United States were MoM procedures (Bozic et al. 2009). That same year also marked the beginning of a dramatic decline in MoM usage. Citing high early failure rates, the US Food and Drug Administration (FDA) recalled the Durom acetabular component (Zimmer, Warsaw, Indiana) and 2 years later, the FDA similarly recalled the ASR Hip Resurfacing System as well as the ASR XL Acetabular System (DePuy, Warsaw, Indiana) (Fig. 3.2). By 2009, MoM procedures comprised only 10% of all primary THA in the United States (Bozic et al. 2009); that percentage has dropped further since.

Hip resurfacing, which was perceived as an evolution from mold arthroplasty, is a subcategory of hip replacement in which the femoral head is capped while maintaining the proximal femoral bone with a stemmed implant. Hip resurfacing was first described in the 1930s and was in use through the 1950s (Fig. 3.3). It was popularized for the treatment of young and active patients in the 1970s through the use of cemented polyethylene acetabular components, but insufficient wear resistance, wear-debris-induced osteolysis, and implant loosening resulted in the

Fig. 3.2 Depuy ASR metal on metal

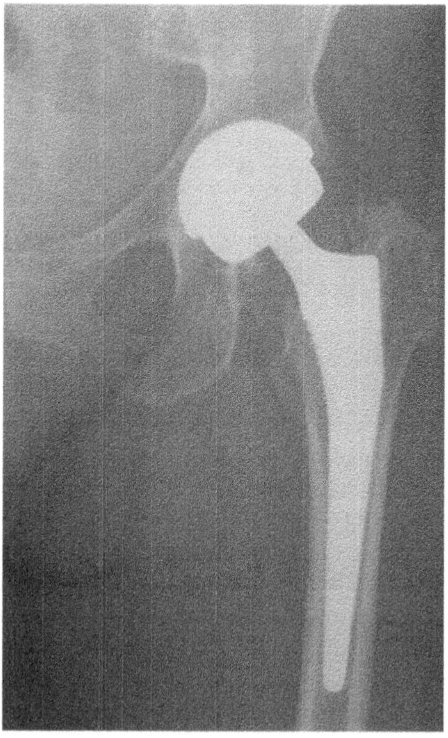

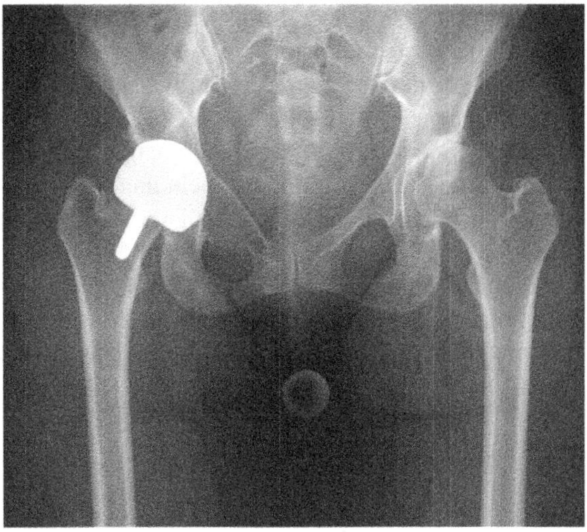

Fig. 3.3 Birmingham hip resurfacing

abandonment of this surgical option. The advent of improved metallurgy led to metal-on-metal hip resurfacing (MoMHR). MoMHR, which gained popularity in the 1990s, is still currently a commonly used technique. In the UK, 8% of all primary total hip arthroplasties and 40% of those performed for patients between the ages of 55 and 64 are MoMHR (Smith et al. 2012a, b).

Proposed advantages of hip resurfacing include bone preservation, conservation of native hip biomechanics, reduced dislocation rates, ease of revision, reduced prevalence of venous thromboembolism (VTE), and prevention of stress shielding in the femur. Disadvantages specific to resurfacing include risk of femoral neck fracture, aseptic loosening, and the release of small, bioreactive cobalt particles over time due to wear (Watanabe et al. 2000). Several MoMHR implants have been marketed over the years. Most implants include a cementless acetabular shell and a cemented femoral cap with the articular bearing surface composed of cobalt-chromium alloys.

Survival rates for hip resurfacing are still being investigated. While there are studies reporting on short and mid-term survival of such implants, there is a paucity of data on long-term outcomes. One single surgeon study reported a 10-year survival rate of 98% in males (Treacy et al. 2011). A large registry-based retrospective study from England identified risk factors for reduced survivorship of MoMHR implants (Smith et al. 2012a, b). The study noted that hip resurfacing resulted in significantly worse outcomes in women when compared to match THA patients, regardless of femoral head size. The authors noted that reduced head size in the setting of MoMHR is linked to worse survivorship in men, and predicted 5-year revision rates, demonstrating a near linear association with head size after the first year. A Finnish registry study confirmed a significant difference in revision risk between men and women following resurfacing, but no difference between MoMHR and MoM THA for matched patients (Seppanen et al. 2012). These findings led surgeons to limit their indications for resurfacing to young active men.

Survival rates in the setting of total hip arthroplasty using metal-on-metal implants are decreased compared to those of alternate bearing surfaces. One recent study out of India suggested a survival rate of 68.9% at 7 years, far lower than quoted for metal-on-polyethylene survival rates. In this series, revisions were most commonly secondary to adverse reactions to metal debris (ARMD). ARMD includes a spectrum of findings, including macroscopic necrosis, osteolysis, large, sterile hip effusions, and periprosthetic solid and cystic masses, also known as pseudotumors (Bolognesi and Ledford 2015). Other studies have quoted even lower survivorship. One large series showed an implant survival of only 51.2% at 6 years (Langton et al. 2010). The alarmingly lower survivorship of metal-on-metal implants has been a driving force in the reduced use of these implants. Given the advancements made in alternate bearing technology with improved ceramic and polyethylene options, surgeons have generally opted out of using MoM implants in the setting of total hip arthroplasty.

3.3 Metal Ion Release

MoM hip implants were reintroduced as a low-wear, high-performance alternative to MoPE, especially in younger, more active patients. There were several perceived positives regarding MoM implants. Compared to conventional MoPE articulation, the volumetric wear rates of large head metal articulation were shown to be significantly decreased (Anissian et al. 1999). MoM articulation also allowed for the use of large-diameter femoral heads and the prospect of both decreased wear and decreased risk of dislocation (Berry et al. 2005). However, national registry data began to reveal significantly higher revision rates (2–3X) in MoM implants in comparison with other hip implants (Australia 2010; England and Wales 2010).

Observed increased revision rates have been attributed to the corrosive metal interaction between cobalt-chromium components of the femoral head and acetabular liner, resulting in release of metal particles and ions into the periprosthetic space. It is widely understood that implant devices undergo a "run-in" period whereby any irregularities on the surfaces of devices are worn down. The vast majority of metal ions are released during this time, and therefore, the highest systemic ion concentrations will be reported during the run-in period, which typically lasts 1 to 3 years (Savarino et al. 2014). While cobalt and chromium are required elements for normal biological function, high concentrations of these ions are toxic and have been shown to interfere with several important biological processes (Anissian et al. 2002). Of particular note are the formation of symptomatic soft-tissue masses including adverse reactions to metal debris (ARMD) and aseptic lymphocytic vasculitis-associated lesions (ALVAL) (Pandit et al. 2008; Langton et al. 2010). Significant effort has been made to better understand the implications of elevated metal ion levels secondary to MoM implantation as well as the threshold metal ion level above which ARMD, ALVAL, and implant failure occur.

3.3.1 Metal Ion Levels

Published information regarding normal levels for trace metals in humans is scarce and variable, as is that of both pre- and postoperative orthopedic patients (Ring et al. 2016). Rodushkin et al. (1999) recorded whole blood chromium levels of 0.4–1.2 ppb and whole blood cobalt levels of 0.022–0.255 ppb among 31 healthy patients. Delaunay et al. reported a far broader range for whole blood chromium (1–35 ppb) and an average whole blood cobalt concentration of 0.8 ppb (Delaunay et al. 2010). Delaunay also reported average serum chromium and cobalt average concentrations of 0.5 ppb and 0.4 ppb, respectively (Delaunay et al. 2010). Choi et al. reported serum chromium levels of 0.19–0.87 ppb and serum cobalt levels of 0.13–0.80 ppb across 51 healthy control subjects (Choi et al. 2015). The association between MoM implants and increased metal ion levels has been investigated extensively. De Smet et al. (2008) reported that patients with well-functioning MoM prostheses have higher concentrations of both serum chromium and cobalt, with ranges of 0.4–21.5 ppb and 1–14 ppb, respectively. In the presence of metallosis (defined as gray discoloration of the hip joint), these concentrations increase dramatically, resulting in serum chromium and cobalt levels rising to 5.3–93 ppb and 4.3–94 ppb, respectively (De Smet et al. 2008). Choi et al. (2015) reported postoperative serum chromium and cobalt concentration in the range of 0.61–116.80 ppb and 0.12–127.80 ppb, respectively. Vendittoli et al. (2007) also reported a significant increase in postoperative metal ion levels, but in whole blood rather than serum. Whole blood chromium and cobalt levels were shown to be 9–10 times that of healthy control subjects. Given the range of metal ion levels found in both well-functioning and symptomatic knees, it was deemed important to establish threshold levels to determine when abnormal wear is occurring. De Smet et al. (2008) suggested that metallosis is indicated when serum chromium and cobalt levels exceed 17 and 19 ppb, respectively. In 2012, the Mayo Clinic issued a communication that proposed serum threshold values of 15 ppb for chromium and 10 ppb for cobalt (Mayo Clinic 2012). Regarding whole blood, the 2010 and 2012 medical device alerts from the Medicines and Healthcare products Regulatory Agency recommended a threshold value for chromium and cobalt metal ion levels of 7 ppb, above which more frequent surveillance and further testing should occur (MHRA 2010, 2012).

3.3.2 Effect of Femoral Head Size

Over the years, there has been a trend toward larger femoral head size in hip arthroplasty in order to improve stability and reduce impingement by increasing the implant's head to neck ratio. The increase in "jump distance" offered by larger heads has been an important factor in reducing instability and short-term dislocation. A recent study noted that head sizes greater than 36 mm led to decreased dislocations at short-term followup. This benefit comes with a cost, however.

The disadvantage of larger femoral head sizes is the resultant increased volumetric wear, which leads to increased serum cobalt levels. The literature reports conflicting data regarding the effect of head size on metal ion production and overall survival. While some studies have found no relationship between head size and serum metal ion levels, others have identified increased ion levels with smaller 28 mm heads as compared with larger 36 mm heads (Engh et al. 2014). Head size has, however, generally been correlated with worse outcomes and higher revision rates in MoM. One study noted that femoral heads less than 47 mm in diameter were more likely to require revision at 5 years. Another study noted that a metal femoral head diameter greater than 50 mm is an independent risk factor for developing ARMDs. However, Australian national registry found no correlation between head size and ARMDs at 5-year followup though there was an increased failure rate with head sizes greater than 32 mm (De Steiger et al. 2011). Complicating matters further is the suggestion that corrosion and fretting at head neck interface (Dyrkacz et al. 2013) or a large head/short taper combination (Donaldson et al. 2014) are significant contributing factors to metal ion levels.

Although maximizing head size is associated with reduced revision rates, improved stability, and decreased impingement, surgeons must remain aware of the increased volumetric wear that may result from larger heads. A study of metalheads revealed that 26 mm heads had a mean total volumetric wear of 88 mm^3, while 36 mm heads resulted in wear of nearly 160 mm^3. Increased particles are associated with increased osteolysis and increased systemic ion levels. Therefore, hypervigilance when placing cobalt-chromium bearing surfaces is paramount in order to maximize mechanical stability and motion while minimizing systemic effects and loosening. Looks fine now that comment was a remnant from much earlier revisions.

3.3.3 *Effect of Acetabular Component Positioning*

Beyond the intrinsic characteristics of components, technical considerations have been associated with increased metal ion release. Ideal component positioning in hip arthroplasty has long been a subject of debate. Originally described by Lewinnek et al. (1978), the component "safe zones" were identified as predictive of instability in the setting of hip arthroplasty following a posterior approach; however, more recent evidence points toward combined anteversion of the femoral component and the acetabular cup. A 2016 prospective series described this "safe zone" for the acetabular component to be 10–25 degrees of anteversion and 30–50 degrees of abduction. In response to concerns regarding MoM implants, efforts have focused on identifying proper component positioning to optimize wear and minimize edge loading, which is thought to be associated with increased ion release. A large study of 214 patients who underwent MoM hip resurfacing found that steeply inclined acetabular components (greater than 55°) were associated with increased serum cobalt and chromium levels at a followup of 1 year. (De Haan et al.

2008). The cause of increased ion levels in the setting of a steeply inclined component is thought to be due to edge loading. Early edge loading is a result of imperfect component positioning and can occur regardless of the bearing surface used. However, this process has much more significant consequences in the setting of MoM devices as the process disrupts fluid film lubrication, which in turn leads to accelerated wear (Udofia and Jin 2003). Meticulous and accurate implant positioning is paramount in preventing abnormal loading, metal particle formation, and associated serum cobaltism and local tissue reaction.

Beyond implant positioning, the amount of head coverage, described as the arc of cover, was identified as a critical factor in reducing the amount of particulate debris produced over time. The arc of cover is defined as the product of the radius of the cup and the acetabular component angle, which varies by implant design. In one study, the arc of cover (Fig. 3.4) showed significant correlation with serum metal ion levels, and to a greater extent than either the abduction angle or the implant size independently (De Haan et al. 2008). Consequently, surgeons planning to utilize MoM implants must combine careful technique with the judicious use of implants in order to position the prostheses in an optimal position to reduce particle production, serum ion concentration, and the resulting physiologic consequences.

Although acetabular component position and its relationship with wear and metal ion levels have been evaluated extensively, there is a paucity of data regarding the impact of femoral component positioning. Proper femoral component position as well as adequate offset and length restoration restore abductor tension reduce joint reactive forces and maintain equal leg lengths. A recent study suggested that femoral component positioning, as measured using CT scanning to identify changes in offset and abductor lever arm length and angle, is not associated

Fig. 3.4 Representation of arc of cover

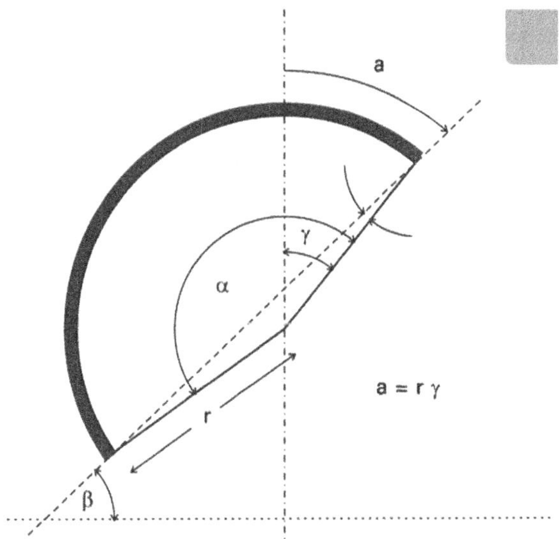

with increased wear, elevated serum levels of cobalt or chromium, or poor functional scores (Mann et al. 2016). Interestingly, the study did not identify a correlation between acetabular component position and activity level with serum ion levels.

3.4 Bioreactivity and ARMD (Adverse Reaction to Metal Debris)

MoM THA has been implicated in both systemic and local physiological effects due to adverse reactions to metal debris (ARMD). While metal particulate debris is smaller than its polyethylene counterpart, the molecules are more numerous and more biologically active. As a result, patients have been observed to experience several physiologic sequelae, both locally and systemically, at long-term followup after MoM THA.

3.4.1 Systemic Concerns

3.4.1.1 Cardiomyopathy

The deleterious cardiac effects of cobalt toxicity were first brought to attention in the 1960s when increased cobalt sulfate in beer resulted in a cardiomyopathy epidemic (Morin 1967). The myocardium of patients afflicted by cobalt toxicity revealed patchy interstitial fibrosis on light microscopy despite appearing macroscopically normal at autopsy. Though the gastrointestinal uptake experienced by these patients differs from the etiology of increased serum cobalt in patients following MoM THA, the propensity for cobalt deposition in myocardial tissue and the resulting interstitial edema, pericardial effusion, and diffuse myocardial degeneration is relevant (Morin 1967).

Large population studies focusing on the cardiac effects of cobalt are limited, and however several case reports exist. One patient sustained a catastrophic failure of a cobalt-chromium femoral head resulting in acute cobalt toxicity which was initially misdiagnosed as hypothyroidism, but was later treated for a diagnosis of dilated cardiomyopathy, left ventricular failure, and a large pericardial effusion. Despite drainage of the pericardial effusion, the patient developed cardiogenic shock requiring vasopressor support at which point elevated serum cobalt levels were detected, as well as elevated serum levels of titanium and chromium. Despite emergent exploration of the hip with prosthesis removal, cobalt chelation therapy, and downward trending cobalt levels, the patient developed multi-organ system failure and died. Autopsy revealed heavy metal toxicity of the tissues characterized by electron-dense deposits in the cardiac mitochondria and significant fibrosis (Zywiel et al. 2013). Another patient developed cobalt toxicity with bilateral

MoM THA, who became symptomatic approximately 11 months after his second operation. The patient had a negative cardiac stress test, an echocardiogram revealing stage II diastolic dysfunction with mildly diminished ejection fraction, and elevated serum cobalt and chromium levels. Cardiac MRI was performed which revealed biventricular dysfunction and diffuse myocardial hyper-enhancement of the anterior, lateral, and apical walls with sparing of the base and mid-septum similar to that seen with amyloidosis and consistent with diffuse, fulminant myocarditis of toxic origin (Mosier et al. 2016). Endomyocardial biopsy was performed during catheterization and revealed myocyte hypertrophy and interstitial fibrosis with scattered myofibers containing large cytoplasmic vacuoles. Further analysis showed replacement of myofibers by collagen, reduced contractile elements, vacuolar spaces, and increased lipofuscin. The patient ultimately required cardiac transplant (Mosier et al. 2016).

The presumed mechanism of cobalt toxicity is multifactorial. It includes inhibition of cellular respiration secondary to the inhibition of mitochondrial dehydrogenase. Damage of the electromechanical matching of myocardial tissue due to altered transmembrane transport induced by cobalt resulting in reduction of calcium concentration also impairs cardiac function. Finally, inhibition of sympathetic tone due to alterations of the beta-adrenergic system and the type IV delayed hypersensitivity reaction affects the myocardium as seen in other tissues.

Despite the lack of dedicated literature on the topic, the onset of cobalt-induced cardiomyopathy is rapid and often lethal with a mortality of up to 50%. Thus, it must be taken very seriously by clinicians treating patients with MoM and vague systemic symptoms such as malaise, fatigue, anorexia, or dyspnea and those resembling heart failure (McDermott et al. 1966; Seghizzi et al. 1994).

3.4.1.2 Carcinogenicity and Genetic Changes

There has been significant concern over whether chronically elevated blood metal ion concentrations lead to carcinogenesis. Chromosomal aberrations and DNA damage have been associated with metal debris following total hip arthroplasty (Case et al. 1996; Bonassi et al. 2000; Daley et al. 2004). Despite these changes, many studies have shown that the overall cancer rate is not increased following metal-on-polyethylene THA, first-generation metal-on-metal arthroplasty, or modern metal-on-metal arthroplasty (Visuri et al. 1996, 2010; Makela et al. 2012; Smith et al. 2012a, b; Brewster et al. 2013). In an analysis of the Finnish registry, it was noted that patients undergoing MoM were at an increased risk of developing skin basal cell carcinoma and soft-tissue sarcomas compared to a non-MoM cohort (Makela et al. 2014). The risks of other cancers including lung, prostate, colon, leukemia, etc. are not significantly different between MoM and non-MoM groups (Makela et al. 2014), and studies suggest there is actually a lower incidence of these cancers in patients who underwent hip resurfacing procedures (Smith et al. 2012a, b). Equivalent or lower cancer risk in MoM patients compared to other bearing surfaces versus the general population may be affected by the inherent selection bias in choosing younger and healthier patients to receive MoM implants, particularly when including resurfacing procedures (Smith et al. 2012a, b). In general, the risk of cancer-related mortality as well as all-cause mortality is actually less in the MoM cohort than in the non-MoM cohort (Smith et al. 2012a, b; Makela et al. 2014).

Despite the clinical evidence against MoM resulting in cancer, it is clear that genetic changes occur at the cellular level. In vitro studies reveal that exposure of fibroblasts to CoCr particles triggered rapid generation of reactive oxygen species which were eliminated through phagocytosis and mitochondrial-mediated processes, but still resulted in aneuploidy, chromosome clumping, fragmentation of mitochondria, and damage to the microtubule network of the cell cytoskeleton (Raghunathan et al. 2013). In periprosthetic tissues of patients with failed MoM hip replacements, Sarhardi et al. reported 5 of 20 patients had at least one hotspot position missense or deletion mutation in one of the genes of the cancer gene panel. Additionally, they found that there were genetic changes (copy number alterations and mutations) in the DNA of the JAK2, NOTCH1, and RUNX2 proteins (Sarhadi et al. 2015), which have previously been implicated in the both hematologic malignancies (JAK2 and NOTCH1) or in osteoblast-related bone dysplasia (RUNX2) (Sarhadi et al. 2015). Of note, the presence of genetic anomalies was associated with longer in situ time of the implant, suggesting a dose-dependent effect, of sorts (Sarhadi et al. 2015).

3.4.1.3 Polyneuropathy

Very little has been published regarding metallosis-induced polyneuropathy following THA; however, deafness following occupational exposure is well known (Seiler et al. 1988; IARC 2006) and several case reports exist. One case report described a patient who developed a progressive sensory disturbance and hearing loss following THA with a CoCr prosthesis. Nerve conduction studies revealed no sensory nerve action potentials, and the patient underwent a sural nerve biopsy confirming axonopathy. The patient's neuropathy resulted in significant dysesthesias and paresthesias, diminished joint position sense of the fingers and feet, distal muscle weakness, loss of deep tendon reflexes, and sensorineural hearing loss with resolution of all symptoms following revision arthroplasty and concordant normalization of her serum cobalt and chromium concentrations (Ikeda et al. 2010). Another case series involved a patient who had a ceramic on ceramic prosthesis which was revised to a ceramic stem and cup but with a metal head, which resulted in elevated serum cobalt and chromium levels and subsequent hearing loss, vision loss, and peripheral neuropathy. Of note, the patient's CSF was sampled and also revealed elevated cobalt concentration. The patient's symptoms gradually resolved over time (Steens et al. 2006). In addition to the aforementioned symptomatology, another case report noted a patient who experienced seizures, dysgeusia, and muscle mass reduction as potential presentation for cobalt and chromium toxicity after getting revised to a metal head (Oldenburg et al. 2009). Metallosis can also result in thyroid abnormalities, and thus the early vague neurologic symptoms can be confused with hypothyroidism; however, given confirmation with nerve conduction studies, nerve biopsy, and CSF analysis, it is highly suggestive that the peripheral neuropathy associated with metallosis following arthroplasty is a separate complication.

3.4.1.4 Renal Effects

Metal particles, unlike most organic chemicals, are unable to be degraded by metabolic means, and thus can only be excreted via the renal or gastrointestinal systems. This poses concern over the potential nephrotoxic effects of the metallosis associated with MoM THA. The urine concentrations of cobalt, chromium, and nickel, as well as their ratio to urinary creatinine, were all elevated in patients with MoM; however, urine values were not strongly correlated with serum values or renal impairment, so the clinical relevance is unclear (Newton et al. 2012). Long-term followup has not revealed any statistically significant elevations of serum creatinine levels or degradation of serum creatinine clearance, and the mean serum cobalt and chromium concentrations remained within normal limits (Marker et al. 2008). It is surmised that the metal released from cobalt-chromium implants is below the total body concentration threshold for the kidneys to result in any lasting deleterious effects in the setting of a baseline healthy renal system (Black 1988; Allen et al. 1997; Marker et al. 2008). However, experimental models have shown that elevated cobalt and chromium levels can stimulate the production of hypoxia-inducible factor (HIF), thus suggesting that these ions promote a state of hypoxia, which is deleterious to the renal tubules. There remains much to be elucidated about the physiologic effect of metal ions in the renal system (Shrivastava et al. 2008; Nangaku 2009; Newton et al. 2012).

3.4.2 Local Tissue Reactions

Adverse reactions to metal debris (ARMD) is a general term to describe all adverse soft-tissue reactions to metal debris, including aseptic lymphocyte-dominated vasculitis-associated lesion (ALVAL) and pseudotumors most commonly discussed in reference to MoM THA (Fig. 3.5). The presence of both of these lesions is an indication for revision, both due to patient discomfort as well as potential detrimental effects of the lesions themselves.

3.4.2.1 Aseptic Lymphocyte-Dominated Vasculitis-Associated Lesion (ALVAL)

Aseptic lymphocyte-dominated vasculitis-associated lesion (ALVAL) is a phenomenon first described in 2005, and it is a part of a spectrum of disorders

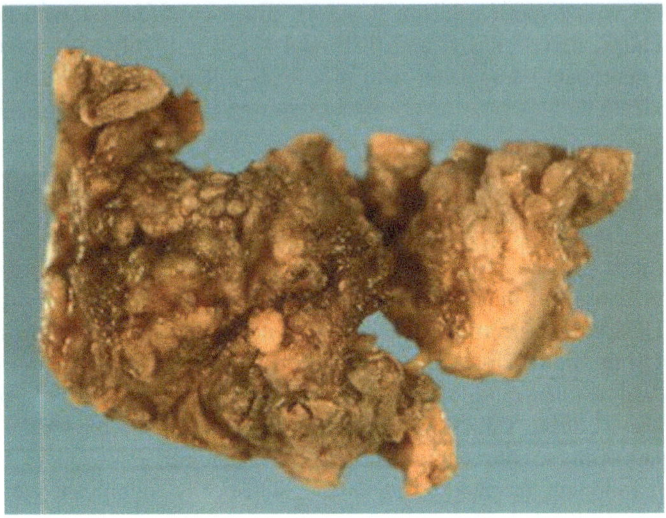

Fig. 3.5 Pseudotumor

encompassing adverse soft-tissue reactions to metal debris (Davies et al. 2005; Duggan 2013). The metal debris triggers a lymphocyte-based inflammatory reaction resulting in chronic inflammation, which in turn causes alterations in the surrounding vasculature. Histopathological features of ALVAL resemble the tissues surrounding a failed THA; however, they also display a dense perivascular inflammatory infiltrate that is unique to the family of lesions (Watters et al. 2010; Duggan 2013). The presence of ALVAL is associated with adverse outcomes, including lymphadenopathy, neurological symptoms, and periprosthetic fracture (Yanny et al. 2012). ALVAL is frequently used interchangeably with pseudotumor in the literature, highlighting the lack of understanding regarding the pathogenesis of lesion formation and their evolution.

3.4.2.2 Pseudotumor

Pseudotumors, while thought to be related to ALVAL, are presumed to be a distinct entity. They are sterile, inflammatory lesions within the tissue, which form as a consequence of a delayed type IV hypersensitivity reaction (Duggan 2013). The tumors themselves are neither infectious nor neoplastic. They more closely resemble granulomatous or cystic lesions consistent with chronic foreign body inflammation, which is progressive (Bosker et al. 2015). Patients with pseudotumor classically present with pain, the degree of which has been shown to correlate with the size of the lesion (Duggan 2013). While swelling and serum cobaltism (≥ 4 ug/l) are correlated with the presence of a pseudotumor, the strongest predictor for this complication is pain. The presence of pseudotumors is associated with implant failure, though the size threshold has yet to be established. Despite these findings, there are still some patients who have asymptomatic pseudotumors and patients who have pseudotumors in the setting of normal metal ion levels (Bosker et al. 2015). However, when pseudotumors are found, they serve as an indication for revision because of the local tissue destruction that can ensue, making subsequent revision surgeries more complicated and associated with poorer outcomes (Grammatopolous et al. 2009; Bosker et al. 2015).

3.4.3 Diagnostic Assessment

3.4.3.1 Clinical Evaluation

Algorithms created by the Hip Society provide a good framework for a systematic evaluation of painful metal-on-metal articulation of the junction. Physical examination and a thorough history are essential in the workup of painful metal-on-metal articulation of the junction. Patients who have a symptomatic metal-on-metal articulation present with hip or groin pain. Persistent pain or early recurrence of preoperative symptoms suggests infection or adverse reactions to metal debris or adverse local tissue reactions. Patients also may present with a palpable mass or fluid collection near the hip, with or without loss of hip abduction. Catching, locking, or crepitus is also common, so it is imperative to assess hip range of motion (Lombardi et al. 2012).

Symptomatic MoM implants require a thorough history and physical examination as well as anteroposterior and lateral radiographs of the hip. Infection should be considered as a cause of pain and appropriate laboratory markers should always be obtained in these patients. Erythrocyte sedimentation rate, C-reactive protein level, and synovial white blood cell (WBC) count can be elevated in the absence of infection in patients with MoM implants. Therefore, these tests have poor predictive value. In these cases, synovial neutrophil percentage is a good diagnostic option, with 80% or higher indicating a diagnosis of infection (Wyles et al. 2013). It is important that the hip aspirate WBC count must be performed manually in order to avoid clogging of the counting machine—an automated count may yield a result of too many cells to count due to metal debris.

3.4.3.2 Metal Ion Levels

Serum ion concentrations of cobalt and chromium are used for screening and diagnosis, but a review of the literature reveals mixed results. Hart et al. evaluated the relationship of serum cobalt and chromium ion levels and their sensitivity and specificity in predicting failure of MoM articulations. The MHRA 2010 cutoff value of 7 ppb showed a specificity of 89% and sensitivity of 52% in detecting preoperative unexplained failed MoM articulation in patients with normal imaging results. Hart suggested that the optimal cutoff value for both serum cobalt and chromium levels was 5 ppb, which had a specificity of 63% and sensitivity of 85% (Hart et al. 2011).

Elevated serum cobalt and chromium ion levels correlate with poor implant positioning, including an Abduction/inclination angle greater than 55° and anteversion less than 5° or greater than 25° (De Haan et al. 2008; Langton et al. 2010). These data support the association of implant malposition, wear, and failure. Hence, implant malposition or an elevated serum cobalt or chromium ion level necessitates revision because implant failure is already occurring in the symptomatic patient and in the asymptomatic patient, implant failure is impending. Langton et al. showed that cobalt and chromium concentrations were indicators of the performance of metal-on-metal implants (Langton et al. 2010). Sidaginamale argued that whole blood testing was a quicker, more accurate representation of systemic metal ion exposure and therefore should be preferred to serum ion level measurement. In addition, Sidaginamale reported cobalt levels to be more a more reliable measure than chromium levels in the assessment of systemic metal ion exposure (Sidaginamale et al. 2013).

If serum metal ion levels are determined to be elevated, the next step is to evaluate radiographs for evidence of osteolysis and component malpositioning. The presence of either of these radiographic findings indicates that revision THA should be strongly considered (Lombardi et al. 2012). If neither finding is present, serum metal ion levels should be closely monitored every 6 months. The track record of the implant should be taken into consideration, even in the asymptomatic patient (Lombardi et al. 2012).

The literature reports conflicting data regarding the effect of head size on metal ion production. Some studies found no relationship between femoral head size and serum metal ion levels in metal-on-metal THA (Bernstein et al. 2011), while others reported increased serum metal ion levels with 28-mm femoral heads compared with 36-mm femoral heads (Engh et al. 2014). Registry data from Australia showed an increased failure rate for MoM THA implants with a femoral head size greater than 32 mm (De Steiger et al. 2011). Complicating matters further is the suggestion that corrosion and fretting at head neck interface (Dyrkacz et al. 2013) or a large head/short taper combination (Donaldson et al. 2014) are contributing factors to metal ion levels.

3.4.3.3 Imaging

Beyond serologic measurements and plain radiographic evaluation, magnetic resonance imaging (MRI) has emerged as a powerful diagnostic tool in the evaluation of the fluid and soft-tissue component surrounding the implant, which is an indication for revision THA. The amount of artifact from the implant on a traditional MRI scan is significant. Adjusting the matrix and receiver bandwidth of a clinical MRI scan can reduce 90% of the metal artifact from THA (Toms et al. 2010). These alterations to a traditional MRI scan produce metal artifact reduction sequence (MARS) MRI.

With the use of MARS MRI, prospective evaluation of 31 patients with painful MoM implants found that fluid collections and severe muscle atrophy were the most likely findings, in addition to muscle edema. MARS MRI is useful in diagnosing and monitoring at-risk metal-on-metal THA implants (Sabah et al. 2011). A case–control study showed that although fluid collections, or pseudotumors, could readily be found in patients with MoM implants, no difference was noted in those with a well-functioning implant versus those with a painful implant. This result called into question the importance of the finding on MARS MRI (Hart et al. 2012). Similar results have been reported in the radiology literature, where conventional sequences with 1.5-Tesla clinical imaging showed no correlation between pseudotumor presence and patient pain (Chang et al. 2012).

A Japanese study on the benefit of ultrasound as a cost-effective means of detecting soft-tissue changes surrounding MoM implants showed promise (Nishii et al. 2012). Hence, a complex cyst or mass (large, heterogeneous, and irregularly shaped) on metal artifact reduction sequence MRI or ultrasound necessitates revision. This finding indicates that implant failure is occurring in the symptomatic patient and that implant failure is impending in the asymptomatic patient. Observation should be considered only in asymptomatic patients with serum cobalt and chromium ion levels less than 5 ppb, with or without a simple cyst on MARS MRI or ultrasound. Yearly observation is suggested because cyst progression has not been observed earlier than 6 months with MARS MRI or ultrasound studies (Lombardi et al. 2012).

3.5 Conclusions

Advances in polyethylene and ceramic technology coupled with the negative attention received by metal-on-metal implants have made it increasingly difficult for surgeons to choose these bearing surfaces in the setting of THA. The medical–legal environment in the United States is such that surgeons using these implants in the face of recalls and less favorable outcomes would place themselves at much increased risk of litigation. Metal-on-metal hip resurfacing, on the other hand, still has a role in the appropriately screened patient. The advantages of resurfacing over THA in young, active males suffering from debilitating degenerative joint disease, mean that the benefits may outweigh the risks in that patient population. Although the role of metal-on-metal bearings is very limited in 2016, the revision burden is anticipated to increase and it is paramount that surgeons in training learn and understand this technology in order to properly diagnose and manage patients suffering from complications of these devices.

References

Allen MJ, Myer BJ, Millett PJ (1997) The effects of particulate cobalt, chromium and cobalt-chromium alloy on human osteoblast-like cells in vitro. J Bone Jt Surg (Br) 79:475–482

Amstutz HC (1996) Editorial comment. Clin Orthop Relat Res. Metal on Metal Hip Protheses: Past Performance and Future Directions 329: S2–S3

Anissian HL, Stark A, Gustafson A, Good V, Clarke IC (1999) Metal-on-metal bearing in hip prosthesis generates 100-fold less wear debris than metal-on-polyethylene. Acta Orthop Scand 70:78e582

Anissian HL, Stark A, Grandberg B, Good V, Bucht E (2002) Cobalt ions influence proliferation and function of human osteoblast-like cells. Acta Orthop Scand 73:369–374

Australian Orthopaedic Association Nation Joint Replacement Registry (2010) Annual report. Australian Orthopaedic Association, Adelaide, SA, Australia

Bernstein M, Walsh A, Petit A, Zukor DJ, Huk OL, Antoniou J (2011) Femoral head size does not affect ion values in metal-on-metal total hips. Clin Orthop Relat Res 469(6):1642–1650

Berry DJ, Von Knoch M, Schleck CD, Harmsen WS (2005) Effect of femoral head diameter and operative approach on risk of dislocation after primary total hip arthroplasty. J Bone Jt Surg Am 87: 2456e2463

Bizot P, Nizard R, Hamadouche M, Hannaouche D, Sedel L (2001) Prevention of wear and osteolysis: alumina-on-alumina bearing. Clin Orthop Relat Res 393:85–93

Black J (1988) Does corrosion matter? J Bone Jt Surg (Br) 70(4):517–520

Bolognesi MP, Ledford CK (2015) Metal-on-metal total hip arthroplasty: patient evaluation and treatment. J Am Acad Orthop Surg 23:724–731

Bonassi S, Hagmar L, Strömberg U, Montagud AH, Tinnerberg H, Forni A, Heikkila P, Wanders S, Wilhardt P, Hansteen IL, Knudsen LE, Norppa H (2000) Chromosomal aberrations in lymphocytes predict human cancer independently of exposure to carcinogens. Eur Study Group Cytogenet Biomark Health Cancer Res 60:1619–1625

Bosker BH, Ettema HB, van Rossum M, Boomsma MF, Kollen BJ, Maas M, Verheyen CC (2015) Pseudotumor formation and serum ions after large head metal-on-metal stemmed total hip replacement: risk factors, time course and revisions in 706 hips. Arch Orthop Trauma Surg 135:417–425

Bozic KJ, Kurtz S, Lau E, Ong K, Chiu V, Vail TP, Rubash HE, Berry DJ (2009) The epidemiology of bearing surface usage in total hip arthroplasty in the United States. J Bone Jt Surg Am 91(7):1614–1620

Brewster DH, Stockton DL, Reekie A, Ashcroft GP, Howie CR, Porter DE, Black RJ (2013) Risk of cancer following primary total hip replacement or primary resurfacing arthroplasty of the hip: a retrospective cohort study in Scotland. Br J Cancer 108(9):1883–1890

Case CP, Langkamer VG, Howell RT, Webb J, Standen G, Palmer M, Kemp A, Learmonth ID (1996) Preliminary observations on possible premalignant changes in bone marrow adjacent to worn total hip arthroplasty implants. Clin Orthop (Suppl) 329:269–279

Chang EY, McAnally JL, Van Horne JR, Statum S, Wolfson T, Gamst A, Chung CB (2012) Metal-on-metal total hip arthroplasty: do symptoms correlate with MR imaging findings? Radiology 265(3):848–857

Charnley J (1961) Arthroplasty of the hip: a new operation. Lancet 1:1129–1132

Choi HJ, Lim SJ, Park YS, Lee SY (2015) Simple and robust ICP-MS method for simultaneous determination of serum Co and Cr in routine clinical practice. Clin Chim Acta 439:91–96

Daley B, Doherty AT, Fairman B, Case CP (2004) Wear debris from hip or knee replacements causes chromosomal damage in human cells in tissue culture. J Bone Jt Surg (Br) 86:598–606

Davies AF, Willert HG, Campbell PA, Learmonth ID, Case CP (2005) An unusual lymphocytic perivascular infiltration in tissues around contemporary metal-on-metal joint replacements. J Bone Jt Surg (Am) 87:18–27

De Haan R, Pattyn C, Gill HS (2008) Correlation between inclination of the acetabular component and metal ion levels in metal-on-metal hip resurfacing replacement. J Bone Jt Surg Br 90 (10):1291–1297

De Smet K, De Haan R, Calistri A, Campbell PA, Ebramzadeh E, Pattyn C, Gill HS (2008) Metal ion measurement as a diagnostic tool to identify problems with metal-on-metal hip resurfacing. J Bone Jt Surg (Am) 90:202–208

De Steiger RN, Hang JR, Miller LN, Graves SE, Davidson DC (2011) Five-year results of the ASR XL acetabular system and the ASR hip resurfacing system: an analysis from the Australian Orthopaedic Association National Joint Replacement Registry. J Bone Jt Surg (Am) 93(24):2287–2293

Delaunay C, Petit I, Learmonth ID, Oger P, Vendittoli PA (2010) Metal-on-metal bearings total hip arthroplasty: the cobalt and chromium ions release concern. Orthop Traumatol Surg Res 96 (8):894–904

Donaldson FE, Coburn JC, Siegel KL (2014) Total hip arthroplasty head-neck contact mechanics: a stochastic investigation of key parameters. J Biomech 47(7):1634–1641

Duggan PJ (2013) Current literature and imaging techniques of aseptic lymphocyte-dominated vasculitis-associated lesions (ALVAL). Clin Radiol 68(11):1089–1096

Dyrkacz RM, Brandt JM, Ojo OA, Turgeon TR, Wyss UP (2013) The influence of head size on corrosion and fretting behaviour at the head-neck interface of artificial hip joints. J Arthroplasty 28(6):1036–1040

Engh CA, MacDonald SJ, Sritulanondha S, Korczak A, Naudie D, Engh C (2014) Metal ion levels after metal-on-metal total hip arthroplasty: a five-year, prospective randomized trial. J Bone Jt Surg Am 96(6):448–455

Grammatopolous G, Pandit H, Kwon YM, Gundle R, McLardy-Smith P, Beard DJ, Murray DW, Gill HS (2009) Hip resurfacings revised for inflammatory pseudotumor have a poor outcome. J Bone Jt Surg Br 91:1019–1024

Hart AJ, Sabah SA, Bandi AS, Maggiore P, Tarassoli P, Sampson BA, Skinner J (2011) Sensitivity and specificity of blood cobalt and chromium metal ions for predicting failure of metal-on-metal hip replacement. J Bone Jt Surg Br 93(10):1308–1313

Hart AJ, Satchithananda K, Liddle AD, Sabah SA, McRobbie D, Henckel J, Cobb JP, Skinner JA, Mitchell AW (2012) Pseudotumors in association with well-functioning metal-on-metal hip prostheses: a case-control study using three-dimensional computed tomography and magnetic resonance imaging. J Bone Jt Surg Am 94(4):317–325

IARC (2006). Metallic cobalt particles. (With or without tungsten carbide). Cobalt metal with tungsten carbide (Group 2A). Cobalt metal without tungsten carbide (group 2B). Cobalt sulfate and other soluble cobalt (II) salts (group 2B). IARC Monographs 2006; 86:37 http://monographs.iarc.fr/ENG/Monographs/vol86/volume86.pdf

Ikeda T, Takahashi K, Kabata T, Sakagoshi D, Tomita K, Yamada M (2010) Polyneuropathy caused by cobalt chromium metallosis after THA. Muscle Nerve 42:140–143

Langton DJ, Jameson SS, Joyce TJ, Hallab NJ, Natu S, Nargol AV (2010) Early failure of metal-on-metal bearings in hip resurfacing and large-diameter total hip replacement: a consequence of excess wear. J Bone Jt Surg Br 92: 38e46

Learmonth ID, Young C, Rorabeck C (2007) The operation of the century: total hip replacement. Lancet 370:1508–1519

Lewinnek GE, Lewis JL, Tarr R, Compere CL, Zimmerman JR (1978) Dislocations after total hip-replacement arthroplasties. J Bone and Jt Surg Am. 60:217–220

Lombardi AV Jr, Barrack RL, Berend KR, Cuckler JM, Jacobs JJ, Mont MA, Schmalzried TP (2012) The hip society: algorithmic approach to diagnosis and management of metal-on-metal arthroplasty. J Bone Jt Surg Br 94(11 suppl A) 14–18

MacDonald SJ, McCalden RW, Chess DG, Bourne RB, Rorabeck CH, Cleland D, Leung F (2003) Metal-on-metal versus polyethylene in hip arthroplasty: a randomized clinical trial. Clin Orthop Rel Res 406:282–296

Makela KT, Visuri T, Pulkkinen P, Eskelinen A, Remes V, Virolainen P, Junnila M, Pukkala E (2012) Risk of cancer with metal-on-metal hip replacements: population based study. Br Med J 345:e4646. https://doi.org/10.1136/bmj.e4646

Makela KT, Visuri T, Pulkkinen P, Eskelinen A, Remes V, Virolainen P, Junnila M, Pukkala E (2014) Cancer incidence and cause-specific mortality in patients with MoM hip replacements in Finland. Acta Orthop 85(1):32–38

Mann SM, Kunz M, Ellis RE, Rudan JF (2016) Component position and metal ion levels in computer-navigated hip resurfacing arthroplasty. J Arthroplasty 32(1):110–124

Marker M, Grubl A, Riedl O, Heinze G, Pohanka E, Kotz R (2008) MoM hip implants: do they impair renal function in the long term? Arch Orthop Trauma Surg 128:915–919

McDermott PH, Delaney RL, Egan JD, Sullivan JF (1966) Myocardosis and cardiac failure in men. JAMA 198:163–166

Mayo Clinic (2012) Evaluation of metal-on-metal wear of orthopaedic implants – the role of serum chromium and cobalt analysis. Mayo Med Lab: Communique 37:1–8

McKee GK, Watson-Farrar J (1966) Replacement of arthritic hips by the McKee-Farrar prosthesis. J Bone Jt Surg Br 48:245–259

Medicine and Healthcare Products Regulatory Agency (2010) Medical device alert: all metal-on-metal (MoM) hip replacements. Tech. Rep. MDA/2012/008

Medicines and Healthcare Products Regulatory Agency (2012) Medical device alert (MDA/2012/036): all metal-on-metal (MoM) hip replacements; 2012

Morin Y (1967) Quebec beer drinkers cardiomyopathy: etiologic associations. Can Med Assoc J 97:926–928

Mosier BA, Maynard L, Sotereanos NG, Sewecke JJ (2016) Progressive cardiomyopathy in a patient with elevated cobalt ion levels and bilateral metal-on-metal hip arthroplasties. Am J Orthop 45(3):E132–E135

Nangaku M (2009) Novel therapeutic approach targeting the HIF-HRE system in the kidney. Adv Exp Med Biol 645:81–86

National Joint Registry for England and Wales (2010) Seventh annual report. National Joint Registry Centre, Hemel Hempstead, Hertfordshire, UK

Newton AW, Ranganath L, Armstrong C, Peter V, Roberts NB (2012) Differential distribution of cobalt, chromium and nickel between whole blood, plasma and urine in patients after metal-on-metal (MoM) hip arthroplasty. J Orthop Res 30(10):1640–1646

Nishii T, Sakai T, Takao M, Yoshikawa H, Sugano N (2012) Ultrasound screening of peri-articular soft tissue abnormality around metal-on-metal bearings. J Arthroplasty 27(6):895–900

Oldenburg M, Wegner R, Baur X (2009) Severe cobalt intoxication due to prosthesis wear in repeated total hip arthroplasty. J Arthroplasty 24(5): 825.e15–e20

Pandit H, Glyn-Jones S, McLardy-Smith P, Gundle R, Whitwell D, Gibbons CL, Ostlere S, Athanasou N, Gill HS, Murray DW (2008) Pseudotumours associated with metal-on-metal hip resurfacings. J Bone Jt Surg Br 90:e847–e851

Raghunathan VK, Devey M, Hawkins S, Hails L, Davis SA, Mann S, Chang IT, Ingham E, Malhas A, Vaux DJ, Lane JD Case CP (2013) Influence of particle size and ROS on cobalt chrome nanoparticle-mediated genotoxicity. Biomaterials 3559–3570

Ring G, O'Mullane J, O'Riordan A, Furey A (2016) Trace metal determination as it relates to metallosis of orthopaedic implants: Evolution and current status. Clin Biochem 49(7–8):617–635

Rodushkin I, Ödman F, Branth S (1999) Multielement analysis of whole blood by high resolution inductively coupled plasma mass spectrometry. Fresen J Anal Chem 364(4):338–346

Sabah SA, Mitchell AW, Henckel J, Sandison A, Skinner JA, Hart AJ (2011) Magnetic resonance imaging findings in painful metal-on-metal hips: a prospective study. J Arthroplasty 26(1):71–76

Sarhadi VK, Parkkinen J, Reito A, Nieminen J, Porkka N, Wirtanen T, Laitinen M, Eskelinen A, Knuutila S (2015) Genetic alterations in periprosthetic soft tissue masses from patients with MoM THA. Mutat Res 781: 1–6

Savarino L, Cadossi M, Chiarello E, Fotia C, Greco M, Baldini N, Giannini S (2014) How do metal ion levels change over time in hip resurfacing patients? a cohort study. Sci World J 29:19–25

Seghizzi P, D'Adda F, Borleri D, Barbic F, Mosconi G (1994) Cobalt myocardiopathy: a critical review of the literature. Sci Total Environ 150:105–109

Seiler HG, Sigel H, Siegel A (eds) (1988) Handbook on the toxicity of inorganic compounds, 259. Marcel Dekker, New York (NY)

Seppanen M, Makela K, Virolainen P, Remes CV, Pulkkinen P, Eskelinen A (2012) Hip resurfacing arthroplasty: short-term survivorship of 4,401 hips from the Finnish Arthroplasty Register. Acta Orthop 83:207

Shrivastava K, Ram MS, Bansal A, Singh SS, Ilavazhagan G (2008) Co-supplementation promotes hypoxic tolerance and facilitates acclimatization to hypobaric hypoxia in rat brain. High Altitude Med Biol 9:63–75

Sidaginamale RP, Joyce TJ, Lord JK, Jefferson R, Blain PG, Nargol AVF, Langton DJ (2013) Blood metal ion testing is an effective screening tool to identify poorly performing metal-on-metal bearing surfaces. Bone Jt Res 2(5):84–95

Smith AJ, Dieppe P, Howard PW, Bolm AW (2012a) Failure rates of metal-on-metal hip resurfacings: analysis of data from the National Joint Registry for England and Wales. Lancet 380(9855):1759–1766

Smith AJ, Dieppe P, Porter M, Blom AW (2012b) Risk of cancer in first seven years after metal-on-metal hip replacement compared with other bearings and general population: linkage study between the National Joint Registry of England and Wales and hospital episode statistics. BMJ 344:2383

Smith-Petersen MN (1948) The classic: evolution of mold arthroplasty of the hip joint. J Bone Joint Surg 30B:L:59

Steens W, Von Foerster G, Katzer A (2006) Severe cobalt poisoning with loss of sight after ceramic-metal pairing in a hip—case report. Acta Orthop 77(5):830–832

Toms AP, Smith-Bateman C, Malcolm PN, Cahir J, Graves M (2010) Optimization of metal artifact reduction (MAR) sequences for MRI of total hip prostheses. Clin Radiol 65(6):447–452

Treacy R, McBryde C, Shears E, Pynsent P (2011) Birmingham hip resurfacing: a minimum follow-up of ten years. J Bone Jt Surg Br. 93(1):27–33

Udofia IJ, Jin ZM (2003) Elastohydrodynamic lubrication analysis of metal-on-metal hip-resurfacing prostheses. J Biomech 36:537–544

Vendittoli PA, Mottard S, Roy AG, Dupont C, Lavigne M (2007) Chromium and cobalt ion release following the Durom high carbon content, forged metal-on-metal surface replacement of the hip. J Bone Jt Surg Br 89(4):441–448

Visuri T, Pukkala E, Paavolainen P, Pulkkinen P, Riska EB (1996) Cancer risk after metal on metal and polyethylene on metal total hip arthroplasty. Clin Orthop (Suppl) 329:S280–S289

Visuri T, Pulkkinen P, Paavolainen P, Pukkala E (2010) Cancer risk is not increased after conventional hip arthroplasty: a natiowide study from the Finnish Arthroplasty Register with follow-up of 24,636 patients for a mean of 13 years. Acta Orthop 81:77–81

Watanabe Y, Shiba N, Matsuo S, Higuchi F, Tagawa Y, Inoue A (2000) Biomechanical study of the resurfacing hip arthroplasty: finite element analysis of the femoral component. J Arthroplasty 15:505–511

Watters TS, Cardona DM, Menon KS, Vinson EN, Bolognesi MP, Dodd LG (2010) Aseptic lymphocyte-dominated vasculitis-associated lesion: a clinicopathologic review of an under recognized cause of prosthetic failure. Am J Clin Pathol 134:886–893

Wiles P (1957) The surgery of the osteo-arthritis hip. Br J Surg 45:488–497

Wyles CC, Larson DR, Houdek MT, Sierra RJ, Trousdale RT (2013) Utility of synovial fluid aspirations in failed metal-on-metal total hip arthroplasty. J Arthroplasty 28(5):818–823

Yanny S, Cahir JG, Barker T, Wimhurst J, Nolan JF, Goodwin RW, Marshall T, Toms AP (2012) MRI of aseptic lymphocyte vasculitis-associated lesions in metal-on-metal hip replacements. Am J Roentgenol 198:1394–1402

Zywiel MG, Brandt JM, Overgaard AC, Turgeon TR, Syed KA (2013) Fatal cardiomyopathy after revision total hip replacement for fracture of a ceramic liner. Bone Jt J 95(B): 31–37

Chapter 4
Copper in Medicine: Perspectives and Toxicity

Avinash P. Ingle, Priti Paralikar, Sudhir Shende, Indarchand Gupta, Jayanta Kumar Biswas, Luiza Helena da Silva Martins and Mahendra Rai

Abstract Copper is one of the most important microelements required by all kind of life forms including human beings for their proper growth, development, and survival. Copper plays an important role in various body functions and regulation of different pathways. Hence, it has been used since pre-Vedic time as potential medicine to cure a number of diseases. Although, copper has significant medicinal value, the maintenance of adequate copper levels in the body is of vital importance because the lack or excess amount of such essential trace elements are known to cause a variety of health problems. The failure in the regulation of copper metabolism is mainly responsible for deficiency and accumulation of copper in different parts of the body. Generally, deficiency of copper leads to several copper deficiency syndromes including Menkes' disease. Similarly, high level of copper due to accumulation results in many diseases like Wilson's diseases, Alzheimer's disease, etc. Considering the key role of copper in human health, the present chapter has been focused on such related aspects, which include uptake and metabolism of copper, and its dietary recommendations. In addition, various disorders caused due to deficiency and excess amount of copper are also discussed in detail.

Keywords Copper · Microelement · Deficiency · Tamra · Medicine
Ayurveda

A. P. Ingle · P. Paralikar · S. Shende · M. Rai (✉)
Nanotechnology Laboratory, Department of Biotechnology,
SGB Amravati University, Amravati, Maharashtra, India
e-mail: pmkrai@hotmail.com

I. Gupta
Department of Biotechnology, Institute of Science, Aurangabad, Maharashtra, India

J. K. Biswas
Pollution, Ecotoxicology and Ecotechnology Research Unit, Department of Ecological Studies, University of Kalyani, Kalyani 741235, West Bengal, India

L. H. da Silva Martins
Center of Natural Sciences and Technology, State University of Pará, UEPA, Belém, Pará, Brazil

M. Rai et al. (eds.), *Biomedical Applications of Metals*,
https://doi.org/10.1007/978-3-319-74814-6_4

4.1 Introduction

Copper (Cu) is an essential microelement required by all living organisms for proper growth, development, and survival (Chellan and Sadler 2015). As far as human health is concerned, copper is involved in numerous body functions necessary for fundamental body processes like respiration, free radical eradication, energy production, formation of connective tissues, metabolism of oxygen and iron, maturation of extracellular matrix and neuropeptide, and neuroendocrine signaling (Fraga 2005; Chellan and Sadler 2015). A healthy, 70 kg body contains about 100 mg of copper. Out of these, about two-thirds of total body copper is located in skeleton and muscles, but the highest concentrations are in the liver, followed by the brain, kidney, and heart (Ward et al. 2003).

Due to progress in medical sciences, copper has gained a great deal of attention. The important role of copper is preliminary catalytic and it acts as cofactor for numerous enzymes like Cu/Zn superoxide dismutase (a cytosolic protein that speeds up the dismutation of superoxide), cytochrome c oxidase (the terminal mitochondrial electron carrier), tyrosinase (located in melanocytes and involved in the conversion of tyrosine into melanin), ceruloplasmin (a plasma glycoprotein, may function as a copper transport and as an antioxidant), lysyl oxidase (responsible for oxidative deamination of peptidyl lysine), etc. Similarly, it also acts as a ligand for various other proteins required for respiration, iron transport and metabolism, cell growth, and hemostasis (Puig and Thiele 2002; Bertini et al. 2010). In addition, copper also plays an important role in many physiological functions of nervous, hematological, cardiovascular, reproduction, and immune systems (Cerone et al. 2000). Sharma et al. (2005) proposed that copper promotes proper development of antibodies and white blood cells, in addition to antioxidant enzyme production.

Overall health benefits of copper are important for healthy life, because copper plays a key role in the normal metabolic process, which is associated with amino acids and vitamins. It is the third most prevalent mineral in the body and is mostly carried by the blood plasma protein, ceruloplasmin. Copper cannot be produced by the body and hence needs to be added from external food sources. The various foods which contain considerable amount of copper mainly includes, meat, seafood, beans, whole grains, soy flour, wheat bran, almonds, avocados, barley, garlic, nuts, oats, blackstrap molasses, beets, and lentils. There are reports suggesting that copper can also enter the human body through drinking water in copper pipes and by using copper cookware. Oysters are the richest source. It was reported that there are chances of loss in copper content due to prolonged storage of food in tin cans and in high acid content (https://www.organicfacts.net/).

As copper is an essential metal for life, the maintenance of its adequate levels according to the standards proposed by various national and international food and health organizations is of vital importance and is highly regulated. Copper is absorbed from diet, mainly in the duodenum, although it was also proposed that some absorption takes place in the stomach and in the distal part of the small intestine. Moreover, a further process of copper metabolism is highly complex and mediated with help of many proteins (Hordyjewska et al. 2014). However, dysfunction of copper metabolism leading to its excess or deficiency results in acute to severe disorders in human beings (Cerpa et al. 2005). Extensive studies performed including most recent ones revealed that deficiency of copper exerts many negative effects on human health which leads to various disorders such as anemia, leucopenia, and myeloneuropathy (Wazir and Ghobrial 2017), Alzheimer's dementia (Xu et al. 2017), etc. However, the excess concentration of copper in the body causes toxicity which results in Wilson's diseases and Menkes disease (Hordyjewska et al. 2014), etc.

The present chapter is aimed to discuss the role of copper in human health. In addition, various other related aspects such as how copper as a pre-Vedic metal used in medicine, dietary recommendations, uptake, transport and metabolism of copper and the diseases due to deficiency and excess of copper are also discussed.

4.2 Copper: A Pre-Vedic Metal Used in Medicine

There are many reports that copper has been used by human civilizations dates back to around 5000 BC. According to an article published in the newspaper "The Telegraph", copper was used to sterilize chest wounds and drinking water in Egypt and it was mentioned in The Smith Papyrus, the Egyptian medical text written around 2600 BC. In addition, Greeks, Romans, and Aztecs also used copper metal or its compounds for the treatment of chronic infections and for hygiene in general.

Similarly, there is a report in ancient Indian Ayurvedic text *Charaka Samhita* (300 BC) that copper kills fatal microbes, including its role in the purification of drinking water (The Telegraph 2012). Since pre-Vedic times, copper is known as *Tamra* and it was a part of day-to-day livelihood functions. Moreover, it is the earlier metal known and used for the preparation of the stronger alloy metals brass and bronze of which it is a component. As described in *Charaka Samhita* various formulations of "*Tamra*" (copper) can be effectively used for the management of a wide range of diseases like Krimi (worms), Sthaulya (stoutness), *Arsha* (hemorrhoids/piles), Ksaya (seizure/fit), Pandu (iron deficiency anemia), Kusta (leprosy), Swasa (asthma), Kasa (cough), Amlapitta (gastritis/acidity), Sotha (oedema), Sula (pain in the sides of the chest), *Yakrit Roga* (liver diseases), etc. In addition, *Charaka* advocates the use of "*Tamra Patra*" (copper vessels) in several pharmaceutical procedures. Moreover, samples with characteristic metallic sheen (*Snigdham*), soft (*Mridulam*), bright reddish in color (*Shonam*), having the high tensile strength (*Ghanaghata Ksamam*), heavy (*Guru*), and devoid of impurities (*Nirvikaram*) are the different forms of copper which are identified as best for medicinal purposes. Also, "*Tamra Bhasma*" is used as an effective medicine in the treatment of many diseases with normal doses in the range of 15–60 mg (Galib et al. 2011).

4.3 Dietary Recommendations for Copper

As mentioned earlier, copper is an essential trace element required in adequate proportions for good human health. In this context, various national and international organizations such as World Health Organization (WHO), U.S. Institute of Medicine (IOM), The European Food Safety Authority (EFSA), etc., concerning with nutrition and human health have proposed certain standards for dietary intake of copper for the maintenance of proper health. The Recommended Dietary Allowance (RDA) and Tolerable upper intake levels (ULs) per day for adults, youths, children, pregnant and lactating women are different. These proposed standards also differ among organizations and countries. According to WHO (1996), the acceptable intake of copper in adults is 1.3 mg/day.

However, as per the standards proposed by IOM, the adequate intakes (AIs) of copper for healthy adult men and women is 0.9 mg/day. Whereas, in case of children aged between 1 and 3 years, 4 and 8 years, 9 and 13 years, and 14 and 18 years are proposed to be 0.34, 0.44, 0.7, and 0.89 mg/day respectively. In addition, for safety, IOM also sets ULs for vitamins and minerals, in case of adults ULs for copper is set at 10 mg/day. However, in case of children between 1 and 3 years, 4 and 8 years, 9 and 13 years, and 14 and 18 years it set to be 1, 3, 5, and 8 mg/day respectively. Moreover, for pregnant and lactating women the proposed AIs are 1.0 and 1.3 mg/day respectively (DRI 2001).

It was observed that full-term and premature infants are more sensitive to copper deficiency than adults. Generally, the last 3 months of pregnancy is the period when fetus accumulates copper, but infants that are born prematurely did not get sufficient time to store adequate reserves of copper in their livers and hence, require more copper at birth than full-term infants. Therefore, as per IOM and WHO standards 0.2 mg/day is the safe and adequate intake for full-term infants, whereas for premature babies it is about 1 mg/day. (https://web.archive.org/web/20101015204256/, http://www.copperinfo.com/health/goodhealth.html).

Similarly, EFSA also defined AIs for copper based on mean observed intakes in several European Union (EU) countries. According to EFSA, the proposed AIs of copper for men is 1.6 mg/day and that for women is 1.3 mg/day. However, in case of children, AIs are 0.7 mg/day for children aged 1–3 years, 1 mg/day for 3–10 years, 1.3 and 1.1 mg/day for boys and girls aged 10–18 years, respectively. For infants aged between 7 and 11 months proposed AIs are 0.4 mg/day, whereas, for pregnant and lactating women it is 1.5 mg/day (EFSA 2006, 2015).

4.4 Copper Uptake, Distribution, and Metabolism

4.4.1 Uptake and Distribution of Copper

In humans, dietary copper is absorbed across the mucosal membrane of stomach to small intestine through a mucous layer which covers intestinal wall (Linder 1991).

Various nutritional and biochemical studies have focused on the mechanism of copper absorption and metabolism. Several genetic and biochemical studies also identified the different proteins that play vital role in copper uptake, export, and distribution (Gupta and Lutsenko 2009). Mostly, the *Saccharomyces cerevisiae* (yeast)-mediated copper transport has been extensively studied. Eide (1998) demonstrated yeast-mediated copper transport with high affinity for uptake of copper. The main route of entry of copper into the cell from the blood is through copper transporters (CTR) (Maryon et al. 2007; Kim et al. 2008). These include CTR1 (high-affinity transporter), CTR2 (low-affinity transporter), copper efflux transporter namely, ATP7A and ATP7B, and copper chaperones (Gupta and Lutsenko 2009). However, the uptake and distribution of copper in persons suffering from Menkes and Wilson's disease is different, it mainly occurs in the presence of ATP7A and ATP7B (Mercer 2001; Lutsenko et al. 2007). The overall distribution of copper in Menkes and Wilson's disease patient is schematically represented in Fig. 4.1.

Zhou and Gitschier (1997) reported that inactivation of CTR1 results in low entry of copper into cell and iron deficiency, because of the limited supply of copper to copper-dependent ferroxidase pathways. Uptake of copper is managed by human CTR (hCTR1) into enterocyte. The process of uptake of copper is mediated by the action of reductase enzyme, which helps to reduce Cu (II) to Cu (I) ions, an acceptable state for the hCTR1 receptor for copper. After absorption into the gut, copper is secreted into blood circulation and bound to albumin, copper histidine complexes (low molecular weight), and transcuprein. Upon reaching the liver, hepatocytes rapidly take up the copper via copper receptor hCTR1 (de Romana et al. 2011; Hordyjewska et al. 2014).

In human, intestinal fluid and blood plasma have a specific and high affinity for copper binding. Albumin is the most abundant plasma protein, around 10–12% of total plasma copper bounds to albumin (Wirth et al. 1985; Barrow et al. 1988;

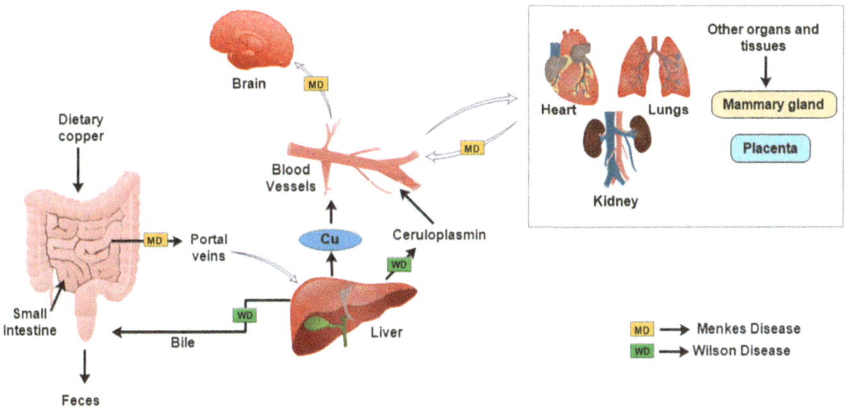

Fig. 4.1 Schematic representation of overall distribution of copper in the body

Tapiero et al. 2003). Copper binds to albumin with the help of three amino acids at N-terminal. This does not eliminate binding but lowers the affinity of copper (Masuoka and Saltman 1994). The solubility and availability of copper are enhanced by milieu acid, nitrate and sulfate anions, histidine, methionine, lactose, and starch, presumably after its hydrolysis to glucose (Aggett 1999; Stern et al. 2007). The copper uptake from foodstuffs is weakened by Maillard reaction products which interact with amino acids, magnesium, and calcium to precipitate copper in the gut lumen. Likewise, vitamin C oxidizes cuprous copper to cupric, which impairs copper uptake in animals. This mechanism does not occur in humans (O'Brien and Morrissey 1997).

4.4.2 Metabolism of Copper

Copper plays a crucial role in metabolism in humans, because it allows many enzymes to function properly (Harris 2001). Copper is important for maintaining epithelial and connective tissues throughout the body, strength of skin and blood vessels. It also plays an important role in the production of melanin, myelin, and hemoglobin, and maintains the functions of thyroid gland normally (Groff et al. 1995; Osredkar and Sustar 2011). Copper is absorbed in the gut and transported to the liver where it binds to albumin. Copper enters into bloodstream via ceruloplasmin (plasma protein), where metabolism of copper is controlled and is excreted in bile (Adelstein and Vallee 1961). A transporter protein namely copper membrane transporter 1 (CMT1) on the cells of small bowel carries copper inside the cell, where some part of copper is carried by copper transporter proteins (ATOX1) to Golgi network and some part of copper binds to metallothioneins. Upon increasing concentration of copper, ATP7A enzymes release copper into the liver. Further, ATP7B enzyme in liver cells gets linked to ceruloplasmin with copper and releases it into bloodstream. The excess of copper is removed by secreting into bile (Harris et al. 1998; Osredkar and Sustar 2011). The proper metabolism of copper requires appropriate balance with zinc and manganese. Zinc can compete with copper in the small intestine and interfere with its absorption.

4.5 Role of Copper in Human Health

It has been observed that copper in adequate concentration acts as traditional medicine for many human diseases, however, the deficiency and excess concentration of copper showed negative effects and cause health problems in human beings. Various diseases and disorders caused due to deficiency and excess concentration of copper are illustrated in Fig. 4.2.

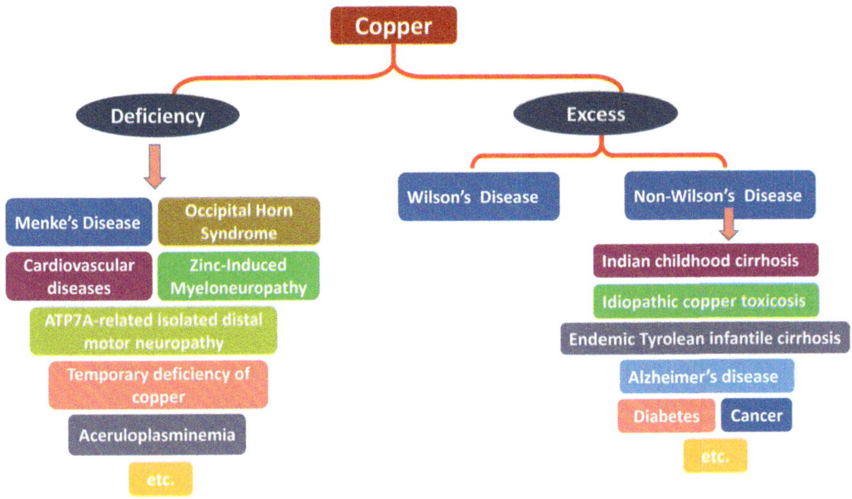

Fig. 4.2 Illustration of various diseases caused due to deficiency and excess concentration of copper

4.5.1 Diseases Related to Copper Deficiency

Several deficiency syndromes occur due to the lack of copper in the animal metabolism. However, in humans, the necessity of copper was noticeably demonstrated by various studies showing anemia, neutropenia, and bone marrow abnormalities particularly in young children with copper deficiencies (Cordano et al. 1964). The children were responsive to copper therapy. In addition, several studies have demonstrated the requirement of copper in immune function, bone formation, red- and white blood cell maturation, lipid metabolism, myocardial contraction, iron transport, and neurological developments (Danks 1988). Klevay (1998) reported that the consumption of diets providing less than 1 mg of copper per day can be associated with adverse health effects. Copper deficiency occurs in a variety of circumstances such as alcoholism, diabetes, hypertension, and total parental nutrition feedings (Tokuda et al. 1986; Danks 1988; Shaw 1992; Olivares and Uauy 1996; Uauy et al. 1998).

There is a substantial dispute, however, on the level to which copper deficiency influences human prenatal development. Buamah et al. (1984) reported that in pregnant women, the finding of low serum copper concentrations during mid-gestation was a risk factor for anencephaly. Morton et al. (1976) reported a noteworthy correlation between low copper content in drinking water and the incidence of neural tube defects in South Wales. Besides this, there are several other copper deficiency syndromes (CDS) such as Menkes' Disease (MS), ATP7A-Related Isolated Distal Motor Neuropathy, Occipital Horn Syndrome, Zinc-Induced Myeloneuropathy, and Aceruloplasminemia, are mentioned associated with a large phenotypic variation in characters and the mutations in the gene encoding for the transporters are implicated in distinct phenotypes (Shibata et al. 1995; Kaler 2014; Manto 2014).

4.5.1.1 Menke's Disease (MD)

MD is characterized by hypothermia neuronal degeneration, mental retardation, abnormal lightly pigmented hair (scalp hair called kinky or steel wool), seizures, aortic aneurysms, and bone fragility (Uriu-Adams and Keen 2005). It is generally caused due to the mutation in the ATP7A gene (ATP7A on the TGN membrane of the placenta, gut, and brain). It is most important in X-linked inherited diseases (Shim and Harris 2003). The gene ATP7A encodes for an enzyme, copper-transporting ATPase which functions as an intracellular pump to transport copper into the trans-Golgi network for integration into copper-requiring enzymes together with dopamine b-hydroxylase and also mediates copper exodus from cells (Hordyjewska et al. 2014). MD is generally found in male individuals (Tümer 2013; Manto 2014). Most ATP7A mutations are partial gene deletions or intragenic mutations (Tümer 2013). The female carriers are mosaics of wild-type and mutant cells because of the random inactivation of X chromosome (Møller et al. 2012). Affected females showed the clinical symptoms, which are milder when compared to males with the same mutations.

MD presents in newborns of 6 weeks to 1 year. Patients have a state of copper deficiency, because the copper accumulates in the intestine which then cannot be absorbed in the blood. A similar process occurs at the level of the blood–brain barrier, which leads to cause a lack of ions within the central nervous system. The typical biochemical examination of urine samples showed the lower serum copper and ceruloplasmin, abnormal plasma, and cerebrospinal fluid (CSF) neurochemicals, and increased concentrations of β-2-microglobulin (Kaler 2014). The superoxide dismutase1 (SOD1) reduces immune-reactivity, unlike the expression of superoxide dismutase 2 (SOD2) (Shibata et al. 1995). The therapy for MD is based on the replacement of copper and the parenteral administration is exercised (Brewer 2003a, b). Gene therapy with adeno-associated viral (AAV) vectors is also hopeful (Haddad et al. 2014).

4.5.1.2 ATP7A-Related Distal Motor Neuropathy

The ATP7A-related distal motor neuropathy is a rare disorder caused due to deficiency of copper, it commonly affects the peripheral motor nerves. The phenotypic appearance of this disease is similar to Charcot–Marie–Tooth disease type 2 (Kaler 2011). The mechanisms of the peripheral neuropathy remain to be explicated. Two unique ATP7A missense mutations (T994I and P1386S) cause subtle defects in ATP7A intracellular trafficking, which results in a preferential accumulation at the plasma membrane (Yi and Kaler 2014). An abnormal interaction between ATP7A and adaptor protein complexes is presumed to be the molecular mechanism (Yi and Kaler 2014).

4.5.1.3 Occipital Horn Syndrome (OHS)

OHS is allelic to MD and is considered as a milder modification. It was found that the associated symptoms were initiated in the first decade. The association of coarse hair and joint hyperlaxity is very reminiscent as well as hammer-shaped clavicular heads and occipital bone exostoses are typical. In some patients a dysautonomia which is related to the reduced activity of the dopamine-β-hydroxylase, whereas the connective tissue abnormalities are attributed to the deficit of lysyl oxidase. Ceruloplasmin and serum copper levels are normal or decreased.

4.5.1.4 Zinc-Induced Myeloneuropathy

Zinc-induced myeloneuropathy is also caused due to copper deficiency (Schleper and Stuerenburg 2001). The syndrome in human is similar to the copper deficiency myelopathy occurring in ruminants (Bennetts and Chapman 1937). This disorder mainly occurs after continued exposure to zinc (Lanska and Remler 2014). Regular use of dental fixatives containing zinc has been identified as an activating factor (Gabreyes et al. 2013). Patients who had undergone gastrojejunal bypass surgeries are also at high risk (Choi and Strum 2010). The first disturbances are sensory symptoms in the feet which then, after a few years, mimics the subacute combined degeneration of the spinal cord. Chronic zinc ingestion may also cause bone marrow suppression with anemia, neutropenia, and thrombocytopenia. By contrast to Wilson's disease (WD), urinary copper levels are typically decreased (Jaiser and Winston 2010). Although copper substitution may perhaps regress cytopenias, neurological discrepancies are permanent in 40% of cases, highlighting the significance of detecting the hypocupremic state immediately as possible.

4.5.1.5 Aceruloplasminemia

Aceruloplasminemia is an autosomal recessive disease caused by mutations in the Cp allele on chromosome 3q, and results in a total absence of ceruloplasmin in blood. As a result, this causes the accumulation of iron in the central nervous system, especially in basal ganglia, in retina, liver, and pancreas (Brewer 2003a, b). Clinically, patients exhibit retinal degeneration, diabetes mellitus and also a progressive neurological syndrome combining cerebellar ataxia, extrapyramidal signs, and dementia, usually between the age of 25 and 60 years (Miyajima 2003; Pan et al. 2011, Kono 2012). The absence of ceruloplasmin does not generate marked changes in copper metabolism but only changes iron metabolism. It produces a gradual accumulation of iron in the liver, pancreas, retina, and central nervous system. The biochemical study showed enhanced lipid peroxidation caused by iron-mediated cellular radical injury in ceruloplasmin knockout mice (Kono 2012). However, the blood examination of a patient suffering from aceruloplasminemia shows low concentrations of copper and iron in serum which is referred to as microcytic anemia. Moreover, brain MRI shows low intensities due to iron accumulation, mainly in striatum, thalamus, and cerebellum. MRI of the liver can also be suggested to these patients. As far as the treatment is concerned, iron chelators, such as desferrioxamine, are routinely recommended (Pan et al. 2011). Fresh frozen human plasma (FFP) decreases iron contents in the liver and may improve neurologic deficits. Antioxidants, such as vitamin E and the oral administration of zinc may be helpful to prevent the tissue damage (Miyajima 2003).

4.5.1.6 Cardiovascular Diseases

The experimental copper deficiency has considerably demonstrated the increase in susceptibility of cardiovascular tissues and lipoproteins to lipid peroxidation, thus increasing the risk of cardiovascular disease (Percival 1998). Particularly, the heart and its vessels are susceptible to copper deficiency, which may alter the cardiac morphology including enlarged myocytes, fragmented basal laminae at capillary–myocyte interfaces, derangement of myofibrils and mitochondrial proliferation, fragmentation and swelling (Uriu-Adams and Keen 2005). In addition, impaired contractile and mitochondrial respiratory functions and electrocardiographic abnormalities are observed in hearts with copper deficiency. Hypertrophic cardiomyopathy is prominent in humans having mutations in cytochrome c oxidase of copper chaperone. Copper deficiency also leads to anemia, because the cytochrome c oxidase is essential for blood formation. Experiments on copper depletion also demonstrate abnormalities in aortic stenosis and blood pressure (Rowland and Schneider 2001; Uriu-Adams and Keen 2005). Many of the adverse histopathological and hemodynamic effects on the heart can be reversed through repletion of copper by dietary copper supplementation, possibly through the normalization of the expression of genes, which are involved in calcium cycling, contractility, extracellular matrix metabolism, and inflammation (Uriu-Adams and Keen 2005). The data showing a correlation between copper deficiency and atherosclerosis is also available, which demonstrated that an increased concentration of total cholesterol and LDL with reduction of HDL was observed in the subjects who were fed with an experimental diet with low copper (Rowland and Schneider 2001; Brewer 2003a, b).

4.5.1.7 Temporary Deficiency of Copper

Copper deficiency has been described typically in newborns with total parenteral nutrition lacking adequate mineral supplementation or in people with a constant nephritic syndrome that enhances copper losses. The low-copper condition has been allied with bone malformation during development, impaired melanin synthesis, increased osteoporosis, and poor immune response; consequently, increasing frequency of infections, alterations with cholesterol metabolism, cardiovascular disease, and disturbance of metabolism of other trace elements, for instance, iron mobilization occurs. Some investigators have recommended that chronic consumption of drinking water with elevated copper concentration may possibly be risky for susceptible populations, including infants, young children, and individuals, who are heterozygotic for Wilson's disease (Uriu-Adams and Keen 2005; Ugarte et al. 2013).

4.5.2 Diseases Resulted Due to Excess Amount of Copper

As the deficiency of copper leads to various disorders, its excess amount in the human body also found to be harmful to human beings. The mechanism of copper homeostasis is properly regulated, however, failure of those regulation results in several abnormalities, causing or supporting the development of the disease. The diseases caused due to excess amount can be categorized into Wilson's diseases, non-Wilson's disease (copper toxicosis) and other life-threatening diseases like Alzheimer's disease, diabetes, and cancer, which are described hereafter.

4.5.2.1 Wilson's Disease (WD)

WD is an autosomal recessive genetic disorder caused by disabling mutations in both copies of the ATP7B gene, which is differentially expressed in tissues (ATP7B is expressed in the TGN membrane of hepatocyte) (Shim and Harris 2003). The gene ATP7B is responsible for copper's transfer into the secretory pathway for the binding into Cp and excretion into the bile (Brewer et al. 2000). Brewer et al. (2000) have studied the 26 pregnancy cases of 19 women with Wilson's disease, which was further treated with zinc as their sole anti-copper drug. Among the 26 infants, 24 were normal, one had a surgically correctable heart defect, and another had anencephaly. Clinical manifestations are neurological damage and liver disease, i.e., patients demonstrate, especially, death of the nervous system (with both the neurological and also psychiatric signs) and the liver. The cornea of the eye is affected, resulting in the hallmark brown discoloration, which is very specific for neurological WD, the "Kayser–Fleischer ring" (Tapiero et al. 2003). Whereas the juvenile form is mainly associated with liver symptoms, the adult presentation tends to manifest mainly with neurological deficits (Lorincz 2010). In WD, copper concentration in the liver is very high; contrastingly in the blood, it has very low levels. The urinary copper levels are typically increased and are used as a biomarker of the disease. In an affected brain, the contents of copper are between two and eight times greater compared to a normal brain (Faa et al. 2001).

4.5.2.2 Non-Wilsonian Disorders (Copper Toxicosis)

The non-Wilsonian disorders caused due to excessive accumulation of copper, occurring in early childhood include Indian childhood cirrhosis, Idiopathic copper toxicosis, and endemic Tyrolean infantile cirrhosis. The increased uptake of copper through food and drinking water is believed to be responsible for the development of these diseases (Brewer 2003a, b; Wu et al. 2016).

Idiopathic copper toxicosis usually results due to the accumulation of high level of copper in the liver. About 138 infants were reported to be dead due to this disease in west Austria, Germany, and Italy during 1900–1980 (Baker et al. 1995). Similarly, as far as Indian scenario is concerned, infants fed with milk stored in brass or copper utensils were found to develop Indian childhood cirrhosis (ICC) due to same reason of high level of copper in the liver. Pathologically it is characterized by the accumulation of Mallory's hyaline in necrotic hepatocytes, micronodular cirrhosis, remarkable lack of regenerative nodule, characteristic orcein positive granules with no chronic biliary disease (Baker et al. 1995). Such condition results from WD gene, wherein it is well-known that mild copper accumulation occurs without showing medical problems with natural intake of copper. This pathologic condition develops when the usual source of nutrition and/or water for infants contains a high level of copper. WD can become dominant and expresses in heterozygote condition (Butler et al. 2001). Another hypothesis states that there is role of the undiscovered gene, which weakens the mechanism of copper excretion thereby resulting in the various disorders (Brewer 2003a, b).

4.5.2.3 Alzheimer's Disease

It is a neural disorder, where multiple alterations in various cellular processes are involved. It is an age-associated disorder, characterized by the presence of several types of amyloid plaques and neurofibrillary tangles, mostly consisting of amyloid-β protein and hyperphosphorylated tau. The disease involves inflammation in the neuron, oxidative stress, impairments in energy metabolism, etc., as far the role of copper in this disease is concerned, alteration in homeostasis of metallic ions including copper plays a key role in the pathogenesis of Alzheimer's disease. Copper checks the excessive activity of N-methyl-d-aspartate receptors, the excitatory neurotransmitter receptors (Eskici and Axelsen 2012; Noda et al. 2013). With aging the copper level rises in blood plasma and serum and it is also found to be elevated in AD brains (Eskici and Axelsen 2012; Noda et al. 2013). The increased copper level thus negatively correlated with the loss of cognition (Arnal et al. 2013). Moreover, a significantly high amount of copper (400 lM) has been reported to be present in senile plaques in AD brain. There are reports suggesting that high concentration of copper causes homodimerisation of amyloid precursor protein (APP), leading to amyloid b aggregation and hyperphosphorylation of tau protein (Atwood et al. 2000; Arnal et al. 2013; Gonzalez-Dominguez et al. 2014). Copper is a redox active metal. Alterations in copper homeostasis may generate conditions favorable for superoxide yielding redox cycling and oxidation stress-mediated damage to membrane polyunsaturated lipids and redox-based neurochemical reactions occurring in the brain (da Silva et al. 2013; Gonzalez-Dominguez et al. 2014).

4.5.2.4 Diabetes

Diabetes is the disease resulting due to alteration in glucose homeostasis. The copper regulation becomes defective in case of nonclinical models of diabetes. It involves advanced-glycation end products (AGEs), which can transform amino acid residues producing pathological copper-binding sites in the extracellular matrix components of the blood vessels walls (Cooper 2012; Squitti et al. 2017). It has been believed to develop due to lack of ferroxidase activity in the tissues, leading to accumulation of high amount of iron in the pancreas (Uriu-Adams and Keen 2005). However, metabolism of copper is also thought to play a direct or indirect role in the development of this disease (Takahashi et al. 1996). In case of a diabetic patient, the liver and kidney were reported to have a high amount of metallothionein concentration. Additionally, copper ions in the blood can increase the rate of advanced glycosylated end product formation, which is associated with the pathogenicity of secondary complications in diabetes. The blood plasma concentration of copper was also reported to be high in the diabetic patient as compared to the nondiabetic persons. The high plasma concentration leads to hypertension, retinopathy, and microvascular disease (Uriu-Adams and Keen 2005).

In the clinical and nonclinical models of disease, urinary copper excretion studies demonstrated the excessive amount of chelatable free copper in diabetes patients (Ito et al. 2001; Cooper et al. 2005). There are reports suggesting that AD and diabetes share common pathways which alter the copper and glucose metabolism. The abnormalities in mitochondrial function, glucose, and copper metabolism have been reported in both diseases. A receptor for AGEs (RAGE), a multi-ligand receptor has been found to play a key role in the development of inflammatory pathways both in diabetes and AD. They transport the circulating Aβ across the blood–brain barrier, thereby generating ROS and abnormalities in cerebral blood flow (Perrone and Grant 2015; Puqazhenthi et al. 2017).

4.5.2.5 Cancer

Alterations in the concentration of trace element produces an adverse effect on cellular metabolism and therefore, can induce carcinogenesis. As mentioned earlier, copper induces the production of ROS, the imbalance between ROS and antioxidant can lead to direct DNA damage, mutation, and development of cancer (Khoshdel et al. 2016). There are evidence suggesting that cancer cells generally require a high amount of copper as compared to normal cells. Therefore, anticancer therapy targeting copper metabolism can be a better option to restrict the cancer growth (Easmon 2002). Patients suffering from leukemia, sarcoma, brain tumor, lung cancer, cervical cancer, liver cancer, and breast cancer has been found to contain high serum copper level. Particularly, in breast and ovarian cancer, the copper level can be elevated as much as two–threefold (Pavlova and Thompson 2016). It is interesting to further note that after recovery from these cancers, the serum copper level returned to its normal level. This fact points toward the importance of high copper level in cancer (Brewer et al. 2000; Nasulewicz et al. 2004).

It has been claimed that disturbance in copper level leads to the mutation in p53 gene. Hence, copper displaces zinc from its normal binding site present on p53, causing its misfolding and finally leading to altered function (Sharif et al. 2012; Khoshdel et al. 2016). Additionally, copper is also suggested to induce cancer by inducing tumor angiogenesis (Khoshdel et al. 2016). However, further in-depth studies about the mechanism of copper-induced development of cancer and angiogenesis need to be performed.

4.6 Conclusions

The previous reports confirmed the involvement of copper in several cellular events and its requirement for normal cell functioning. Moreover, due to the vital role of copper in human health, it has considerably attracted a great deal of attention from researchers. It is proved that maintenance of an adequate level of copper in the body is essentially required, because the imbalance of copper level in human body results in many diseases like Wilson's disease, Menke's disease, childhood copper toxicosis syndromes, aceruloplasminemia, Alzheimer's disease, etc. In addition, it also promotes the development of many other life-threatening diseases like cardiovascular diseases, diabetes, and cancer. Moreover, it is now evident that deficiency of copper during all stages of life may have hematological manifestations. Therefore, a healthy diet is of utmost importance for the optimization of health. Copper is required in small amounts and it is considered as a trace element, but its role in the body is challenging. Unfortunately, yet copper often does not get the recognition, even after knowing that dietary supplements often lack copper and presence of a large amount of zinc and iron can also disturb the copper balance in the body.

References

Adelstein SJ, Vallee BL (1961) Copper metabolism in man. N Engl J Med 265:892–897

Aggett PJ (1999) An overview of the metabolism of copper. Eur J Med Res 4(6):214–216

Arnal N, Morel GR, de Alaniz MJT, Castillo O, Marra CA (2013) Role of copper and cholesterol association in the neurodegenerative process. Int J Alzheimer's Dis 10:1–15

Atwood CS, Scarpa SC, Huang X, Moir RD, Jones WD, Fairlie DP, Tanzi RE, Bush AI (2000) Characterization of copper interaction with Alzheimer amyloid b peptides: identification of an attomolar-affinity copper binding site on amyloid b1-42. J Neurochem 75:1219–1233

Baker A, Gormally S, Saxena R, Baldwin D, Drumm B, Bonham J, Portmann B, Mowat AP (1995) Copper-associated liver disease in childhood. J Hepatol 23:538–543

Barrow L, Tanner MS (1988) Copper distribution among serum proteins in paediatric liver disorder and malignancies. Eur J Clin Invest 18:555–560

Bennetts HW, Chapman FE (1937) Copper deficiency in sheep in Western Australia: a preliminary account of the aetiology of enzootic ataxia of lambs and anaemia of ewes. Aust Vet J 13: 138–149

Bertini I, Cavallaro G, McGreevy KS (2010) Cellular copper management-a draft user's guide. Coord Chem Rev 254:506–524

Brewer GJ (2003a) Copper in medicine. Curr Opin Chem Biol 7:207–212

Brewer GJ (2003b) Copper-lowering therapy with tetrathiomolybdate for cancer and diseases of fibrosis and inflammation. J Trace Elem Exp Med 16:191–199

Brewer GJ, Johnson VD, Dick RD, Fink KJ, Kluin KJ, Hedera P (2000) Treatment of Wilson's disease with zinc XVII: Treatment during pregnancy. Hepatology 31(2):364–370

Buamah PK, Russell M, Milford-Ward A, Taylor P, Roberts DF (1984) Serum copper concentrations significantly less in abnormal pregnancies. Clin Chem 30(10):1676–1677

Butler P, McIntyre N, Mistry PK (2001) Molecular diagnosis of Wilson disease. Mol Genet Metab 72:223–230

Cerone SI, Sansinanea AS, Streitenberger SA, Garcia MC, Auza NJ (2000) Cytochrome c oxidase, Cu, Zn-superoxide dismutase, and ceruloplasmin activities in copper-deficient bovines. Biol Trace Elem Res 73:269–278

Cerpa W, Varela-Nallar L, Reyes AE, Minniti AN, Inestrosa NC (2005) Is there a role for copper in neurodegenerative diseases? Mol Aspects Med 26:405–420

Chellan P, Sadler PJ (2015) The elements of life and medicines. Philosophical Transactions of the Royal Society A: Mathematical, Physical and Engineering Sciences 373:20140182. https://doi.org/10.1098/rsta.2014.0182

Choi EH, Strum W (2010) Hypocupremia-related myeloneuropathy following gastrojejunal bypass surgery. Ann Nutr Metab 57:190–192

Cooper GJ (2012) Selective divalent copper chelation for the treatment of diabetes mellitus. Curr Med Chem 19:2828–2860

Cooper GJ, Chan YK, Dissanayake AM, Leahy FE, Keogh GF, Frampton CM, Gamble GD, Brunton DH, Baker JR, Poppitt SD (2005) Demonstration of a hyperglycemia-driven pathogenic abnormality of copper homeostasis in diabetes and its reversibility by selective chelation: Quantitative comparisons between the biology of copper and eight other nutritionally essential elements in normal and diabetic individuals. Diabetes 54:1468–1476

Cordano A, Baertl JM, Graham GG (1964) Copper deficiency in infants. Pediatrics 34:324–326

da Silva SL, Vellas B, Elemans S, Luchsinger J, Kamphuis P, Yaffe K, Sijben J, Groenendijk M, Stijnen T (2013) Plasma nutrient status of patients with Alzheimer's disease: systematic review and meta-analysis. Alzheimer's Dement 10:1–18

Danks DM (1988) Copper deficiency in humans. Annu Rev Nutr 8:235–257

de Romana L, Olivares M, Uauy R, Araya M (2011) Risks and benefits of copper in light of new insights of copper homeostasis. J Trace Elem Med Biol 25:3–13

DRI (2001) Dietary Reference Intakes (DRI) for vitamin A, vitamin K, arsenic, boron, chromium, copper, iodine, iron, manganese, molybdenum, nickel, silicon, vanadium and zinc. National Academies Press (US), pp. 224-257

Easmon J (2002) Copper and iron complexes with antitumor activity. Expert Opin Ther Pat 12:789–818

EFSA (2006) Tolerable upper intake levels for vitamins and minerals, European Food Safety Authority

EFSA (2015) Scientific opinion on dietary reference values for copper. EFSA Panel on Dietetic Products, Nutrition and Allergies (NDA). EFSA J 13(10): 4253

Eide DJ (1998) The molecular biology of metal ion transport in *Saccharomyces cerevisiae*. Annu Rev Nutr 18:441–469
Eskici G, Axelsen PH (2012) Copper and oxidative stress in the pathogenesis of Alzheimer's disease. Biochemistry 51:6289–6331
Faa G, Lisci M, Caria MP, Ambu R, Sciot R, Nurchi VM, Silvagni R, Diaz A, Crisponi G (2001) Brain copper, iron, magnesium, zinc, calcium, sulfur and phosphorus storage in Wilson's disease. J Trace Elem Med Biol 15:155–160
Fraga CS (2005) Relevance, essentiality and toxicity of trace elements in human health. Mol Aspects Med 26:235–244
Gabreyes AA, Abbasi HN, Forbes KP, McQuaker G, Duncan A, Morrison I (2013) Hypocupremia associated cytopenia and myelopathy: a national retrospective review. Eur J Haematol 90:1–9
Galib Barve M, Mashru M, Jagtap C, Patgiri BJ, Prajapati PK (2011) Therapeutic potentials of metals in ancient India: a review through Charaka Samhita. J Ayurveda Integr Med 2:55–63
Gonzalez-Dominguez R, Gracia-Barrera T, Gomez-Ariza JL (2014) Characterization of metal profiles in serum during the progression of Alzheimer's disease. Metallomics 6:292–300
Groff JL, Gropper SS, Hunt SM (1995) Advanced nutrition and human metabolism. West Publishing Company, New York
Gupta A, Lutsenko S (2009) Human copper transporters: mechanism, role in human diseases and therapeutic potential. Futur Med Chem 1(6):1125–1142
Haddad MR, Choi EY, Kaler S (2014) AAVrh10-ATP7A administration to the cerebrospinal fluid, in combination with subcutaneous copper, normalizes neurological outcomes in a mouse model of Menkes disease. Mol Ther 22(1):S99–S100
Harris ED (2001) Copper homeostasis: the role of cellular transporters. Nutr Rev 59:281–285
Harris ED, Qian Y, Tiffany-Castiglioni E, Lacy AR, Reddy MC (1998) Functional analysis of copper homeostasis in cell culture models: a new perspective on internal copper transport. Am J Clin Nutr 67(5 Suppl):988S–995S
Hordyjewska A, Popiołek Ł, Kocot J (2014) The many faces of copper in medicine and treatment. Biometals 27(4):611–621
https://web.archive.org/web/20101015204256/, http://www.copperinfo.com/health/goodhealth.html. Accessed 07 Nov 2017
https://www.organicfacts.net. Accessed 07 Nov 2017
Ito S, Fujita H, Narita T, Yaginuma T, Kawarada Y, Kawagoe M, Sugiyama T (2001) Urinary copper excretion in type 2 diabetic patients with nephropathy. Nephron 88:307–312
Jaiser SR, Winston GP (2010) Copper deficiency myelopathy. J Neurol 257:869–881
Kaler SG (2011) ATP7A-related copper transport diseases-emerging concepts and future trends. Nat Rev Neurol 7:15–29
Kaler SG (2014) Translational research investigations on ATP7A: an important human copper ATPase. Ann N Y Acad Sci 1314:64–68
Khoshdel Z, Naghibalhossaini F, Abdollahi K, Shojaei S, Moradi M, Malekzadeh M (2016) Serum copper and zinc levels among iranian colorectal cancer patients. Biol Trace Elem Res 170(2):294–299
Kim BE, Nevitt T, Thiele DJ (2008) Mechanisms for copper acquisition, distribution and regulation. Nat Chem Biol 4(3):176–185
Klevay LM (1998) Lack of a recommended dietary allowance for copper may be hazardous to your health. J Am Coll Nutr 17(4):322–326
Kono S (2012) Aceruloplasminemia. Curr Drug Targets 13:1190–1199
Lanska DJ, Remler B (2014) Myelopathy among zinc-smelter workers in Upper Silesia during the late 19th century. Neurology 82:1175–1179
Linder MC (1991) Biochemistry of copper. Plenum Press, NewYork
Lorincz MT (2010) Neurologic Wilson's disease. Ann N Y Acad Sci 1184:173–187
Lutsenko S, Barnes NL, Bartee MY, Dmitriev OY (2007) Function and regulation of human copper-transporting ATPases. Physiol Rev 87(3):1011–1046
Manto M (2014) Abnormal copper homeostasis: mechanisms and roles in neurodegeneration. Toxics 2:327–345

Maryon EB, Molloy SA, Zimnicka AM, Kaplan JH (2007) Copper entry into human cells: progress and unanswered questions. Biometals 20(3–4):355–364
Masuoka J, Saltman P (1994) Zinc(II) and copper (II) binding to serum albumin. A comparative study of dog, bovine, and human albumin. Biol Chem 269:25557–25561
Mercer JFB (2001) The molecular basis of copper-transport diseases. Trends Mol Med 7(2):64–69
Miyajima H (2003) Aceruloplasminemia. In: Pagon RA, Adam MP, Ardinger HH, Bird TD, Dolan CR, Fong CT, Smith RJH, Stephens K (eds), Gene Reviews. University of Washington, Seattle, 1993–2014
Møller LB, Lenartowicz M, Zabot MT, Josiane A, Burglen L, Bennett C, Riconda D, Fisher R, Janssens S, Mohammed S, Ausems M, Tümer Z, Horn N, Jensen TG (2012) Clinical expression of Menkes disease in females with normal karyotype. Orphanet J Rare Dis 7:6
Morton MS, Elwood PC, Abernethy M (1976) Trace elements in water and congenital malformations of the central nervous system in South Wales. Br J Prev Soc Med 30(1):36–39
Nasulewicz A, Mazur A, Opolski A (2004) Role of copper in tumour angiogenesis clinical implications. J Trace Elem Med Biol 18:1–8
Noda Y, Asada M, Kubota M, Maesako M, Watanabe K, Uemura M, Kihara T, Shimohama S, Takahashi R, Kinoshita A, Uemura K (2013) Copper enhances APP dimerization and promotes Ab production. Neurosci Lett 547:10–15
O'Brien J, Morrissey PA (1997) Metal ion complexation by products of the Maillard reaction. Food Chem 58(1–2):17–27
Olivares M, Uauy R (1996) Copper as an essential nutrient. Am J Clin Nutr 63(5 Suppl.): 791S–796S
Osredkar J, Sustar N (2011) Copper and zinc, biological role and significance of copper/zinc imbalance. J Clin Toxicol S 3:001. https://doi.org/10.4172/2161-0495.S3-001
Pan PL, Tang HH, Chen Q, Song W, Shang HF (2011) Desferrioxamine treatment of aceruloplasminemia: long-term follow-up. Mov Disord 26:2142–2144
Pavlova NN, Thompson CB (2016) The emerging hallmarks of cancer metabolism. Cell Metab 23 (1):27–47
Percival SS (1998) Copper and immunity. Am J Clin Nutr 67:1064S–1068S
Perrone L, Grant WB (2015) Observational and ecological studies of dietary advanced glycation end products in national diets and Alzheimer's disease incidence and prevalence. J Alzheimer's Dis 45:965–979
Puig S, Thiele D (2002) Molecular mechanism of copper uptake and distribution. Curr Opin Chem Biol 6:171–180
Puqazhenthi S, Qin L, Reddy PH (2017) Common neurodegenerative pathways in obesity, diabetes, and Alzheimer's disease. Biochimica et Biophysica 1863(5):1037–1045
Rowland LP, Schneider NA (2001) Amyotrophic lateral sclerosis. N Engl J Med 344:1688–1700
Schleper B, Stuerenburg HJ (2001) Copper deficiency-associated myelopathy in a 46-year-old woman. J Neurol 248:705–706
Sharif R, Thomas P, Zalewski P, Fenech M (2012) The role of zinc in genomic stability. Mutat Res 733:111–121
Sharma MC, Joshi C, Pathak NN, Kaur H (2005) Copper status and enzyme, hormone, vitamin and immune function in heifers. Res Vet Sci 79:113–123
Shaw JCL (1992) Copper deficiency in term and preterm infants. In Nestle Nutrition Workshop Series, Nutritional Anemias, Fomon SJ, and Zlotkin S, eds. New York: Raven Press 30: 105–119
Shibata N, Hirano A, Kobayashi M, Umahara T, Kawanami T, Asayama K (1995) Cerebellar superoxide dismutase expression in Menkes' kinky hair disease: an immunohistochemical investigation. Acta Neuropathol 90:198–202
Shim H, Harris ZL (2003) Genetic defects in copper metabolism. J Nutr 133:1527S–1531S
Squitti R, Mendez AJ, Simonelli I, Ricordi R (2017) Diabetes and Alzheimer's disease: can elevated free copper predict the risk of the disease? J Alzheimer's Dis 56(3):1055–1064
Stern BR, Solioz M, Krewski D, Aggett P, Aw TC, Baker S, Crump K, Dourson M, Haber L, Hertzberg R, Keen C, Meek B, Rudenko L, Schoeny R, Slob W, Starr T (2007) Copper and

human health: biochemistry, genetics, and strategies for modelling dose-response relationships. J Toxicol Environ Heal Part B 10:157–222

Takahashi Y, Miyajima H, Shirabe S, Nagataki S, Suenaga A, Gitlin JD (1996) Characterization of a nonsense mutation in the ceruloplasmin gene resulting in diabetes and neurodegenerative disease. Hum Mol Genet 5:81–84

Tapiero H, Townsend DM, Tew KD (2003) Trace elements in human physiology and pathology. Copper. Biomed Pharmacother 57:386–398

The Telegraph (2012) The kiss of copper. Published on May 7, 2012. Available at: https://www.telegraphindia.com/1120507/jsp/knowhow/story_15458385.jsp

Tokuda Y, Yokoyama S, Tsuji M, Sugita T, Tajima T, Mitomi T (1986) Copper deficiency in an infant on prolonged total parenteral nutrition. Journal of Parenteral Enteral Nutrition 10(2):242–244

Tümer Z (2013) An overview and update of ATP7A mutations leading to Menkes disease and occipital horn syndrome. Hum Mutat 34:417–429

Uauy R, Olivares M, Gonzalez M (1998) Essentiality of copper in humans. Am J Clin Nutr 67(5 Suppl.):952S–959S

Ugarte M, Osborne NN, Brown LA, Bishop PN (2013) Iron, zinc, and copper in retinal physiology and disease. Surv Ophthalmol 58:585–609

Uriu-Adams JY, Keen CL (2005) Copper, oxidative stress, and human health. Mol Aspects Med 26:268–298

Ward EM, Keen CL and McArdle HJ (2003) The impact of copper on human health. International Copper Association Ltd., New York. Available at: www.copperinfo.com

Wazir SM, Ghobrial I (2017) Copper deficiency, a new triad: anemia, leucopenia, and myeloneuropathy. J Comm Hosp. Intern Med. Perspect 7(4):265–268

WHO (1996) Trace elements in human nutrition and health. World Health Organization, Geneva

Wirth PL, Linder MC (1985) Distribution of copper among multiple components of human serum. J the Natl Cancer Inst 75:277–284

Wu X, Leegwater PAJ, Fieten H (2016) Canine models for copper homeostasis disorders. Int J Mol Sci 17(2):196. https://doi.org/10.3390/ijms17020196

Xu J, Church SJ, Patassini S, Begley P, Waldvogel HJ, Curtis MA, Faull RLM, Unwin RD, Cooper GJS (2017) Evidence for widespread, severe brain copper deficiency in Alzheimer's dementia. Metallomics 9(8):1106–1119

Yi L, Kaler S (2014) ATP7A trafficking and mechanisms underlying the distal motor neuropathy induced by mutations in ATP7A. Ann N Y Acad Sci 1314:49–54

Zhou B, Gitschier J (1997) hCTR1: a human gene for copper uptake identified by complementation in yeast. Proc Natl Acad Sci 94(14):7481–7486

Chapter 5
Silver: Biomedical Applications and Adverse Effects

Luiza Helena da Silva Martins, Mahendra Rai, João Moreira Neto, Paulo Weslem Portal Gomes and Júlia Helena da Silva Martins

Abstract Silver metal has been used by humanity for about 7000 years. The use of this metal was observed in objects such as coins and cutlery that was used due to the corrosion resistance of this noble metal. Due to slow corrosion, the silver ions are continuously released from the materials. Silver is a metallic transition element, which has a shiny and white appearance. This metal can be found widely in the human environment. The use of silver in various branches of medicine has increased significantly as antibacterial, antiviral, antimycotic, and chemotherapeutic agents. In addition, this metal is very effective in medical devices, textile, cosmetic, and even household appliance. Silver can act as a drug in its most varied forms, whether in ionic, colloidal, combined, or nanoparticle form, this element has demonstrated potential in a series of treatments of diseases, including cancer, malaria, and inflammation, mainly in the uterine region. Silver can also be used in the treatment of wounds, burns, presenting high potential as human medication. The therapeutic potential of metal complexes in the treatment of cancer has attracted interest because the metals have peculiar characteristics (redox activity, modes of variable coordination, and reactivity in relation to the organic substrate). In addition, although silver

L. H. da Silva Martins (✉)
Center of Natural Sciences and Technology, State University of Pará—UEPA, Belém, Pará, Brazil
e-mail: luhelemarte@gmail.com

M. Rai
Nanobiotechnology Lab, Department of Biotechnology, SGB Amravati University, Amravati 444602, Maharashtra, India

J. M. Neto
School of Chemical Engineering, University of Campinas—UNICAMP, Campinas, São Paulo, Brazil

P. W. P. Gomes
Center of Social Sciences and Education, State University of Pará—UEPA, Salvaterra, Pará, Brazil

J. H. da Silva Martins
Faculty of Electrical Engineering, Federal University of Pará—UFPA, Belém, Pará, Brazil

M. Rai et al. (eds.), *Biomedical Applications of Metals*,
https://doi.org/10.1007/978-3-319-74814-6_5

may have an adverse effect on the body and the environment, if used in an excessive concentration. But, if used in an ideal concentration, it may be a good approach for current medicine.

Keywords Silver · Antimicrobial · Toxicity · Medicine · Adsorption

5.1 Introduction

Silver is a metallic transition element, has a glossy and white appearance, and can be found widely in the human environment. At low concentrations, silver may be present in the human body due to inhalation of particles in the air and contamination of diet and drinking water, but silver has no trace metal value in the human body. The use of silver has significantly increased due to its antibacterial, antimycotic, and chemotherapeutic activity, as well as being very effective in wound care products, medical devices, textiles, cosmetics, and even home appliances (Lansdown 2010).

Silver compounds have been widely exploited because of their medicinal properties for centuries. Silver-based compounds were used as popular remedies for tetanus and rheumatism in the nineteenth century and for colds and gonorrhea before the advent of antibiotics in the early twentieth century. Silver was widely used for skin burns, but interest in the salts silver or silver salt solutions in the treatment of burns, eventually disappeared after World War II (Atiyeh et al. 2007).

The threat posed by the possible outbreak of antibiotic-resistant microbes is growing globally and requires the introduction and production of new, more advanced platforms for the study and development of more potent antimicrobial agents against strains resistant to different drugs. Thus, the antimicrobial activity of silver nanoparticles (AgNPs) is widely recognized, although its activity may change with physical characteristics of the nanoparticle, such as its shape, mass, size, and composition, and conditions of its synthesis, such as pH, ions, and macromolecules. Their forms may be relevant to antibacterial activity. Compared with larger AgNPs, smaller AgNPs have a higher binding surface and show more intense bactericidal activity. The variation in the thickness and molecular composition of the membrane structures of Gram-positive and Gram-negative bacteria explains the difference in their sensitivities to AgNPs. The bactericidal activity presumably occurs due to changes in the bacterial cell wall structure as a result of interactions with incorporated AgNP, leading to a greater permeability of the membrane and consequently to the death of the cells. AgNPs also interact with biomaterials rich in sulfur and phosphorus, which include intracellular components such as proteins or DNA, and extracellular components such as membrane proteins. These components influence respiration, division, and ultimately the survival of cells. By compromising the bacterial cell wall, silver ions can enter the cells, leading to damaged DNA accumulation and effect on protein synthesis, being highly effective as antimicrobial agents (Chung et al. 2016).

In order to have a better antimicrobial efficacy of silver, it is necessary for this element to undergo ionization because the silver ion is a highly reactive species, it reacts rapidly with negatively charged proteins, RNA, DNA, chloride ions, and so on. This property explains the mechanisms of antibacterial action. And this action is what has been the basis of the silver use as a medicine in the health area (Atiyeh et al. 2007).

In the 1990s, there was a resurgence of the promotion of silver in the form of colloidal silver, which was used as an alternative medicine treatment. The affirmation for its use is that it was an essential mineral supplement or it could treat various diseases. Although colloidal silver products are legally available as health supplements, these are illegal in the USA. The commercial product termed "colloidal silver" includes solutions containing various concentrations of silver ion compounds, silver colloids, or protein-bound silver compounds. Unlike the clinical production of drugs, the manufacture of these products is not standardized, and therefore, results in various concentrations and also in particle sizes (Wong and Liu 2010).

AgNPs showed promising antitumor effects, as reported in the study by Zhang et al. (2014), where a low concentration of AgNPs caused DNA damage and genotoxicity, although no significant cytotoxicity was recorded (Zhang et al. 2014; Wei et al. 2015). However, the toxicity of the silver nanoparticles itself may be useful for therapies against cancer because it is highly sought after. Positive results were achieved by incorporating AgNPs into cancer treatments. They not only can passively interact with cells, but also actively meditate on molecular processes to regulate cellular functions (Wei et al. 2015).

Malaria is one of the most common infectious diseases, and has become a public health problem in many tropical countries. The ineffectiveness of treatment against this available disease is the main reason behind its threat. Current malaria treatment strategies have failed due to drug resistance in *Plasmodium falciparum* and drug toxicity in humans. Thus, the development of effective antimalarial drugs is something that is needed. Silver as discussed in the course of this chapter, presents several applications in the medical field, for the treatment of malaria; the form of silver nanoparticles (AgNPs) demonstrated significant activity against the malaria parasite called *P. falciparum* and its vector female Anopheles mosquito. AgNPs may be a solution for the control of this disease (Rai et al. 2017).

In this chapter, we have discussed the various applications of silver and its derivatives in medicine.

5.2 Silver in Medicine History

Silver metal has been used by humanity for a long time (about 7000 years). The use of silver was observed in objects such as coins and cutlery, it was used due to the corrosion resistance of this noble metal. In addition, its use was emphasized due to antibacterial effect. Owing to the slow corrosion, the silver ions are continuously released from the materials. As many bacterial strains today are resistant to antibiotics, silver is used in many cases for disinfection, as coatings, as well as in ionic or nanoparticulate form. In addition, application in many products consumed outside the medical sector is found, for example, in textiles or sprays to avoid bad odors of sweat. Moreover, increasingly it has been used in the cosmetics industry (Chernousova and Epple 2013).

Silver was already known and widely used by the Chaldeans in the mid-4000 BCE, was the third metal most used by these ancient peoples, the first was gold and the second copper. Thus, at the turn of the millennium, silver had several applications in the medical area, first because this metal has antimicrobial character, and at that time, there was not enough knowledge for the perception that the microorganisms were the cause of diseases like infections. The metal has been used for a number of functions, including vessels, liquid containers, coins, trimmings, sheets, sutures, solutions such as nitrate, oxide, bromide, chloride, and iodide, colloids providing fine particles and electric colloids. Silver electrical colloids became the primary supporter of antimicrobial therapy in the early part of the twentieth century until the introduction of antibiotics in the early 1940s (Alexander 2009).

Herodotus reported that the Persian kings never drank the water that was not transported in silver containers, which keeps the water fresh for years. This was particularly important in military conflicts, where freshwater from natural sources was not readily available. The ancient Phoenicians, Greeks, Romans, Egyptians, and other peoples also used silver in one way or another to preserve food and water, and this was practiced during World War II. The Macedonians perhaps were the first who attempted to prevent or treat surgical infections, and used the application of silver plaques for better healing. Hippocrates used silver preparations for the treatment of ulcers and to promote healing of wounds. It is likely that silver nitrate has also been used as a medication since it has already been mentioned in a pharmacopeia published in Rome in 69 BCE. By the mid-1800s, there was a widespread acceptance that wine, water, milk, and vinegar remained pure for long periods when stored in silver pots. Silver nitrate has also been used successfully to treat skin ulcers, compound fractures, and wounds (Alexander 2009).

Over time, well-established indications for the effective use of silver were for water purification, wound dressings for healing promotion, infection prevention and treatment, dental hygiene (prevention and correction of pyorrhea, gingivitis, and bad breath), ocular conditions (mainly the prevention of neonatal ophthalmia), and other infectious complications. There is less clear evidence of (possibly effective) efficacy for use in epilepsy and central nervous system disorders, a variety of digestive disorders such as advanced age or disability, and for the treatment of arthritis, hemorrhoids, dandruff, and warts. Silver was also recommended for a wide variety of other diseases, where effectiveness was questionable. These included diabetes mellitus, obesity, colds, psoriasis, allergies, and many others (Alexander 2009).

Nowadays, there are still several studies for the use of silver in medicine, among the studies one has tried to find a better remedy for the topical treatment of burns than the silver sulfadiazine so far have been unsuccessful (Klasen 2000). Its use as a disinfectant is already more restricted mainly to silver sulfadiazine cream due to the development of more modern antibiotics for the treatment of infectious diseases, and silver sulphadiazine has topical use only for the treatment of wounds from burns. From the 1990s, there was a resurgence of silver in its colloidal out as an alternative medicine treatment. Silver was also marketed with claims that it would be an essential mineral supplement capable of treating various diseases. However, although colloidal silver products are legally available as health supplements, this component is illegal in the US, and the country is making some claims about the medical effectiveness of this colloidal silver (Wong and Liu 2010).

Gopiraman et al. (2016) reported the efficacy of AgNPs/CMC on antibacterial activity in Gram-negative bacteria (*Escherichia coli*) and Gram-positive bacteria (*Stalpylococcus aureus*). Nanocellulose fibers were prepared by deacetylation of electrospun cellulose acetate nanofibers, which were then treated with sodium chloroacetate to prepare nano anionic cellulose fibers (CMC). Aqueous silver nitrate ($AgNO_3$) solution with different concentrations was used to produce nanofiber composites. To obtain the AgNPs/CMC, the resulting Ag/CMC nanofibers were chemically reduced with $NaBH_4$. The nanocomposites were characterized by FE-SEM, FTIR, XPS, and SEM-EDS. The antimicrobial tests were performed using *S. aureus* and *E. coli* bacteria following the standard test method JIS L1902, 2008. EDS results confirmed higher silver content in CMC–Ag nanofibers than AgNPs/CMC nanofibers. The antimicrobial test and EDS results showed higher silver release (greater halo width) by the first compared to the later, which gives better antimicrobial activity for the CMC–Ag nanofibers. This comparative study of the antibacterial performance between CMC–Ag nanofibers and AgNPs/CMC nanofibers was conducted and the antibacterial tests demonstrated better silver release characteristics by the CMC–Ag nanofibers.

Wu et al. (2017) studied the incorporation of Ag in nano-zeolite grafted onto the membrane surface of this nanocomposite, which demonstrated that this material presented sustainable and regenerable antimicrobial activity. In this study, two new methods of forming antimicrobial coating based on zeolite with polyvinyl alcohol (PVA) and polydopamine (PDA), respectively, were examined. Both methods achieved a wide range of Ag loading. Silver release and bacterial exposure experiments showed that increased accelerated Ag, released Ag-zeolite, which led to higher antimicrobial activity. The reduction of Ag^+ to Ag (0), however, stabilized the Ag, decreasing the rate of Ag release and significantly prolonging the antimicrobial efficacy against bacterial growth on the membrane surface. These results showed that polymer/zeolite nanocomposite coatings present potential as a versatile approach to the antimicrobial activity.

5.3 Absorption of Silver in the Human Body

Metals are substances that exhibit high electrical conductivity, malleability, and brightness, and which can lose their electrons to form cations. Metals are found naturally in the Earth's crust and their compositions vary between different locations. The distribution of metal in the atmosphere is monitored by the properties of the given metal and by various environmental factors (Khlifi and Hamza-Chaffai 2010; Jaishankar et al. 2014).

Toxicity to xenobiotic materials is directly related to the amount absorbed in the body, its metabolism and accumulation in the target organs, and the cellular vulnerability to toxic irreversible changes. Clinical and experimental studies have shown that metals absorbed in the body interacts and compete for binding sites in carrier proteins and that when the protective mechanisms offered by the major metal binding proteins such as metallothioneins and epidermal barrier function become saturated, toxic changes occur (Lansdown 2010). There are several silver metal absorption forms in the human body, such absorption may be through ingestion, inhalation, intraparenteral insertion of medical devices, and even through dermal contact, however, the literature on the absorption of silver by all routes in beings remain poor, poorly correlated, and not statistically stable. Metabolic pathways are the same irrespective of the pathway of absorption (Landsdown 2006, 2010). Several information on the absorption of silver as a cause of argyria and increased blood flow are derived from occupational health studies, where workers were exposed to silver compounds over a long period (years) (Rosenman et al. 1979; DiVincenzo et al. al. 1985; Rosenman et al. 1987; Drake and Hazelwood 2005; Lansdown 2010). On the basis of these studies, it is not so rare and impossible to identify the amount of silver that can be absorbed into the circulation of the gastrointestinal tract, lungs, or percutaneous absorption or how much is retained, but silver urine or fecal excretion may be informative (Klaassen 1979; DiVincenzo et al. 1985; Wan et al. 1991; Williams and Gardner 1995; Lansdown 2010).

There is still much controversy regarding the routes that predominate in the metabolism of silver in the human body. Its transient or long-term accumulation in kidney, liver, and bone, and its excretion patterns in bile, urine, hair, and nails are a matter of great concern (Wan et al. 1991; Zheng et al. 2003; Lansdown 2010). The biliary excretion pathway predominates over the urinary tract, but the urinary measure of silver can provide a convenient index of silver absorption across all routes and serve as a guide to the body's total silver content at blood levels of 100 gL^{-1} (Skog and Wahlberg 1964; Wan et al. 1991; Lansdown 2010). At higher concentrations, urinary excretion patterns are irregular. Biological monitoring of workers exposed to long-term silver environmental waste showed elevated silver concentrations in hair, blood, urine, and feces (DiVincenzo et al. 1985; Williams and Gardner 1995; Lansdown 2010), but fecal silver represents the excretion in bile plus 90% or more ingested with food and not absorbed into the circulation. With the examination of 37 silver workers, Di Vincenzo et al. (1985) concluded that at recommended environmental concentrations of 0.1 mg/m^3 (TLV), fecal silver excretion would be about 1 mg per day (DiVincenzo et al. 1985; Lansdown 2010). The critical evaluation of reported clinical and experimental studies showed that silver is not absorbed into neurological tissue, but is linked as inert precipitation in lysosomal vacuoles of the blood–brain barrier and CSF–blood barrier (Zheng et al. 2003; Lansdown 2007, 2010).

5.4 Anti-inflammatory Effects of Silver Metal

Inflammation is defined as an early protective homeostatic immune response when tissue trauma occurs. This is due to the production of proinflammatory cytokines and the activation of cells in the immune system. It is important to keep in mind the elucidation of pro-and anti-inflammatory pathways that are important for the development of protective strategies for regenerative tissue against damage caused by imbalances in cytokines, oxidants, and antioxidants that may occur within the wound (Wong et al. 2009).

An example of an inflammatory process is the formation of abdominal adhesions, which consist of abnormal fibrous bands that form between the organs or structures of the body, which is part of the healing process in response to tissue trauma after abdominal surgery. Among the complications that may occur, the most frequent is intestinal obstruction. Being this mechanism already known and consolidated in the literature and in practice (Wong et al. 2009).

In addition to being an excellent antibacterial agent, Wong and Liu (2010) showed how the silver action model works on burn wounds, as well as on a model of peritoneal adhesion in mice, where AgNPs had anti-inflammatory properties. In the model for burns, significantly lower levels of proinflammatory cytokine (Interleukin 6) IL-6 were found in AgNP-treated animals using real-time quantitative RT-PCR. On the other hand, IL-10 mRNA levels, an anti-inflammatory cytokine, remained higher in the AgNP group compared to other silver compounds at all time points monitored during healing.

According to studies by Wong and Liu (2010) polymorphonuclear cells (PMNs) and fibroblasts produced IL-6, which was recognized as an initiator of events in the physiological changes of inflammation; the decrease in IL-6 expression may result in fewer neutrophils and macrophages being recruited into the wound and fewer cytokines being released into the wound with subsequently less paracrine stimulation of cell proliferation, migration of fibroblasts and keratinocytes, and production of extracellular matrix.

Interleukin 10 (IL-10) could inhibit the synthesis of proinflammatory cytokines, and also inhibits the migration of leukocytes to the site of inflammation, in part inhibiting the synthesis of various chemokines, including the monocyte-1 chemoattractant protein (MCP-1) and the macrophages inflammatory protein-1α (MIP-1a). The differences found in mRNA levels of various cytokines further confirmed that AgNPs can effectively modulate cytokine expression during the suppression of inflammation (Wong and Liu 2010).

The anti-inflammatory action of silver nanoparticles has been suggested in several studies previously described. On the other hand, it has been observed that inflammation plays a significant role in the formation of postoperative adhesions. In animal models, Wong and Liu (2010) reported that intraperitoneal injection of silver nanoparticles significantly reduced the degree of postoperative fibrous adhesion. Anti-inflammatory effects have also been found in other models of inflammatory diseases by other researchers. Taken together, Wong and Liu (2010) suggested that silver nanoparticles can effectively reduce inflammation and its use in other inflammatory conditions is anticipated in advance.

5.5 The Antimicrobial Mechanisms of Silver

The use of silver as a disinfectant agent is not new and the silver compounds have been shown to be effective against aerobic and anaerobic bacteria by the precipitation of bacterial cellular proteins, which results in the blockade of the microbe respiratory system. Prior to the advent of silver nanoparticles, silver nitrate was an effective antibacterial agent used clinically. Then the use of silver agents was subsided as antibiotics had come to the forefront of the past century. However, the use of silver has recently returned due to the emergence of antibiotic-resistant bacteria because of excessive use of these compounds (Rai et al. 2009; Wong and Liu 2010).

In recent years, silver nanoparticles (AgNPs) have been increasingly used in medical and consumer products as an effective silver-based antibacterial agent. The use of these nanoparticles has aroused great interest among scientists because of the AgNPs' antibacterial mechanism. An interesting question regarding the antibacterial mechanism of AgNPs is whether they exert the same antibacterial action on bacterial cells as Ag^+ ions. In fact, this issue has been under discussion for more than a decade and is not yet fully consolidated (Li et al. 2016).

Ivask et al. (2013) reported studies showing the magnitude of the charged nanomaterials' toxicity correlated with the amount of silver (Ag^+) ions dissolved in solution and demonstrated that the positively charged silver capacity interacted strongly with the bacterial surface resulting in high concentrations of Ag^+ bioavailable from these particles. The positively charged particles also interfered with the normal function of the bacterial electron transport chain and were responsible for the formation of Reactive Oxygen Species (ROS) in the cell membrane.

Reactive oxygen production and flagellar activity were observed in a wide range of silver species. In contrast, the effects on lipopolysaccharides on the outer surface of the cells appear to be specific to the nanoparticles. These data suggest that although the AgNPs toxicity is large-scale Ag^+ media mediated, the way the particles interact with bacterial cells and some of the pathways involved in the toxicity of the particles are highly dependent on the physicochemical properties of the nanoparticles. These results have important implications for understanding the toxicity mechanisms of silver nanomaterials (Ivask et al. 2013).

Li et al. (2016) performed the first comparative study of the antibacterial mechanism of silver ions (Ag^+) and AgNPs using Fourier-transform infrared spectroscopy (FTIR). These authors described a multifaceted silver antibacterial mechanism for Ag^+ and AgNPs at the molecular level. For both Ag^+ and AgNPs, it was found that silver complexes with thiol groups induce the destruction of proteins, causing the loss of Lipopolysaccharide (LPS) from the bacterial membrane, which led to the conformation of the DNA of the microorganisms. In addition, through the time-dependent FTIR study, the authors found that when interacting with the bacterial cell, Ag^+ and AgNPs present different kinetic behaviors, implying the presence of the "particle-specific" indirect effect of AgNPs. The authors concluded that the observed similarities and differences of Ag^+ and AgNP with respect to their antibacterial behaviors might promote a better knowledge about the antibacterial mechanism of silver.

Panáček et al. (2009) studied the antifungal activity of silver nanoparticles (NPs) prepared by the modified Tollens process using pathogenic *Candida* spp by determining minimum inhibitory concentration (MIC), minimum fungicidal concentration (MFC), and time dependence of inhibition of yeast growth. The cytotoxicity of silver NP to human fibroblasts was determined simultaneously. Silver NPs exhibited an inhibitory effect against the yeasts tested at the concentration of 0.21 mg/L Ag. The inhibitory effect of silver NPs was increased through their stabilization and the lower MIC equal to 0.05 mg/L was determined for silver NPs stabilized by sodium dodecyl sulfate against *Candida albicans* II. The MICs obtained from the silver NPs and in particular from the stabilized silver NPs were comparable and in some cases even better than the MICs of the conventional antifungal agents determined by the E test. Silver NPs effectively inhibited yeast growth tested at concentrations below the cytotoxic limit against the human fibroblasts tested, determined at a concentration equal to 30 mg/L Ag. In contrast, ionic silver inhibited the growth of tested yeasts at concentrations comparable to the cytotoxic level (approximately 1 mg/L) of ionic silver against the human fibroblasts tested.

There are different silver delivery systems, which include those that provide silver from ionic compounds such as silver calcium phosphate and silver chloride, and those that provide silver from metallic compounds such as nanocrystalline silver. However, the difficulties with many current silver antimicrobial topics are in their low levels of silver release, the limited number of silver species released the lack of penetration, the rapid consumption of silver ions and the presence of nitrate bases or creams that are proinflammatory which adversely affects the healing of wounds. Other issues include blemishes, electrolyte imbalance, and patient discomfort. Over the past few years, there has been a rapid increase in the number of silver dressings available to physicians to address these issues (Atiyeh et al. 2007).

The interactions of the silver complex molecules can best be understood by Fig. 5.1, which shows the Hirshfeld surface modeled on the cation molecule, $[Ag(2,6\text{-di}(CH_2OH)py)_2]^+$ and corresponding two-dimensional fingerprints showing all types of contacts and how they are reduced and selected: Ag···O/O···Ag, O···H/H···O, C···H/H···C. As expected, the contacts H···H comprise 39% of the surface area due to the small van der Waals radius of hydrogen and packaging effects on molecular structures, so the distances H···H observed are typical without extremely short ones. In addition, O···H/H···O contacts play a dominant role with a significant contribution of 33.7%. It has been found that the arms of the compound CH_2OH of the 2,6-di(CH_2OH)py bonds are mainly involved in hydrogen bonds of OH quite strongly, where the shorter interactions are shown as long peaks and the interactions of CH are the lowest. Another type of contact C···H/H···C weak, contain only

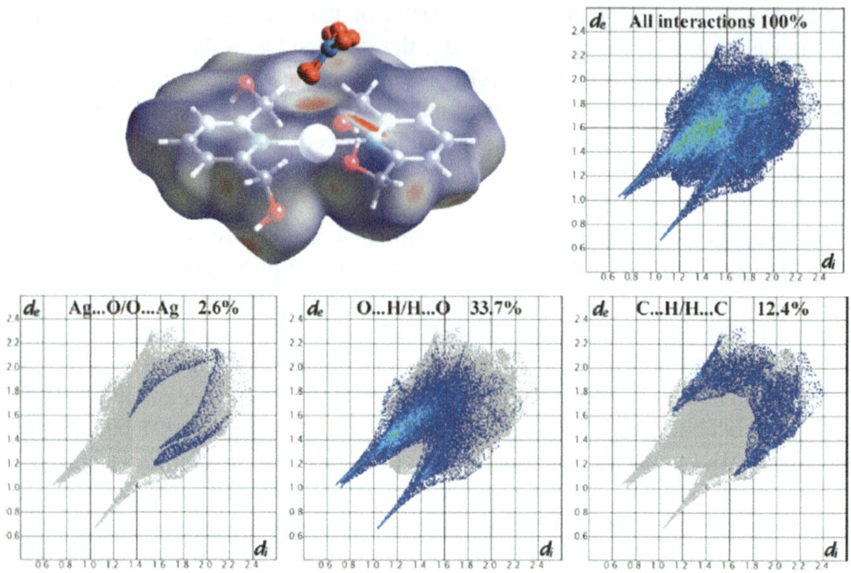

Fig. 5.1 Hirshfeld surface of Ag(I) complex-cation molecule with the geometrical function d_{norm} mapped onto it (a color scale from red to blue: –0.75 Å–1.2 Å) and corresponding finger plots indicating all types of contacts and these reduced to contact types as following Ag···O/O···Ag, O···H/H···O, C···H/H···C [the distances from a surface point to the nearest interior/exterior atoms ($d_{i/e}$) are given in Å]. (*Source* Kalinowska-Lis et al. 2016, with permission of MDPI Open Access)

12.4% of the surface. The interactions of the aromatic compound π-π represented mainly by C···C/C···N (4.4 and 1.4%, respectively), as well as N···H/H···N (3.5%) contribute to the Hirshfeld surface comparable to all interactions with the metal atom Ag1 (4.2%). Among the short contacts of Ag···X, X (X = O, N, C, H) dominate the Ag···O (2.6%) (Kalinowska-Lis et al. 2016).

AgNPs can have their sustained release of Ag^+ since, within the bacterial cells, where a lowering of the pH of the medium occurs, this can end up causing the creation of free radicals that induce oxidative stress, and this causes the bacterial activity of AgNPs more intense (Wong and Liu 2010). In addition, a recent study showed that yeast and *Escherichia coli* were inhibited at a low concentration of AgNP, the study of mechanisms revealed that free radicals and oxidative stress were responsible for antibacterial activities (Kim et al. 2007).

5.6 Silver as Virucidal Agent

According to Wei et al. (2015), Silver in AgNPs form have been shown to inhibit viruses such as HIV-1, Tacaribe (TCRV), and hepatitis B (HBV), recombinant respiratory syncytial virus (RSV), monkeypox virus, murine norovirus (MNV)-1, and the influenza A/H1N1 virus. Park et al. (2014) have recently developed and evaluated a novel multi-sized AgNP-decorated micron-sized magnetic hybrid colloid (MHC) that could be used to inactivate viral pathogens with minimal chances for potential release into the environment.

5.7 Silver Metal in Cancer Medication

In general, metals are essential components of the cells chosen by nature. They are often found in the catalytic domain of enzymes and are involved in biological process processes, ranging from electron exchange to catalysis, in addition to having structural roles. Metals are widely used in cellular activities. The metals of zinc, cobalt, silver, vanadium, strontium, manganese, and copper are examples of metals involved in catalytic processes (Ndagi et al. 2017).

The therapeutic potential of metal complexes for the treatment of cancer has attracted great interest in recent years, since these metals have peculiar characteristics, such as redox activity, variable coordination modes, and reactivity in relation to the organic substrate. These properties become attractive in the design of metal complexes that bind selectively to the biomolecular target with a resulting alteration in the cellular mechanism of proliferation (Frezza et al. 2010).

In the past, silver complexes have not received much attention compared to other metals, although these complexes have shown good cytotoxic activity against many cancer cell lines. Recently, the cytotoxic properties of the silver (I) complexes have attracted a great deal of interest, since they showed greater cytotoxic activity than cisplatin with relatively low toxicity and greater selectivity toward cancer cells. In an in vitro study conducted to evaluate the cytotoxic properties of silver (I) complexes against B16 (murine melanoma) and noncarcinogenic 10T1/2 (murine fibroblast) cell lines, silver complexes containing hydroxymethylene group showed higher cytotoxic activity against B16 (murine melanoma) than silver nitrate ($AgNO_3$), silver sulfadiazine (AgSD), and cisplatin. These complexes showed relatively low toxicity against noncancerous 10T1/2 (murine fibroblast). Similarly, it was disclosed in a study set to determine the anticancer properties of the gold (I) and silver (I) N-heterocyclic complexes that these compounds, along with cisplatin, exhibited similar anticancer activity as the lung cancer H460. In a related development, the silver complexes of 2,6-disubstituted pyridine ligands were synthesized. Binders and complexes were evaluated in vitro with doxorubicin (reference compound) in hepatocellular carcinoma (HepG2), pulmonary adenocarcinoma (A549), colon carcinoma (HT29), and mammary adenocarcinoma (MCF7) using MMT (multimodal therapy). All of the synthesized complexes showed more significant activity than the corresponding ligands, and most of the prepared silver complexes exhibited excellent cytotoxic activity against the cancer cell line tested in comparison to doxorubicin. All of these properties have placed silver complexes as a promising metal complex to achieve the future of chemotherapy (Ndagi et al. 2017).

In terms of cancer detection, Au–Ag nanorods were used in a recent study as the form of a nanoplatform for multivalent binding by multiple aptamers, in order to increase the signal and binding forces of aptamers in cancer cell recognition. The molecular assembly of aptamers in the nanorods showed the authors 26 times greater affinity than the original aptamer probes (Huang and Chang 2008). Thus, these nanorod-aptamer conjugates have been shown to be highly promising for use in cell-specific targeting, as well as the detection and targeting capability required for cell studies, disease diagnosis, and therapy (Wong and Liu 2010).

5.8 Adverse Effects of Silver in the Human Body

Among metals, silver is classified as part of xenobiotic metals (chemical compounds foreign to an organism or biological system) in the human body, since there is evidence to suggest that much of the liberated silver ion can precipitate with chloride anions or phosphate and this may cause strong binding in the form of inert complexes with albumins or macroglobulins; some may be binding or may be deposited in tissue debris. There are no limits to this material available for antibiotic purposes; however, this is of potential significance in relation to toxic factors (Lansdown 2010).

There are many factors that can influence a metal to produce toxic effects on the body, which are metal solubility, the ability of the metal to bond with the biomolecules, and the degree to which the metal complexes formed are metabolized and excreted. A toxic effect is defined as an undesirable or adverse effect on human health. Ingestion is seen as the main entryway for silver compounds and colloidal silver proteins. Inhalation of dust or fumes containing silver occurs primarily in occupational environments. Contact with the skin occurs in occupational environments, from the application of creams that are used as topics to combat burns and there is also the issue of contact by the use of jewelry. Silver can also enter the body through the use of acupuncture needles, catheters, dental amalgams, or wounds caused by accidents (Drake and Hazelwood 2005).

Soluble silver compounds can be readily absorbed when compared to metallic silver or insoluble have great potential in the production of adverse effects on the human body. Acute symptoms of overexposure to silver nitrate, for example, are decreased blood pressure, diarrhea, irritation of the stomach, and decreased respiration. Chronic symptoms of prolonged ingestion of low doses of silver salts may impair degenerating organs. Soluble silver compounds are also able to accumulate in small amounts in the brain and muscles. Silver in any form is not considered toxic to the immune, cardiovascular, nervous, or reproductive systems and is not considered carcinogenic. However, caution should be exercised over the excessive use of this metal (Drake and Hazelwood 2005).

Silver allergy is also one of the well-known adverse effects of exposure to silver in cosmetics, and in patients treated with silver nitrate in the treatment of infected wounds, but in addition a portion of predisposed silver workers such as jewellers, photographers, and other persons exposed to metallic silver (Ag) or silver salts may exhibit symptoms of late hypersensitivity due to this contact (Bosseti et al. 2002; Lansdown 2010). The true extent of the problem is not known as in diagnostic patch test 2% aqueous silver is used. And silver nitrate is not routinely performed except in health risk situations (Lansdown 2010).

Evidence but still poor (as there is a need for further studies) are currently available to show that the use of silver or silver compounds in their ionizable form during pregnancy may be one of the causes of infertility, impairment of fetal growth, or abnormal development in any species. Silver nitrate [1% (m/v)] administered by intrauterine injection in 13 cynomolgus monkeys between 27 and 43 days of pregnancy caused early vaginal bleeding and miscarriage, but two of the seven reassigned animals reconceived and delivered healthy children (McCauley et al. 2010; Lansdown 2010). It is not known if Ag^+ passes transplacentally to accumulate in the fetus (Lansdown 2010).

According to Drake and Hazelwood (2015), some adverse effects that may be caused by exposure and exacerbated use in silver are argyria and argyrosis, respiratory effects, tissues and organs, metabolism problems, according to the same authors, the Occupational Safety and Health Administration (OSHA) and the Safety Administration and Mine Health (MSHA) today apply the Permissible Exposure Limit (PEL) of 0.01 mg/m3 to metallic and soluble silver compounds. The National Institute for Occupational Safety and Health (NIOSH) has established a Recommended Exposure Limit (REL) of 0.01 mg/m^3 for soluble silver compounds and silver metal powder, which is not as different from the value established by OSHA PEL.

5.9 Conclusions

It is concluded that silver was already well known. There have been historical reports of the medicinal use of this metal since a long time, as the years passed and with evolution, a range of researches could be made with medicinal use. The silver has an antimicrobial effect against bacteria, fungi, and viruses. Silver has demonstrated inhibitory activity malaria which is a dreaded disease especially in tropical and developing countries, where public health is still a problem. Depending on how silver is used, in the ionic form, in complex, colloidal, nanoparticles, etc., it may have a specific function. Adverse effects caused by silver should not be overlooked and more rigorous studies must be carried out so that this metal can have its safer use in medicine.

References

Alexander JW (2009) History of the medical use of silver. Surg Infections 10(3):289–292

Atiyeh BS, Costagliola M, Hayek SN, Dibo SA (2007) Effect of silver on burn wound infection control and healing: review of the literature. Burns 33(2):139–148

Bosetti M, Masse A, Tobin E, Cannas M (2002) Silver coated materials for external fixation devices: in vitro biocompatibility and genotoxicity. Biomaterials 23(3):887–892

Chernousova S, Epple M (2013) Silver as antibacterial agent: ion, nanoparticle, and metal. Angew Chem Int Ed 52(6):1636–1653

Chung IM, Park I, Seung-Hyun K, Thiruvengadam M, Rajakumar G (2016) Plant-mediated synthesis of silver nanoparticles: their characteristic properties and therapeutic applications. Nanoscale Res Lett 11(1):40

DiVincenzo GD, Giordano CJ, Schriever LS (1985) Biologic monitoring of workers exposed to silver. Int Arch Occup Environ Health 56(3):207–215

Drake PL, Hazelwood KJ (2005) Exposure-related health effects of silver and silver compounds: a review. Anal Occupational Hygiene 49(7):575–585

Frezza M, Hindo S, Chen D, Davenport A, Schmitt S, Tomco D, Ping-Dou Q (2010) Novel metals and metal complexes as platforms for cancer therapy. Curr Pharm Des 16(16):1813–1825

Gopiraman M, Jatoi AW, Hiromichi S, Yamaguchi K, Jeon HY, Chung IM, Soo KI (2016) Silver coated anionic cellulose nanofiber composites for an efficient antimicrobial activity. Carbohyd Polym 149:51–59

Huang YF, Chang HT, Tan W (2008) Cancer cell targeting using multiple aptamers conjugated on nanorods. Anal Chem 80(3):567–572

Ivask AE, Badawy A, Kaweeteerawat C, Boren D, Fischer H, Ji Z, Chang CH, Liu R, Toylamat T, Telesca D, Zink JI, Cohen Y, Holden PA, Godwin AW (2013) Toxicity mechanisms in *Escherichia coli* vary for silver nanoparticles and differ from ionic silver. ACS Nano 8(1): 374–386

Jaishankar M, Tseten T, Anbalagan N, Mathew BB, Beeregowda KN (2014) Toxicity, mechanism and health effects of some heavy metals. Interdiscip Toxicol 7(2):60–72

Kalinowska-Lis U, Felczak A, Chęcińska L, Szabłowska-Gadomska I, Patyna E, Małecki M, Lisowska K, Ochocki J (2016) Antibacterial activity and cytotoxicity of silver (I) complexes of pyridine and (Benz)imidazole derivatives. X-ray crystal structure of [Ag (2,6-di(CH_2OH) py$)_2$] NO_3. Molecules 21(2):87

Khlifi R, Hamza-Chaffai A (2010) Head and neck cancer due to heavy metal exposure via tobacco smoking and professional exposure: A review. Toxicol Appl Pharmacol 248:71–88

Kim JS, Kuk E, Yu KN, Kim JH, Park SJ, Lee HJ, Kim YK (2007) Antimicrobial effects of silver nanoparticles. Nanomed Nanotechnol Biol Med 3(1):95–101

Klaassen CD (1979) Biliary excretion of silver in the rat, rabbit, and dog. Toxicol Appl Pharmacol 50(1):49–55

Klasen HJ (2000) A historical review of the use of silver in the treatment of burns II. Renewed interest for silver. Burns 26(2):131–138

Lansdown AB (2006) Silver in health care: antimicrobial effects and safety in use. In: Biofunctional textiles and the skin, vol 33. Karger Publishers, pp 17–34

Lansdown AB (2007) Critical observations on the neurotoxicity of silver. Crit Rev Toxicol 37(3):237–250

Lansdown AB (2010) A pharmacological and toxicological profile of silver as an antimicrobial agent in medical devices. Adv Pharmacol Sci, Article ID 910686, https://dx.doi.org/10.1155/2010/910686

Li H, Gao Y, Li C, Ma G, Shang Y, Sun Y (2016) A comparative study of the antibacterial mechanisms of silver ion and silver nanoparticles by Fourier transform infrared spectroscopy. Vib Spectrosc 85:112–121

McCauley RL, Li YY, Chopra V, Herndon DN, Robson MC (1994) Cytoprotection of human dermal fibroblasts against silver sulfadiazine using recombinant growth factors. J Surg Res 56(4):378–384

Ndagi U, Mhlongo N, Soliman ME (2017) Metal complexes in cancer therapy–an update from drug design perspective. Drug Design Develop Therapy 11:599–616

Panáček A, Kolář M, Večeřová R, Prucek R, Soukupová J, Kryštof V, Hamal P, Zbořil R, Kvítek L (2009) Antifungal activity of silver nanoparticles against *Candida* spp. Biomaterials 30(31): 6333–6340

Park S, Park HH, Kim SY, Kim SJ, Woo K, Ko G (2014) Antiviral properties of silver nanoparticles on a magnetic hybrid colloid. Appl Environ Microbiol 80(8):2343–2350

Rai M, Yadav A, Gade A (2009) Silver nanoparticles as a new generation of antimicrobials. Biotechnol Adv 27(1):76–83

Rai M, Ingle AP, Paralikar P, Gupta I, Medici S, Santos CA (2017) Recent advances in use of silver nanoparticles as antimalarial agents. Int J Pharm 526(1–2):254–270

Rosenman KD, Moss A, Kon S (1979) Argyria: clinical implications of exposure to silver nitrate and silver oxide. J Occup Environ Med 21(6):430–435

Rosenman KD, Seixas N, Jacobs I (1987) Potential nephrotoxic effects of exposure to silver. Occup Environ Med 44(4):267–272

Skog E, Wahlberg JE (1964) A comparative investigation of the percutaneous absorption of metal compounds in the guinea pig by means of the radioactive isotopes: ^{51}Cr, ^{58}Co, ^{65}Zn, ^{110}Ag, ^{115}Cd, ^{203}Hg. J Invest Dermatol 43:187–192

Wan AT, Conyers RA, Coombs CJ, Masterton JP (1991) Determination of silver in blood, urine, and tissues of volunteers and burn patients. Clin Chem 37(10):1683–1687

Wei L, Lu J, Xu H, Patel A, Chen ZS, Chen G (2015) Silver nanoparticles: synthesis, properties, and therapeutic applications. Drug Discovery Today 20(5):595–601

Williams N, Gardner I (1995) Absence of symptoms in silver refiners with raised blood silver levels. Occup Med 45(4):205–208

Wong KK, Liu X (2010) Silver nanoparticles—the real "silver bullet" in clinical medicine? Med Chem Comm 1(2):125–131

Wong KK, Cheung SO, Huang L, Niu J, Tao C, Ho CM, Tam PK (2009) Further evidence of the anti-inflammatory effects of silver nanoparticles. Chem Med Chem 4(7):1129–1135

Wu J, Yu C, Li Q (2017) Novel regenerable antimicrobial nanocomposite membranes: Effect of silver loading and valence state. J Membr Sci 531:68–76

Zhang T, Wang L, Chen Q, Chen C (2014) Cytotoxic potential of silver nanoparticles. Yonsei Med J 55(2):283–291

Zheng W, Aschner M, Ghersi-Egea JF (2003) Brain barrier systems: a new frontier in metal neurotoxicological research. Toxicol Appl Pharmacol 192(1):1–11

Chapter 6
The Potential of Metals in Combating Bacterial Pathogens

Natalie Gugala and Raymond J. Turner

Abstract The progression of antimicrobial resistance and the presence of microbial biofilms pose serious threats, which have prompted the development of novel antimicrobials such as metals and metal-based compounds. Whereas the use of metals has historical foundations, metal antimicrobials are presently found in numerous consumer products since they demonstrate effective broad-spectrum activity that enables the eradication of pathogenic microorganisms. Nonetheless, much is yet to be understood regarding the mechanisms by which metals are able to kill microbes. Metal antimicrobial use can cause environmental contamination resulting in altered microbial communities and the propagation of resistance. Furthermore, of primary concern, is the toxicity of metals to humans. Upon the onset of antibiotic resistance, is the use of metals worth the risk? Or are we past the point of consideration, since metal antimicrobials are now routinely used and developed as a means of eliminating threatening microorganisms?

Keywords Metals · Metalloids · Bacteria · Pathogen · Antimicrobial Resistance

6.1 Introduction

Before we think toward metal ions as biocides, we must consider their prevalence in biology. With the occurrence of various metals, metalloids, and transition metals in the environment, it is not surprising that organisms have adapted to accommodate these elements for imperative cellular functions (Waldron and Robinson 2009). Inorganic ions are fundamental to the biochemistry and physiology of all living organisms. Ninety-one elements can be considered metals which have the properties that when pure, are malleable and ductile with good electrical and thermal conductivity. Many metal elements are essential including iron, copper, zinc,

N. Gugala · R. J. Turner (✉)
Biofilm Research Group, University of Calgary, Calgary, Canada
e-mail: turnerr@ucalgary.ca

M. Rai et al. (eds.), *Biomedical Applications of Metals*,
https://doi.org/10.1007/978-3-319-74814-6_6

nickel, magnesium, cobalt, molybdenum, calcium, manganese, and selenium, with unique enzymes being discovered that use or act on elements such as tungsten, arsenic, tellurium, cadmium, and gold. The more common essential metals in the biochemistry of both microbes and mammals are metals such as iron and copper, commonly found in electron-transferring proteins, and those involved in respiratory metabolism such as cytochrome *c* oxidase (Tsukihara et al. 1994). Zinc, which only has a single oxidation state at physiological reduction potentials, is used to organize protein structure such as DNA and RNA polymerase (Wu and Wu 1987) and drive catalysis by acting as a Lewis acid. Manganese is found within the active sites of several proteins including superoxide dismutases and catalases (Keele et al. 1970), while magnesium and calcium are required for a number of roles, including maintaining protein structure and regulating myosin motor activity (Swenson et al. 2014), among others. Overall, it has been predicted that at least one-quarter of all proteins require metal ions (Dupont et al. 2006; Andreini et al. 2004) with elegantly coordinated binding sites, that in turn, define many metals as part of the essentialities for life's survival.

Despite the obligatory roles that essential metals fulfill, elevated concentrations result in cellular toxicity. This consequence is not limited to essential metals, in fact, nonessential metals such as silver, mercury, and tellurium are exceedingly toxic at low concentrations, particularly to microorganisms (Harrison et al. 2004; Teitzel and Parsek 2003). Hence, the toxicity of both essential and nonessential metals has led to their use as antimicrobial agents against a variety of pathogenic bacteria and fungi.

The use of metal compounds as antimicrobial agents is a practice that stretches back thousands of years and well into the twentieth century, only to be replaced by the introduction of organic antibiotics (Hobman and Crossman 2015). Nonetheless, the emergence of metals as antimicrobials has regained attention in the past several decades, largely due to the progression of bacterial resistance to conventional antibiotics, new opportunistic nosocomial and community-acquired pathogens, and microbial biofilms—inherently resistant bacteria aggregated to surfaces that are surrounded by a complex biomolecular matrix offering enhanced protection. In addition, with paucity in the development of new antibiotics, the use of alternative compounds—such as metals—is further enticing and must be explored. Metal compounds can now be found in wound dressings (Kostenko et al. 2010), liquid formulations for hand-washing (Gant et al. 2007), impregnated into textiles such as shirts (Reed et al. 2016) and socks (Borkow et al. 2009) and on medical devices like catheters (Ewald et al. 2006).

In this chapter, we will discuss why the use of metal antimicrobials is rapidly gaining popularity. We will present past and current applications of metals in agriculture, medicine, and in consumer products. Next, we will examine the proposed mechanisms of toxicity for several metals. Finally we will discuss underlying challenges associated with studying metal antimicrobials and their use, including mechanisms of metal microbial resistance, and whether these antimicrobials have a potential future as alternatives to antibiotics.

6.1.1 The Reemergence of Metal Compounds as Antimicrobials

The colonization of microorganisms, where it is not wanted, commonly leads to infectious disease and even death. Hence the control, and ultimately the obliteration of these organisms, is desirable. This can be accomplished through the inhibition of DNA replication, and the inhibition of RNA, cell wall, protein, and membrane synthesis, and inhibition of specific enzymes (Kohanski et al. 2010). The aforementioned mechanisms are in fact, standard classifications of natural and synthetic antibiotics. The classification of antibiotics can also be based on the general mode of action, as either bacteriostatic, in which growth is inhibited, and bactericidal resulting in cell death (Kohanski et al. 2010).

With no question, the introduction of antibiotics in the 1940s was a key achievement in modern medical history (Rodecka et al. 2014). A *New York Times* report on penicillin in 1940 called the drug "the most powerful germ killer ever discovered" (Bakalar 2009). Not long after this discovery however, researchers came to recognize that bacteria could develop resistance to antibiotics over time. Since then, a positive correlation between the use of antimicrobials and the generation of resistance has led researchers to believe that the overuse of antibiotics in agriculture and the misuse in human medicine is to blame (Aminov 2010). This provides an apparent example of Darwinian selection, in which the abuse of antibiotics has led to adaptive pressures (French 2010), thus permitting the colonization of the naturally fit. Resistance can also be an inherent characteristic (Fleming 1929). As it happens, the most obvious generation of resistance occurs upon mutation in the microbial chromosome, singular or sequential. The next response to antimicrobial exposure is the replacement of the inherently susceptible or sensitive microorganisms with the inherently resistant (French 2010). Surviving inherently sensitive organisms acquire resistance mechanisms novel to their genome usually, but not always, from less virulent bacteria. This becomes particularly dangerous when the inherently sensitive are pathogenic or opportunistic bacteria. Exchanging genetic information via plasmids transposons or bacteriophages (French 2010) are common modes of transference. These elements were acquired as a result of environmental pressures, such as the existence of natural antibiotics excreted by residing microbes, primarily through mutations (Bush et al. 2011). Hence, with the application of antibiotic pressures, bacteria once sensitive to antibiotics can easily acquire elements that permit resistance, a process that can occur a number of times resulting in the emergence of multidrug-resistant bacteria.

Unfortunately, the progression of antibiotic resistance is not our only threat. In fact, biofilms, structured assemblies of bacteria surrounded by a self-produced extracellular polymeric substance, contribute an additional layer of difficulty. While the formation of a biofilm is a natural process, the presence of these communities affects industrial productivity, and the health of humans and livestock (Hall-Stoodley et al. 2004). Microbial biofilms contaminate industrial and clinical surfaces (including indwelling devices), and are responsible for numerous chronic infections (Hall-Stoodley et al. 2004). They are capable of mobilizing toxic elements, depleting oxygen reserves, causing biofouling and biocorrosion, and contaminating surfaces (Costerton et al. 1999). The biofilm is an innate state of microbial growth with the fossil record showing evidence of this mode of bacterial existence approximately 3.3–3.4 billion years ago (Wit et al. 2001). It was not until the 1970s that an appreciation for biofilms as a major—if not the most substantial—mode of bacterial subsistence took place (Hall-Stoodley et al. 2004). Growth as a biofilm provides enhanced resistance to traditional antibiotics, which are commonly designed for use against planktonic cells. Consequently, traditional antibiotics cannot eradicate cells that dwell in acute wounds as biofilms. The development of novel antibiotics, a struggle in itself, will not subside antibiotic resistance particularly in the absence of stewardship and stagnation in the drug development industries, rather, it will only contribute to the development of untreatable diseases.

As a result of the aforementioned threats, in the past several decades researchers have begun investigating the use of novel antimicrobials, including bacteriophages (Donlan 2009), antimicrobial peptides (Hancock and Sahl 2006), ozone (Azarpazhooh and Limeback 2008), and metals, such as Cu, Ag, Ga, Ni, Te, Sn and Zn (Harrison et al. 2004). Overall, the metals that are being increasingly considered for antimicrobial agents are typically within the transition metals of the d-block (V, Ti, Cr, Co, Ni, Cu, Zn, Tb, W, Ag, Cd, Au, Hg) and a few other metals and metalloids from groups 13–16 of the periodic table comprising Al, Ga, Ge, As, Se, Sn, Sb, Te, Pb, and Bi.

6.2 Uses of Metals as Antimicrobials

6.2.1 Historic

For thousands of years, metals have been used for their antimicrobial properties in agriculture and medicine. Prior to WWII, travelers would often use water vessels made of Cu and Ag, or drop Ag coins into containers for disinfection and preservation purposes (Alexander 2009; Borkow and Gabbay 2009). The use of Cu as an antiseptic for the treatment of wounds and infections, and in contraceptive intrauterine devices dates back more than 4000 years, and the Egyptians first reported the use of Cu as an astringent in 1500 BC (Borkow and Gabbay 2009). The Macedonians produced silver plates in order to facilitate better wound healing. Silver nitrate was used to treat ulcers and burns and administered internally as a counterirritant in the seventeenth century (Alexander 2009), and later for the management of gonorrheal eye infections in newborns and children (Klasen 2000). In the eighteenth century, As was used for a number of purposes—such as a sedative, an antiseptic for skin infections, or for the treatment of malaria, ulcers, and syphilis (Liu et al. 2008). Inorganic salts of Hg were commonly used in agriculture to prevent plant diseases, as wood preservatives, in animal feed additives, and rodenticides (Huisingh 1974). Mercury has also been used in laxatives and diuretics, and as an antiseptic, antifungal, and biocidal agent since the fifteenth century (Hobman and Brown 1997). In fact, the popular antiseptic Mercurochrome was used up to 1998 when it was finally banned due to the neural toxicity of Hg.

6.2.2 Present Day

In the past several decades, consumers have seen a rise in the use of metals as antimicrobials. Studies have documented the efficacy and performance of metal ions in association with a number of medical devices and products. For example, wound dressings containing Ag have proven to be quite effective, demonstrating a 99% reduction in cell viability within 4 h (Boonkaew et al. 2014). Urinary catheters coated in Ag display a significant benefit to patients with urinary tract infections, when compared to traditional alloy-coated catheters (Saint et al. 1998; Rupp et al. 2004). Combination coatings produced through the deposition of Ag and Ti, have also demonstrated decreased cell viability against *Staphylococcus aureus* and *Klebsiella pneumoniae*, while displaying no cytotoxicity to epithelial and osteoblast cells (Ewald et al. 2006).

Studies have confirmed that hospital surfaces can be contaminated with isolates such as methicillin-resistant *S. aureus* (MRSA), vancomycin-resistant *Enterococci* (VRE), and spores of *Clostridium difficile*, among others, that may be transmitted to other innate objects or patients (Curtis 2008). As a result of this, various Cu surfaces have been examined for their potential in decreasing the viability of pathogenic microorganisms. Reports have demonstrated a reduction in *Listeria monocytogenes* (Wilks et al. 2006), *Escherichia coli*, including a verocytotoxic-genic *E. coli* (Wilks et al. 2005), *Mycobacterium tuberculosis* (Mehtar et al. 2008), *Salmonella enterica*, *Camplylobacter jejuni* (Faúndez et al. 2004), VRE (Warnes and Keevil 2011), MRSA (Noyce et al. 2006), *Bacillus cereus*, and *Deinococcus radiodurans* (Santo et al. 2011) viability on time scales of only minutes to a few hours upon Cu surface exposure, when compared to other surfaces such as stainless steel, PVC, aluminum bronze, and silicon bronze. Protective respiratory face masks impregnated with copper oxide exhibit enhanced anti-influenza biocidal activity (Borkow et al. 2010) and Cu-impregnated socks have been shown to improve the healing of minor wounds and cuts in diabetic patients (Borkow et al. 2009). Copper-impregnated fibers, latex, and polyester resulted in a 2 log reduction in *E. coli*, *S. aureus* MRSA, and VRE numbers after less than 2 h exposure (Borkow and Gabbay 2004). Furthermore, encapsulated Bi-based compounds, in combination with other antibiotics, have been developed in order to eradicate *Helicobacter pylori* (Laine et al. 2003).

Presently, metal containing compounds can be purchased in stores and on the web, in fact, Ag has found its way in numerous consumer products, such as clothing (http://info.lululemon.com/design/fabrics-technology/silverescent), deodorant (http://www.niveamen.in/products/SILVER-PROTECT) (https://toppcock.com/product/toppcock-silver), and even glass (http://www.agc-glass.eu) or toothbrushes (https://nano-b.com/products/nano-b-silver-toothbrush). Companies are now offering silver coating services for a range of products, from flooring to kitchen utensils, even food storage containers (http://www.biocote.com; http://www.silverclear.ca), and medical devices (http://coatings2go.com); similarly for copper (http://www.antimicrobialcopper.org/uk). Product advertisement includes confidence in the safety of metal use as an antimicrobial still, despite the wealth of information published on the mechanisms of metal toxicity, in many cases the precise methods by which they kill microbes, and their effect on human cells for that matter, still remain unclear.

While Cu and Ag make up the majority of available and tested metals of antimicrobial activity, other metals such as Ni, Zn, Al, Cd, Te, Tb, Se, and Ga are increasingly being investigated (Lemire et al. 2013), hence their use is likely to see an increase as the onset of antimicrobial resistance proceeds.

6.3 Mechanisms of Metal Toxicity

In this section, we explore the mechanisms of toxicity in several microorganisms by commonly used past and present metal antimicrobials. Before we begin however, it is imperative that we briefly describe a number of common mechanisms of cell toxicity that can occur. We have already mentioned several ways by which antibiotics are capable of inhibiting cell growth, and these mechanisms can be extrapolated to metals, with no doubt however, variations in the precise modes of action. Nonetheless, indirect effects of antimicrobials, including antibiotics, include the generation of Reactive Oxygen Species (ROS) and propagation of Fenton chemistry, reduction in the total reduced thiol content of the cell, and antioxidant depletion.

Oxygen is a fundamental molecule for aerobic organisms that permits the formation of energy, or ATP, and has a central role in the evolution of multicellular species. Despite this, oxygen can also pose several toxic and mutagenic effects through the generation of Reactive Oxygen Species (ROS) (Thannickal 2009). Single oxygen atoms are unstable hence, the formation of molecular oxygen (O_2) is favorable. Molecular oxygen is a free biradical since one pair of electrons is shared, while two electrons remain unpaired (Buonocore et al. 2010). Reaction with a single electron, originating from the electron transport chain or NADH/NADPH, for example, generates superoxide ($^{\cdot}O_{2^-}$). Dismutation may result in hydrogen peroxide formation, followed with hydroxyl radical ($^{\cdot}OH$) production. Free radicals, whether oxygen-, nitrogen-, carbon- or sulfur-centered, are capable of individual existence and are highly reactive species that propagate undesired reactions within biomolecules (Buonocore et al. 2010). The over-production of ROS results in oxidative stress, a general term encompassing the deleterious process of DNA damage, protein and enzyme inactivation, oxidation of lipid membranes and other biomolecules (Thannickal 2009), in addition to the catalysis of Fenton reactions (Imlay 2013). During aerobic respiration, the formation of radical species is a natural process, however via Fenton chemistry, oxygen toxicity may be intensified, damaging biomolecules and causing antioxidant depletion.

The thiol group of cysteine is ionizable, with a pKa of ~8.5, and upon deprotonation, this amino acid is very reactive. Cysteine can react with electrophiles and is susceptible to ROS (Ritz and Beckwith 2001). These reactions occur endogenously to regulate protein function, and control radical levels, however nonspecific oxidization can lead to uncoordinated functional changes that are both reversible and nonreversible. The occurrence of cysteine residues is fairly uncommon compared to other amino acids, comprising only approximately 2.3% of the human proteome (Rudyk and Eaton 2014a). Within *E. coli* proteins, the frequency of this amino acid is approximately 2% (Turner unpublished). In addition to its occurrence in proteins, cysteine is found within the redox regulatory peptide glutathione (GSH) at a concentration of 10 mM—in most Gram-negative bacteria and in the analogous compound mycothiol in several Gram-positive bacteria. Furthermore, coenzyme A, a substrate found in all genomes sequenced to date (Marino and Gladyshev 2010), contains a thiol group. Although one of the least abundant amino acids, cysteine residues play several important and versatile roles therefore, unintended reactions with ROS may be threatening to the cell (Fig. 6.1).

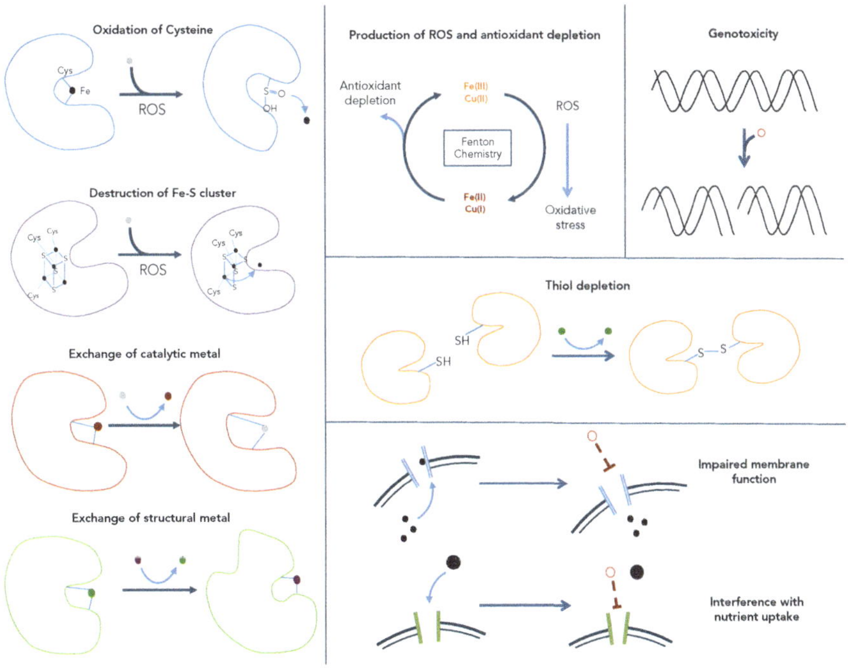

Fig. 6.1 Mechanisms of metal toxicity in bacteria. Metals can cause protein dysfunction via several mechanisms, including oxidation of important residues such as cysteine, the destruction of Fe–S clusters, and the exchange of catalytic and structural metals. Metals can also indirectly result in the production of reactive oxygen species (ROS) causing antioxidant and thiol depletion; a direct outcome of metal exposure as well. Interference with nutrient uptake as well as the impairment of membrane function is additional mechanisms of metal toxicity. Furthermore, some metals have been found to cause genotoxicity, both directly and indirectly

Responses to environmental stress are commonly associated with the expression of several stress response genes. In particular, these genes are under the control of oxido-responsive signal transduction systems, in which the propagation of a signal in the form of a series of biochemical events occurs after the binding of superoxide or other radicals (Pomposiello et al. 2001). In addition to enzymatic defenses such as superoxide dismutase, hydroperoxidases, glutathione reductase, thioredoxin, and catalases non-enzymatic defenses include GSH, NADPH, and NADH pools, β-carotene, ascorbic acid, and α-tocopherol (Cabiscol et al. 2000). Depletion of these defense mechanisms can ultimately lead to cell death through endogenously produced radicals. Below, we briefly explore what is known about some of the more common metal antimicrobials with medical potential.

6.3.1 Copper

Copper has the ability to cycle between Cu(II) and Cu(I) at biologically relevant redox potentials, and in higher organisms this element is a cofactor for over 30 known enzymes (Karlin 1993). Two examples include cytochrome *c* oxidase and NADH dehydrogenase, enzymes that are ubiquitous to aerobic organisms. Regardless of importance, accumulated levels of Cu can lead to cell toxicity. The harm inflicted by this metal is traditionally attributed to the over-production of ROS through Fenton reactions (Solioz et al. 2010). Research has demonstrated that Cu catalyzes the formation of the hydroxyl radical within the periplasm of *E. coli* (Macomber et al. 2007) and several studies have reported the upregulation of genes involved in the elimination of ROS after Cu addition (Teitzel et al. 2006). In spite of this, recent findings suggest that there are alternative mechanisms responsible for the primary effects of Cu-mediated death. In fact, many Gram-positive organisms are resistant to H_2O_2, such as *Lactococcus lactis* (Rochat et al. 2006), and Cu supplementation has been found to decrease the rate of H_2O_2-induced DNA damage in *E. coli* (Macomber et al. 2007). Ligand field theory, a branch of coordination chemistry, is used to predict the electronic arrangements of transition metal complexes with donor ligands. There is a universal order of preference for donor ligands, in which the fourth row of the periodic table gives rise to the Irving–Williams series (Waldron and Robinson 2009). In this series, Cu is the most competitive metal and is expected to bind tightly to ligands, particularly to sulfur and nitrogen. In fact, it has been demonstrated in *E. coli* under in vitro and in vivo conditions that Cu is capable of disrupting the activity of isopropylmalate dehydratase by replacing iron as it coordinates with thiolate or inorganic sulfur ligands (Macomber and Imlay 2009). More recently, researchers have shown that *c*-type cytochrome assembly is a target of Cu toxicity in *Rubrivivax gelatinosus* (Durand et al. 2015). Whether these are the primary sources of cell toxicity in other Gram-negative and Gram-positive organisms, and how this mechanism translates into a cell-wide effect is yet to be explored.

6.3.2 Silver

Compared to Cu, the mechanisms of Ag toxicity have been documented to a lesser extent. The most widely proposed mechanism of Ag is inactivation of enzymes via interaction with the thiol groups of the amino acid cysteine (Liau et al. 1997; Donnell 1999). It has also been suggested that Ag may interact with membrane-bound proteins involved in the electron transport chain. This action uncouples the membrane and renders it permeable to protons. In *E. coli,* it has been observed that Ag interacts with thiol groups found in solvent-exposed iron–sulfur clusters of dehydratases, resulting in the release of Fe and the generation of ROS through Fenton chemistry (Xu and Imlay 2012). Similarly, treatment with silver nitrate results in the coordination of Ag within superoxide dismutase and replacement of the Cu ion in *S. cerevisiae* (Ciriolo et al. 1994). It has also been proposed, using in vitro Fourier-transform infrared spectroscopy, that Ag is capable of interacting with DNA (Arakawa et al. 2001). Finally, using electron microscopy, images of the cell membranes in *E. coli* and *S. aureus* under Ag stress have revealed morphological changes, possibly due to the detachment of the plasma membrane (Jung et al. 2008).

6.3.3 Gallium

To date Ga has not been observed to be significant for cellular maintenance, in fact, the redox potential of this metal is not biologically relevant for most organisms. Gallium, which is Fenton inactive, has been observed to generate ROS as it induces the release of Fe from donor ligands (Kaneko et al. 2007). This occurs because unlike Fe(III), Ga(III) cannot be reduced or oxidized, which is the function of Fe within these enzymes at biologically significant redox potentials (Chitambar and Narasimhan 1991). In *P. aeruginosa,* Ga has been observed to inhibit the uptake of Fe(III) in a concentration-dependent manner by repressing the transcriptional regulator PvdS (Kaneko et al. 2007). This Fe-induced regulator is responsible for the expression of genes involved in the uptake of Fe(III). Compounds or complexes of Ga have been found to be promising therapeutic agents since they have broad-spectrum activity against Gram-negative and Gram-positive bacteria (Banin et al. 2008; Olakanmi et al. 2010). However, the ranges of efficacy for these compounds vary, indicating the mechanisms of this metal are not entirely understood.

6.3.4 Arsenic

It has been Arsenic (As) observed that Astoxicity depends greatly on speciation and the presence of adjacent organic compounds. For example, inorganic As has been found to inhibit metabolic enzymes allosterically (Cooksey 2012). Arsenate enters cells through phosphate uptake systems, and as a result of its close resemblance, and disrupts metabolic pathways that use phosphate. Arsenite binds thiol groups and has been observed to bind oxoglutarate dehydrogenase and pyruvate dehydrogenase. Similarly, as for Cu and Ag, there is evidence that through intermediate thiol radicals, As is capable of generating ROS, leading to the disruption of signal transduction pathways (Valko et al. 2005). Reports have also noted that when As is uncharged influx occurs via aqua-glycerol porins (Rosen 2002).

6.3.5 Mercury

There is no known cellular function of mercury, and the toxicity of this metal to humans has been observed for several centuries (Betts 2010). This metal has been demonstrated, similarly to Ag, to bind tightly to thiol and imine nitrogen groups, hence inactivating the protein and interfering with function. In vitro, this metal has been demonstrated to damage purified dehydratases, whereas in vivo Hg causes bacteriostasis (Xu and Imlay 2012). Hg has also been observed to bind to nucleotides and lipids, causing DNA mutations and possibly contributing to lipid peroxidation. Furthermore, Hg and Hg complexes, which are quite soluble when organic, have the ability to pass through membranes rapidly, providing further insight into the mechanism of action of this metal (Clarkson and Magos 2007).

6.4 Challenges of Studying Metal Antimicrobial Properties

One of the most apparent challenges of metal antimicrobial use lies with the difficulty in understanding the mechanisms of toxicity in bacteria and fungi.

ROS are short-lived entities that react rapidly with biomolecules, oxygen, water, thiols, and inorganic compounds. Therefore, tracking the origin and subsequent downstream consequences of ROS is a difficult task (Gomes et al. 2005). There are many analytical techniques for measuring ROS and reduced thiols, each with its own drawbacks. Several fluorescent probes do not react with ROS or reduced thiols directly, while others are only sensitive to a single species or favor particular reactants over others. Furthermore, since detection may involve several intermediates, isolated chemical events such as reactions with proteins, inorganics, and lipids may occur (Imlay 2015). Additionally, the cell membrane can influence the amount of dye capable of penetrating the cell. Several efflux systems dependent on the proton motive force may cause dye excretion (Wardman 2007), a parameter that may be difficult to control if appropriate controls are not included. Older methods of detection, such as spin trapping, react with radicals at a slow rate and have difficulty in detecting superoxide (Zhao et al. 2005), and nonspecific interactions.

Nearly all probes take a snapshot picture in time, with limited abilities to monitor in real time. Furthermore, exact quantification of reduced or radical species is difficult to obtain. Probes usually deliver a net readout as opposed to monitoring flux through a defined pathway (Rudyk and Eaton 2014b). This misses additional information regarding turnover and the redox state of a particular biomolecule. While reactive oxygen species and reactions with thiols are proposed mechanisms of metal toxicity in microorganisms, detection is limited and caution must be used when analyzing data and drawing conclusions of direct versus indirect outcomes.

The activity of metals as antimicrobials, such as Ag, was initially studied as coatings on catheters and various medical devices. In vitro studies demonstrated decreased cell viability, however, several in vivo studies have failed to display increased cell death. These results were found in Ag-coated fixation pins (Massè et al. 2000) and Ag-coated catheters (Bologna et al. 1999). Reviews have been published examining the effectiveness of coated medical devices (Rupp et al. 2004; Davenport and Keeley 2005), and many have determined that their use reduces the growth of pathogenic bacteria. An explanation for this discrepancy most likely lies in the speciation or release of the metal ions. Our group at the University of Calgary has found that changes in bacterial growth media can alter the efficacy of metal compounds. This is likely due to differences in metal coordination, chelation, and speciation within the assorted culture conditions with parallel changes in the microbe's physiological state(s). In addition, mechanisms of toxicity are commonly studied in one organism under particular growth conditions. Yet the nature of metal ions leads us to believe that mechanisms of toxicity may be different between bacterial families and even strains (Gugala et al. 2017). For example, one study found that the primary targets of Cu in *E. coli* are iron–sulfur clusters of dehydratases (Macomber and Imlay 2009) and that radical formation was not the result of bacterial toxicity since experiments were conducted under anaerobic conditions (Macomber et al. 2007). Yet another study suggested that hydroxyl radicals were involved in bacterial death (Warnes et al. 2012). The various indirect effects that metal ions are capable of generating may influence the rationalization for these differences. In fact, the reactivity of metals with biomolecules is determined by several factors, such as pH and the reduction potential. Hence, metal replacement and coordination in one iron–sulfur center is not identical to another, despite similarities in protein sequence and structure.

What is clear is that determining the direct and subsequent downstream effects of metal exposure is not a trivial task. Studies concerning the mechanisms of metal toxicity and resistance require comprehension of the intricate interplay between metal speciation and elemental characteristics, cell physiology and metabolic diversity, in vivo and in vitro experimental conditions, and direct and indirect targets. While the precise mechanisms of metal toxicity in microorganisms are not entirely understood, it has not arrested the accumulation of numerous reports that illustrate the efficacy and wide use of various metal compounds (Hobman and Crossman 2015).

6.5 The Prevalence of Resistance Toward Metal-Based Antimicrobials

The overuse and misuse of antibiotics against microorganisms have resulted in resistance. The lack of stewardship and the deficiency of novel antibiotics have contributed to this problem. However, the development of resistance represents evolution, signifying a key survival strategy of microorganisms. In fact, antibiotic resistance is best described as antimicrobial resistance. This is because the use of antiseptics, biocides, and other antimicrobials used against bacteria, fungi, viruses, and parasites has also seen a decrease in efficacy. As noted above, microorganisms can acquire resistance through mutations. These organisms are selected and propagate elements of resistance to susceptible bacteria that lack resistance. Mutations may result in the upregulation of proteins that remove, modify, or inactivate the antimicrobial, cause alterations to the antimicrobial target, and/or use biochemical pathway diversions to diminish the threat (Tenover 2006).

Since the 1960s, researchers have explored bacterial resistance to toxic metals, and since then a number of genes conferring metal resistance have been revealed. Whereas no single mechanism delivers total metal resistance, several simplified strategies can be generalized from the appreciable amount of literature that has interpreted physiological adaptations of metal stress (Harrison et al. 2007). First, many microorganisms will restrict the influx of metal ions by regulating the expression and activity of proteins involved in metal uptake. Similarly, metal ions that trigger cell stress can be removed from the cell through the activation of several efflux systems. Third, organic biomolecules, deliberately secreted in the extracellular and intracellular environment, can trap and sequester metal ions. Bacterial cells are also capable of repairing damaged biomolecules following reaction with metal species. Similarly, several bacteria are adapted to chemically modify metal ion species, altering their reactivity and toxicity in the cell. Lastly, once a metabolic protein is inactivated, bacterial cells are capable of using alternative pathways to bypass such damage (see reviews Harrison et al. 2004, 2007; Hobman and Crossman 2015; Reed et al. 2016).

Evidently, the mechanisms of antibiotic resistance and metal resistance are comparable. Metal resistance mechanisms are also found on transferable plasmids and transposons (Brown et al. 1995; Gupta et al. 1998; Kuenne et al. 2010). Research has shown that wastewater treatments plants are ecosystems with a high rate of gene transfer, mainly because human waste contains numerous antibiotics. These systems are reservoirs for antibiotic and metal resistance gene transfers (Szczepanowski et al. 2008). Searching against an antibiotic and metal resistance database, researchers have found that the plasmid metagenomes revealed broad-spectrum antibiotic and metal resistance, 323 out of a total 618 subtypes and 23 out of 23 types, respectively (Li et al. 2015). Whether there is a correlation between antibiotic and metal resistance is still up to debate, however, studies have concluded that metal ion resistance elements were carried on bacteria from the "pre-antibiotic era" (Hughes and Datta 1983), and share linked gene carriage

(Davies and Davies 2010). Furthermore, several metal resistance elements can now be found in new emerging and reemerging pathogenic organisms (Hobman and Crossman 2015).

6.6 Further Considerations

6.6.1 The Development of Metal-Based Antimicrobials

In the past 20 years, material-based science has seen an increase in the use of nanomaterials for advancements in technology. Inorganic antimicrobial nanomaterials, particularly nanoparticles, are no exception to this. These particles, which range from 1 to 100 nm, have the potential to deliver a controlled release of metal ions (Sotiriou and Pratsinis 2010; Gunawan et al. 2011), generate ROS (Zhao et al. 2005), disrupt membranes (Applerot et al. 2012), and can be targeted against specific bacterial or fungal cells (Ranghar et al. 2014). Nanoparticles that are embedded and impregnated into medical devices (Roe et al. 2008), textiles (Perelshtein et al. 2008), and food packaging (Echegoyen and Nerín 2013), are currently being investigated with promising potentials, and we are likely to see a steep increase in their use in the coming decades (Sondi and Salopek-Sondi 2004).

Studies have shown that the effectiveness of metals can be additive and synergistic when combined with other antimicrobials (Bayramov and Neff 2016). Combinations of quaternary cationic compounds and metals are used in industrial settings and for agricultural use (Harrison et al. 2008). Antiseptics such as chlorhexidine and sulfadiazine along with Ag have been impregnated into catheters, demonstrating a reduction in catheter-related bloodstream infections (Lorente et al. 2015). Sulfur crystalline structures of Sb and Bi have been synthesized and demonstrated to be effective antimicrobials against fungal and bacterial species (Joshi et al. 2017). Additionally, natural polysaccharide carbohydrate derivatives of sodium alginate surfactant-metal(II) complexes have been combined and evaluated against Gram-negative bacteria and fungi (Tawfik and Hefni 2016). In these complexes, the polyguluronic chains in the alginate form electronegative cavities that enable metal coordination, permitting for excellent antimicrobial activity and good biocompatibility (Shao et al. 2015). Furthermore, Ag adducts of branched histidine peptides have been synthesized and targeted for use against fungi such as *Candida albicans* and *Aspergillus fumigatus* with minimal antibacterial activity (Leng et al. 2016). Likewise, hydrogels, networks of hydrophilic polymers, have been combined with chitosan, a naturally abundant polymer in sea vertebrates, fungi, and other organisms, and Ag nitrate to produce solutions with antimicrobial properties that can be applied to textiles and other innate surfaces (Kozicki et al. 2016).

The aforementioned compounds demonstrate only a few of the possible antimicrobials produced and currently being developed; the possibilities are essentially endless. We are likely to see an increase in the production of nanoparticles and combination drugs in the near future. In fact, the use of these compounds has several advantages over traditional antibiotics and metal ions, some of which include, the ability to target species, controlled release, increased efficacy with less existing resistance, and greater biocompatibility and bioavailability.

6.6.2 Human Toxicity

In this chapter, we discussed the toxicity of metal compounds to microorganisms however, of the primary concern when considering their use is the toxicity to human cells. The toxicological profile of several metals such as Pb, Hg, As, and Cd have been well documented (Järup 2003). With the widespread use of Cu and Ag, and advancements of Ga and Ti-based products in human and animal medicine along with the agricultural industry, the toxicity of metals to humans makes for concern (Lemire et al. 2013). In the past several years, we have only just begun appreciating the complexity and importance of the human microbiome (Huttenhower et al. 2012). As a result, we must ask ourselves what role do metal antimicrobials play in disrupting this natural flora and how will their use impact our health? While identifying the targets of metal ions and metal compounds may assist in overcoming the uncertainties coupled to human toxicity, is current use warranted despite the potential risk?

6.6.3 Environmental Impact

Antibiotics consumed by animals and humans eventually find their way into the environment, polluting bodies of water and ecosystems. Researchers have observed increased levels of bacterial resistance downstream of municipal treatment plants (Lapara et al. 2011). Furthermore, a study concluded that elevated levels of antibiotic-resistant organisms could also be found downstream of animal feeding facilities, when compared to samples collected elsewhere (Pruden et al. 2012). Although the presence of metals such as Ag, Cu, Cd, Te, and other elements occurs naturally, metal environmental contamination continues to increase as a result of mining and smelting, domestic, medical and agricultural use, and industrial production. This has implications for human health, resulting in cancer, organ failure, and neurological damage, as well as environmental contamination (Tchounwou et al. 2014). We must consider if the use of metals in consumables, such as socks and shirts, is worth contaminating natural environments, altering microbial communities, and eventually our own food supplies as crops and produce accumulate these elements.

We know and understand more about antibiotic resistance than we have in the past. Yet, we are no closer to eradicating resistant bacteria; the numbers of species displaying resistance are on the rise and the development of novel antibiotics has essentially come to a halt. The propagation of resistance is an ecological problem, however, understanding the role of genes involved in resistance is a key component that we repeatedly overlook. One strategy that can be employed to reduce antibiotic resistance is to delay the evolution of resistance for novel antimicrobials, such as metals, by being more vigilant with their use. Unfortunately, we may already be late, as genetic determinants for resistance toward most metal antimicrobials exist. Furthermore, research has demonstrated that there is evidence for carry over between metal and antibiotic resistance genes (Davies and Davies 2010).

6.7 Conclusions

A survey of the use of metals in medicine and agriculture demonstrates that metals are promising. Some metals, such as Ga and Ag, have widespread use against bacteria and fungi, permitting for effective blanket treatments against unidentified microorganisms. For example, Ag has been shown to be effective in vitro and in vivo against Gram-positive (Ip et al. 2006), Gram-negative (Lemire et al. 2015), pathogenic and antibiotic-resistant bacteria (Kostenko et al. 2010), bacterial biofilms (Harrison et al. 2004; Bjarnsholt et al. 2007; Lemire et al. 2015), and fungi (Jung et al. 2007). Generally, low concentrations of metals display microbe toxicity. Combination treatments are further enticing, particularly as target specificity guarantees host safety.

With the current prevalence of antimicrobial resistance and the presence of microbial biofilms, the threat of pathogenic bacteria has developed into a standard healthcare and political concern; we are currently in the post-antibiotic era. With this in mind, we must reconsider if metal antimicrobials have a place on our tabletops, in our food containers, washing machines, air-filters, body washes, clothes, and lotions. Although far more research is required to understand precisely how metals induce killing and accompanying resistance mechanisms, we cannot help but ask ourselves if we are failing to recall history in our modernity by taking two steps backward after our perceived step forward.

References

Alexander JW (2009) History of the medical use of silver. Surgery 10:289–292

Aminov RI (2010) A brief history of the antibiotic era: lessons learned and challenges for the future. Front Microbiol 1:134

Andreini C, Bertini I, Rosato A (2004) A hint to search for metalloproteins in gene banks. Bioinformatics 20:1373–1380

Applerot G, Lellouche J, Lipovsky A, Nitzan Y, Lubart R (2012) Understanding the antibacterial mechanism of CuO nanoparticles: revealing the route of induced oxidative stress. Small 8:3326–3337

Arakawa H, Neault J, Tajmir-Riahi H (2001) Silver(I) complexes with DNA and RNA studied by Fourier transform infrared spectroscopy and capillary electrophoresis. Biophys J 81:1580–1587

Azarpazhooh A, Limeback H (2008) The application of ozone in dentistry: a systematic review of literature. J Dent 36:104–116

Bakalar N (2009) Penicillin, 1940. New York Times 6–7

Banin E, Lozinski A, Brady KM, Berenshtein E, Butterfield PW, Moshe M, Chevion M, Greenberg EP, Banin E (2008) The potential of desferrioxamine-gallium as an anti-*Pseudomonas* therapeutic agent. Proc Natl Acad Sci USA 105:16761–16766

Bayramov DF, Neff JA (2016) Beyond conventional antibiotics—New directions for combination products to combat biofilm. Adv Drug Deliv Rev (in press). https://doi.org/10.1016/j.addr.2016.07.010

Betts KS (2010) Body of proof: biomonitoring data reveal widespread bisphenol A exposures. Environ Health Perspect 118:a353

Bjarnsholt T, Kirketerp-Møller K, Kristiansen S, Phipps R, Nielsen AK, Jensen PØ, Høiby N, Givskov M (2007) Silver against *Pseudomonas aeruginosa* biofilms. APMIS 115:921–928

Bologna RA, Tu LM, Polansky M, Fraimow HD, Gordon DA, Whitmore KE (1999) Hydrogel/silver ion-coated urinary catheter reduces nosocomial urinary tract infection rates in intensive care unit patients: a multicenter study. Urology 54:982–987

Boonkaew B, Kempf M, Kimble R, Supaphol P, Cuttle L (2014) Antimicrobial efficacy of a novel silver hydrogel dressing compared to two common silver burn wound dressings: Acticoat and PolyMem Silver. Burns 40:89–96

Borkow G, Gabbay J (2009) Copper, an ancient remedy returning to fight microbial, fungal and viral infections. Curr Chem Biol 3:272–278

Borkow G, Gabbay J (2004) Putting copper into action: copper-impregnated products with potent biocidal activities. FASEB J 18:1–20

Borkow G, Zatcoff RC, Gabbay J (2009) Reducing the risk of skin pathologies in diabetics by using copper impregnated socks. Med Hypotheses 73:883–886

Borkow G, Zhou SS, Page T, Gabbay J (2010) A novel anti-influenza copper oxide containing respiratory face mask. PLoS ONE 5:e11295

Brown NL, Barrett SR, Camakaris J, Lee BT, Rouch DA (1995) Molecular genetics and transport analysis of the copper-resistance determinant (pco) from *Escherichia coli* plasmid pRJ1004. Mol Microbiol 17:1153–1166

Buonocore G, Perrone S, Tataranno ML (2010) Oxygen toxicity: chemistry and biology of reactive oxygen species. Semin Fetal Neonatal Med 15:186–190

Bush K, Courvalin P, Dantas G, Davies J, Eisenstein B, Huovinen P, Jacoby GA, Kishony R, Kreiswirth BN, Kutter E, Lerner SA, Levy S, Lewis K, Lomovskaya O, Miller JH, Mobashery S, Piddock LJV, Projan S, Thomas CM, Tomasz A, Tulkens PM, Walsh TR, Watson JD, Witkowski J, Witte W, Wright G, Yeh P, Zgurskaya HI (2011) Tackling antibiotic resistance. Nat Rev Microbiol 9:894–896

Cabiscol E, Tamarit J, Ros J (2000) Oxidative stress in bacteria and protein damage by reactive oxygen species. Int Microbiol 3:3–8

Chitambar CR, Narasimhan J (1991) Targeting iron-dependent DNA synthesis with gallium and transferrin-gallium. Pathobiology 59:3–10

Ciriolo MR, Civitareale P, Carrì MT, De Martino A, Galiazzo F, Rotilio G (1994) Purification and characterization of Ag, Zn-superoxide dismutase from *Saccharomyces cerevisiae* exposed to silver. J Biol Chem 269:25783–25787

Clarkson T, Magos L (2007) The toxicology of mercury and its chemical compounds. Crit Rev Toxicol 36:609–662

Cooksey C (2012) Health concerns of heavy metals and metalloids. Sci Prog 95:73–88

Costerton JW, Stewart PS, Greenberg EP (1999) Bacterial biofilms: a common cause of persistent infections. Science 284:1318–1322

Curtis LT (2008) Prevention of hospital-acquired infections: review of non-pharmacological interventions. J Hosp Infect 69:204–219

Davenport K, Keeley FX (2005) Evidence for the use of silver-alloy-coated urethral catheters. J Hosp Infect 60:298–303
Davies J, Davies D (2010) Origins and evolution of antibiotic resistance. Microbiol Mol Biol Rev 74:417–433
De Wit MJ, Dann J, Van Der Gaast S, De Ronde CEJ, Gerneke D (2001) Early Archean fossil bacteria and biofilms in hydrothermally-influenced sediments from the Barberton greenstone belt, South Africa. Precambr Res 106:93–116
Donlan RM (2009) Preventing biofilms of clinically relevant organisms using bacteriophage. Trends Microbiol 17:66–72
Donnell GMC (1999) Antiseptics and disinfectants: activity, action, and resistance. Clin Microbiol Rev 12:147–179
Dupont CL, Yang S, Palenik B, Bourne PE (2006) Modern proteomes contain putative imprints of ancient shifts in trace metal geochemistry. PNAS 103:17822–17827
Durand A, Azzouzi A, Bourbon ML, Steunou AS, Liotenberg S, Maeshima A, Astier C, Argentini M, Saito S, Ouchane S (2015) C-type cytochrome assembly is a key target of copper toxicity within the bacterial periplasm. mBio 6:1–10
Echegoyen Y, Nerín C (2013) Nanoparticle release from nano-silver antimicrobial food containers. Food Chem Toxicol 62:16–22
Ewald A, Glückermann SK, Thull R, Gbureck U (2006) Antimicrobial titanium/silver PVD coatings on titanium. Biomed Eng 5:22
Faúndez G, Troncoso M, Navarrete P, Figueroa G (2004) Antimicrobial activity of copper surfaces against suspensions of *Salmonella enterica* and *Campylobacter jejuni*. BMC Microbiol 4:1–7
Fleming A (1929) on the antibacterial action of cultures of a penicillium. Br J Exp Pathol 10:226–236
French GL (2010) The continuing crisis in antibiotic resistance. Int J Antimicrob Agents 36:S3–S7
Gant VA, Wren MWD, Rollins MSM, Jeanes A, Hickok SS, Hall TJ (2007) Three novel highly charged copper-based biocides: safety and efficacy against healthcare-associated organisms. J Antimicrob Chemother 60:294–299
Gomes A, Fernandes E, Lima JLFC (2005) Fluorescence probes used for detection of reactive oxygen species. J Biochem Biophys Methods 65:45–80
Gugala N, Lemire JA, Turner RJ (2017) The efficacy of different anti-microbial metals at preventing the formation of, and eradicating bacterial biofilms of pathogenic indicator strains. J Antibiot (in press). https://doi.org/10.1038/ja.2017.10
Gunawan C, Teoh WY, Marquis CP, Amal R (2011) Cytotoxic origin of copper (II) oxide nanoparticles: comparative studies and metal salts. ACS Nano 5:7214–7225
Gupta A, Maynes M, Silver S (1998) Effects of halides on plasmid-mediated silver resistance in *Escherichia coli*. Appl Environ Microbiol 64:5042–5045
Hall-Stoodley L, Costerton J, Stoodley P (2004) Bacterial biofilms: from the natural environment to infectious diseases. Nat Rev Microbiol 2:95–108
Hancock REW, Sahl HG (2006) Antimicrobial and host-defense peptides as new anti-infective therapeutic strategies. Nat Biotechnol 24:1551–1557
Harrison JJ, Ceri H, Stremick CA, Turner RJ (2004) Biofilm susceptibility to metal toxicity. Environ Microbiol 6:1220–1227
Harrison JJ, Ceri H, Turner RJ (2007) Multimetal resistance and tolerance in microbial biofilms. Nat Rev Microbiol 5:928–938
Harrison JJ, Turner RJ, Joo DA, Stan MA, Chan CS, Allan ND, Vrionis HA, Olson ME, Ceri H (2008) Copper and quaternary ammonium cations exert synergistic bactericidal and antibiofilm activity against *Pseudomonas aeruginosa*. Antimicrob Agents Chemother 52:2870–2881
Hobman JL, Brown NL (1997) Bacterial mercury-resistance genes. Met Ions Biol Syst 34:527–568
Hobman JL, Crossman LC (2015) Bacterial antimicrobial metal ion resistance. J Med Microbiol 64:471–497
Hughes VM, Datta N (1983) Conjugative plasmids in bacteria of the "pre-antibiotic" era. Nature 302:725–726
Huisingh D (1974) Heavy metals: implications for agriculture. Ann Rev Phytopathol 12:375–388

Huttenhower C, Fah Sathirapongsasuti J, Segata N, Gevers D, Earl AM, Fitzgerald MG, Young SK, Zeng Q, Alm EJ, Alvarado L, Anderson S, Arachchi HM, Bloom T, Ciulla DM, Erlich RL, Feldgarden M, Fisher S, Friedrich DC, Giannoukos G, Goldberg JM, Griggs A, Gujja S, Haas BJ, Hepburn TA, Howarth C, Huang KH, Kells C, Lennon N, Mehta T, Nusbaum C, Pearson M, Priest ME, Russ C, Shenoy N, Sykes SM, Tabbaa DG, Ward DV, Yandava C, Zucker JD, Birren BW, Knight R, Clemente JC, Lozupone CA, McDonald D, Abubucker S, Chinwalla AT, Fulton RS, Hallsworth-Pepin K, Lobos EA, Magrini V, Martin JC, Mitreva M, Sodergren EJ, Wollam AM, Appelbaum E, Bhonagiri V, Chen L, Clifton SW, Delehaunty KD, Dooling DJ, Farmer CN, Fronick CC, Fulton LL, Gao H, Herter B, Kota KC, Mardis ER, Mihindukulasuriya KA, Minx PJ, Oglaughlin M, Pohl C, Tomlinson CM, Walker J, Wang Z, Warren W, Wylie KM, Wylie T, Ye L, Zhou Y, Weinstock GM, Wilson RK, Badger JH, Madupu R, Bihan M, Busam DA, Scott Durkin A, Foster L, Goll J, Li K, McCorrison JM, Miller JR, Rogers Y-HH, Sanka RK, Singh I, Sutton GG, Thiagarajan M, Torralba M, Methé BA, Nelson KE, Creasy HH, Giglio MG, Wortman JR, Abolude OO, Arze CA, Cantarel BL, Crabtree J, Davidovics NJ, Felix VM, Jordan C, Mahurkar AA, Orvis J, Ravel J, Schriml L, White JR, White O, Muzny DM, Worley KC, Buhay CJ, Ding Y, Dugan SP, Holder ME, Jiang H, Joshi V, Kovar CL, Lee SL, Lewis L, Liu Y, Newsham I, Qin X, Reid JG, Wilczek-Boney K, Wu Y, Zhang L, Zhu Y, Gibbs RA, Highlander SK, Petrosino JF, Versalovic J, Aagaard KM, Allen-Vercoe E, Andersen GL, Armitage G, Ayvaz T, Keitel WA, Ross MC, Youmans BP, Baker CC, Begg L, Belachew T, Campbell JL, Deal C, Di Francesco V, Giblin C, Giovanni MY, Blaser MJ, Bonazzi V, Chhibba S, McEwen J, Peterson J, Proctor LM, Schloss JA, Wang L, Wellington C, Wetterstrand KA, Paul Brooks J, Buck GA, Rivera MC, Sheth NU, Canon SR, Chain PSG, Lo C-CC, Scholz M, Kyrpides NC, Liolios K, Markowitz VM, Mavromatis K, Pagani I, Chen I-MAMA, Chu K, Palaniappan K, Cutting MA, Hamilton HA, Harris EL, Dwayne Lunsford R, McInnes P, Davis CC, Desantis TZ, Dewhirst FE, Izard J, Lemon KP, Deych E, La Rosa PS, Shannon WD, Michael Dunne W, Watson MA, Edgar RC, Farrell RM, Sharp RR, Faust K, Raes J, Fodor AA, Forney LJ, Friedman J, Smillie CS, Garcia N, Gonzalez A, Knights D, Kinder Haake S, Hoffmann DE, Huse SM, Jansson JK, Katancik JA, Kelley ST, Rodriguez-Mueller B, King NB, Kong HH, Koren O, Ley RE, Koren S, Liu B, Pop M, Sommer DD, Lewis CM, Spicer P, Madden T, Mannon PJ, McGuire AL, Patel SM, Podar M, Vishnivetskaya TA, Pollard KS, Sharpton TJ, Truty RM, Rho M, Ye Y, Rhodes R, Riehle KP, Sankar P, Schloss PD, Schubert AM, Schmidt TM, Simone GA, Sobel JD, Treangen TJ, Yooseph S, Zoloth L, Conlan S, Segre JA, Chinwalla AT, Creasy HH, Earl AM, Fitzgerald MG, Fulton RS, Giglio MG, Hallsworth-Pepin K, Lobos EA, Madupu R, Magrini V, Martin JC, Mitreva M, Muzny DM, Sodergren EJ, Versalovic J, Wollam AM, Worley KC, Wortman JR, Young SK, Zeng Q, Aagaard KM, Abolude OO, Allen-Vercoe E, Alm EJ, Alvarado L, Andersen GL, Anderson S, Appelbaum E, Arachchi HM, Armitage G, Arze CA, Ayvaz T, Baker CC, Begg L, Belachew T, Bhonagiri V, Bihan M, Blaser MJ, Bloom T, Bonazzi V, Paul Brooks J, Buck GA, Buhay CJ, Busam DA, Campbell JL, Canon SR, Cantarel BL, Chain PSG, Chen I-MAMA, Chen L, Chhibba S, Chu K, Ciulla DM, Clemente JC, Clifton SW, Conlan S, Crabtree J, Cutting MA, Davidovics NJ, Davis CC, Desantis TZ, Deal C, Delehaunty KD, Dewhirst FE, Deych E, Ding Y, Dooling DJ, Dugan SP, Michael Dunne W, Scott Durkin A, Edgar RC, Erlich RL, Farmer CN, Farrell RM, Faust K, Feldgarden M, Felix VM, Fisher S, Fodor AA, Forney LJ, Foster L, Di Francesco V, Friedman J, Friedrich DC, Fronick CC, Fulton LL, Gao H, Garcia N, Giannoukos G, Giblin C, Giovanni MY, Goldberg JM, Goll J, Gonzalez A, Griggs A, Gujja S, Kinder Haake S, Haas BJ, Hamilton HA, Harris EL, Hepburn TA, Herter B, Hoffmann DE, Holder ME, Howarth C, Huang KH, Huse SM, Izard J, Jansson JK, Jiang H, Jordan C, Joshi V, Katancik JA, Keitel WA, Kelley ST, Kells C, King NB, Knights D, Kong HH, Koren O, Koren S, Kota KC, Kovar CL, Kyrpides NC, La Rosa PS, Lee SL, Lemon KP, Lennon N, Lewis CM, Lewis L, Ley RE, Li K, Liolios K, Liu B, Liu Y, Lo C-CC, Lozupone CA, Dwayne Lunsford R, Madden T, Mahurkar AA, Mannon PJ, Mardis ER, Markowitz VM, Mavromatis K, McCorrison JM, McDonald D, McEwen J, McGuire AL,

McInnes P, Mehta T, Mihindukulasuriya KA, Miller JR, Minx PJ, Newsham I, Nusbaum C, O'Laughlin M, Orvis J, Pagani I, Palaniappan K, Patel SM, Pearson M, Peterson J, Podar M, Pohl C, Pollard KS, Pop M, Priest ME, Proctor LM, Qin X, Raes J, Ravel J, Reid JG, Rho M, Rhodes R, Riehle KP, Rivera MC, Rodriguez-Mueller B, Rogers Y-HH, Ross MC, Russ C, Sanka RK, Sankar P, Fah Sathirapongsasuti J, Schloss JA, Schloss PD, Schmidt TM, Scholz M, Schriml L, Schubert AM, Segata N, Segre JA, Shannon WD, Sharp RR, Sharpton TJ, Shenoy N, Sheth NU, Simone GA, Singh I, Smillie CS, Sobel JD, Sommer DD, Spicer P, Sutton GG, Sykes SM, Tabbaa DG, Thiagarajan M, Tomlinson CM, Torralba M, Treangen TJ, Truty RM, Vishnivetskaya TA, Walker J, Wang L, Wang Z, Ward DV, Warren W, Watson MA, Wellington C, Wetterstrand KA, White JR, Wilczek-Boney K, Wu Y, Wylie KM, Wylie T, Yandava C, Ye L, Ye Y, Yooseph S, Youmans BP, Zhang L, Zhou Y, Zhu Y, Zoloth L, Zucker JD, Birren BW, Gibbs RA, Highlander SK, Methé BA, Nelson KE, Petrosino JF, Weinstock GM, Wilson RK, White O (2012) Structure, function and diversity of the healthy human microbiome. Nature 486:207–214

Imlay JA (2015) Diagnosing oxidative stress in bacteria: not as easy as you might think. Curr Opin Microbiol 24:124–131

Imlay JA (2013) The molecular mechanisms and physiological consequences of oxidative stress: lessons from a model bacterium. Nat Rev Microbiol 11:443–454

Ip M, Lui SL, Poon VKM, Lung I, Burd A (2006) Antimicrobial activities of silver dressings: an in vitro comparison. J Med Microbiol 55:59–63

Järup L (2003) Hazards of heavy metal contamination. Br Med Bull 68:167–182

Joshi S, Chauhan HPS, Carpenter N (2017) Preparation, spectroscopic characterization and antimicrobial activities of mixed metal (Sb and Bi) bridged derivatives with mixed sulfur donor ligands. J Mol Struct 1128:221–229

Jung WK, Kim SH, Koo HC, Shin S, Kim JM, Park YK, Hwang SY, Yang H, Park YH (2007) Antifungal activity of the silver ion against contaminated fabric. Mycoses 50:265–269

Jung WK, Koo HC, Kim KW, Shin S, Kim SH, Park YH (2008) Antibacterial activity and mechanism of action of the silver ion in *Staphylococcus aureus* and *Escherichia coli*. Appl Environ Microbiol 74:2171–2178

Kaneko Y, Thoendel M, Olakanmi O, Britigan BE, Singh PK (2007) The transition metal gallium disrupts *Pseudomonas aeruginosa* iron metabolism and has antimicrobial and antibiofilm activity. J Clin Invest 117:877–888

Karlin KD (1993) Metalloenzymes, structural motifs, and inorganic models. Science 261:701–708

Keele BB, McCord JM, Fridovich I (1970) Superoxidase dismutase from *Escherichia coli* B. J Biol Chem 245:6175–6181

Klasen HJ (2000) Historical review of the use of silver in the treatment of burns. I. Early uses. Burns 26:117–130

Kohanski AM, Dwyer JD, Collins JJ (2010) How antibiotics kill bacteria: from targets to networks. Nat Rev Microbiol 8:423–435

Kostenko V, Lyczak J, Turner K, Martinuzzi RJ (2010) Impact of silver-containing wound dressings on bacterial biofilm viability and susceptibility to antibiotics during prolonged treatment. Antimicrob Agents Chemother 54:5120–5131

Kozicki M, Kołodziejczyk M, Szynkowska M, Matusiak A, Adamus A, Karolczak A (2016) Hydrogels made from chitosan and silver nitrate. Carbohyd Polym 140:74–87

Kuenne C, Voget S, Pischimarov J, Oehm S, Goesmann A, Daniel R, Hain T, Chakraborty T (2010) Comparative analysis of plasmids in the genus *Listeria*. PLoS ONE 5:e12511

Laine L, Hunt R, El-Zimaity H, Nguyen B, Osato M, Spénard J (2003) Bismuth-based quadruple therapy using a single capsule of bismuth biskalcitrate, metronidazole, and tetracycline given with omeprazole versus omeprazole, amoxicillin, and clarithromycin for eradication of *Helicobacter pylori* in duodenal ulcer patients. Am J Gastroenterol 98:562–567

Lapara TM, Burch TR, McNamara PJ, Tan DT, Yan M, Eichmiller JJ (2011) Tertiary-treated municipal wastewater is a significant point-source of antibiotic resistance genes into duluth-superior harbor. Environ Sci Technol 45:9543–9549

Lemire JA, Harrison JJ, Turner RJ (2013) Antimicrobial activity of metals: mechanisms, molecular targets and applications. Nat Rev Microbiol 11:371–384

Lemire JA, Kalan L, Alexandru B, Turner RJ (2015) Silver oxynitrate has antimicrobial and antibiofilm efficacy. Antimicrob Agents Chemother 59:4031–4039

Leng Q, Woodle MC, Liu Y, Mixson AJ (2016) Silver adducts of four-branched histidine rich peptides exhibit synergistic antifungal activity. Biochem Biophys Res Commun 477:957–962

Li AD, Li LG, Zhang T (2015) Exploring antibiotic resistance genes and metal resistance genes in plasmid metagenomes from wastewater treatment plants. Front Microbiol 6:1025

Liau SY, Read DC, Pugh WJ, Furr JR, Russell D (1997) Interaction of silver nitrate with readily identifiable groups: relationship to the antibacterial action of silver ions. Lett Appl Microbiol 25:279–283

Liu J, Lu Y, Wu Q, Goyer R, Waalkes MP (2008) Mineral arsenicals in traditional medicines: orpiment, realgar, and arsenolitle. Perspect Pharmacol 326:363–368

Lorente L, Lecuona M, Jiménez A, Lorenzo L, Santacreu R, Ramos S, Hurtado E, Buitrago M, Mora ML (2015) Efficiency of chlorhexidine-silver sulfadiazine-impregnated venous catheters at subclavian sites. Am J Infect Control 43:711–714

Macomber L, Imlay JA (2009) The iron-sulfur clusters of dehydratases are primary intracellular targets of copper toxicity. PNAS 106:8344–8349

Macomber L, Rensing C, Imlay JA (2007) Intracellular copper does not catalyze the formation of oxidative DNA damage in *Escherichia coli*. J Bacteriol 189:1616–1626

Marino SM, Gladyshev VN (2010) Cysteine function governs its conservation and degeneration and restricts its utilization on protein surfaces. J Mol Biol 404:902–916

Massè A, Bruno A, Bosetti M, Biasibetti A, Cannas M, Gallinaro P (2000) Prevention of pin track infection in external fixation with silver coated pins: clinical and microbiological results. J Biomed Mater Res 53:600–604

Mehtar S, Wiid I, Todorov SD (2008) The antimicrobial activity of copper and copper alloys against nosocomial pathogens and *Mycobacterium tuberculosis* isolated from healthcare facilities in the Western Cape: an in vitro study. J Hosp Infect 68:45–51

Noyce JO, Michels H, Keevil CW (2006) Potential use of copper surfaces to reduce survival of epidemic meticillin-resistant *Staphylococcus aureus* in the healthcare environment. J Hosp Infect 63:289–297

Olakanmi O, Gunn JS, Su S, Soni S, Hassett DJ, Britigan BE (2010) Gallium disrupts iron uptake by intracellular and extracellular *Francisella* strains and exhibits therapeutic efficacy in a murine pulmonary infection model. Antimicrob Agents Chemother 54:244–253

Perelshtein I, Applerot G, Perkas N, Guibert G, Mikhailov S, Gedanken A (2008) Sonochemical coating of silver nanoparticles on textile fabrics (nylon, polyester and cotton) and their antibacterial activity. Nanotechnology 19:245705

Pomposiello PJ, Bennik MHJ, Demple B (2001) Genome-wide transcriptional profiling of the *Escherichia coli* responses to superoxide stress and sodium salicylate. J Bacteriol 183:3890–3902

Pruden A, Arabi M, Storteboom HN (2012) Correlation between upstream human activities and riverine antibiotic resistance genes. Environ Sci Technol 46:11541–11549

Ranghar S, Sirohi P, Verma P, Agarwal V (2014) Nanoparticle-based drug delivery systems: promising approaches against infections. Braz Arch Biol Technol 57:209–222

Reed RB, Zaikova T, Barber A, Simonich M, Lankone R, Marco M, Hristovski K, Herckes P, Passantino L, Fairbrother DH, Tanguay R, Ranville JF, Hutchison JE, Westerhoff PK (2016) Potential environmental impacts and antimicrobial efficacy of silver- and nanosilver-containing textiles. Environ Sci Technol 50:4018–4026

Ritz D, Beckwith J (2001) Roles of thiol-redox pathways in bacteria. Ann Rev Microbiol 55:21–48

Rochat T, Gratadoux JJ, Gruss A, Corthier G, Maguin E, Langella P, Van De Guchte M (2006) Production of a heterologous nonheme catalase by *Lactobacillus casei*: an efficient tool for removal of H_2O_2 and protection of *Lactobacillus bulgaricus* from oxidative stress in milk. Appl Environ Microbiol 72:5143–5149

Rodecka I, Martin C, Hill D (2014) The problem of microbial drug resistance. In: Phoenix AD, Fredrick H, Dennison RS (eds) Novel antimicrobial agents and strategies. Wiley VCH, p 439
Roe D, Karandikar B, Bonn-savage N, Gibbins B, Roullet J (2008) Antimicrobial surface functionalization of plastic catheters by silver nanoparticles. J Antimicrob Chemother 61: 869–876
Rosen BP (2002) Biochemistry of arsenic detoxification. FEBS 529:86–92
Rudyk O, Eaton P (2014a) Biochemical methods for monitoring protein thiol redox states in biological systems. Redox Biol 2:803–813
Rudyk O, Eaton P (2014b) Biochemical methods for monitoring protein thiol redox states in biological systems. Redox Biol 2:803–813
Rupp ME, Fitzgerald T, Marion N, Helget V, Puumala S, Anderson JR, Fey PD (2004) Effect of silver-coated urinary catheters: efficacy, cost-effectiveness, and antimicrobial resistance. Am J Infect Control 32:445–450
Saint S, Elmore JG, Sullivan SD, Emerson SS, Koepsell TD (1998) The efficacy of silver alloy-coated urinary catheters in preventing urinary tract infection: a meta-analysis. Am J Med 105:236–241
Santo CE, Lam EW, Elowsky CG, Quaranta D, Domaille DW, Chang CJ, Grass G (2011) Bacterial killing by dry metallic copper surfaces. Appl Environ Microbiol 77:794–802
Shao W, Liu H, Liu X, Wang S, Wu J, Zhang R, Min H, Huang M (2015) Development of silver sulfadiazine loaded bacterial cellulose/sodium alginate composite films with enhanced antibacterial property. Carbohyd Polym 132:351–358
Solioz M, Abicht HK, Mermod M, Mancini S (2010) Response of Gram-positive bacteria to copper stress. J Biol Inorg Chem 15:3–14
Sondi I, Salopek-Sondi B (2004) Silver nanoparticles as antimicrobial agent: a case study on *E. coli* as a model for Gram-negative bacteria. J Colloid Interface. Sci 275:177–182
Sotiriou GA, Pratsinis SE (2010) Antibacterial activity of nanosilver ions and particles. Environ Sci Technol 44:5649–5654
Swenson AM, Trivedi DV, Rauscher AA, Wang Y, Takagi Y, Palmer BM (2014) Magnesium modulates actin binding and ADP release in myosin motors. J Biol Chem 289:23977–23991
Szczepanowski R, Bekel T, Goesmann A, Krause L, Krömeke H, Kaiser O, Eichler W, Pühler A, Schlüter A (2008) Insight into the plasmid metagenome of wastewater treatment plant bacteria showing reduced susceptibility to antimicrobial drugs analysed by the 454-pyrosequencing technology. J Biotechnol 136:54–64
Tawfik SM, Hefni HH (2016) Synthesis and antimicrobial activity of polysaccharide alginate derived cationic surfactant-metal(II) complexes. Int J Biol Macromol 82:562–572
Tchounwou PB, Yedjou CG, Patlolla AK, Sutton DJ (2014) Heavy metals toxicity and the environment. In: Luch A (ed) Experientia supplementum. pp 133–164
Teitzel GM, Geddie A, De Long SK, Kirisits MJ, Whiteley M, Parsek MR (2006) Survival and growth in the presence of elevated copper: transcriptional profiling of copper-stressed *Pseudomonas aeruginosa*. J Bacteriol 188:7242–7256
Teitzel GM, Parsek MR (2003) Heavy metal resistance of biofilm and planktonic *Pseudomonas aeruginosa* heavy metal resistance of biofilm and planktonic *Pseudomonas aeruginosa*. Appl Environ Microbiol 69:2313–2320
Tenover FC (2006) Mechanisms of antimicrobial resistance in bacteria. Am J Infect Control 34: S1–S10
Thannickal VJ (2009) Oxygen in the evolution of complex life and the price we pay. Am J Respir Cell Mol Biol 40:507–510
Tsukihara T, Aoyama H, Yamashita E, Tomizaki T, Yamaguchi H, Shinzawa-itoh K, Nakashima R, Yaono R, Yoshikawa S (1994) Structures of metal sites of oxidized bovine heart cytochrome *c* oxidase at 2.8 A. Science 269:1069–1074
Valko M, Morris H, Cronin MTD (2005) Metals, toxicity and oxidative stress. Curr Top Med Chem 12:1161–1208
Waldron KJ, Robinson NJ (2009) How do bacterial cells ensure that metalloproteins get the correct metal? Nat Rev Microbiol 7:25–35

Wardman P (2007) Fluorescent and luminescent probes for measurement of oxidative and nitrosative species in cells and tissues: Progress, pitfalls, and prospects. Free Radicals Biol Med 43:995–1022

Warnes SL, Caves V, Keevil CW (2012) Mechanism of copper surface toxicity in *Escherichia coli* O157: H7 and *Salmonella* involves immediate membrane depolarization followed by slower rate of DNA destruction which differs from that observed for Gram-positive bacteria. Environ Microbiol 14:1730–1743

Warnes SL, Keevil CW (2011) Mechanism of copper surface toxicity in vancomycin-resistant enterococci following wet or dry surface contact. Appl Environ Microbiol 77:6049–6059

Wilks SA, Michels H, Keevil CW (2005) The survival of *Escherichia coli* O157 on a range of metal surfaces. Int J Food Microbiol 105:445–454

Wilks SA, Michels HT, Keevil CW (2006) Survival of *Listeria* monocytogenes Scott A on metal surfaces: implications for cross-contamination. Int J Food Microbiol 111:93–98

Wu FYH, Wu CW (1987) Zinc in DNA replication and transcription. Ann Rev Nutr 7:251–257

Xu FF, Imlay JA (2012) Silver(I), mercury(II), cadmium(II), and zinc(II) target exposed enzymic iron-sulfur clusters when they toxify *Escherichia coli*. Appl Environ Microbiol 78:3614–3621

Zhao H, Joseph J, Fales HM, Sokoloski EA, Levine RL, Vasquez-Vivar J, Kalyanaraman B (2005) Detection and characterization of the product of hydroethidine and intracellular superoxide by HPLC and limitations of fluorescence. PNAS 102:5727–5732

Chapter 7
Platinum in Biomedical Applications

Olga Sinitsyna, Priti Paralikar, Raksha Pandit and Mahendra Rai

Abstract For a long time, platinum (Pt) is used in medicine because of its outstanding properties such as biocompatibility, electrical conductivity, radiopacity, and durability. Despite the high cost of the noble metal, its unique properties were exploited in a large number of medical devices. These include stents, catheters, pacemakers, defibrillators, cochlear implants, and many others. Pt compounds play an important role in cancer therapy. In the age of nanotechnology, the horizon of the potential applications of Pt was substantially expanded. Nanostructured Pt-based materials were proposed for producing electrodes with advanced characteristics embedded in implantable electronic devices and sensors for detection of biologically important molecules. Pt nanoparticles (PtNPs) are perspective for the treatment of the diseases related to oxidative stress. It is expected that nanoparticle formulations will reduce adverse effects of Pt-based anticancer drugs. In this chapter, we review the traditional and new fields of Pt application in medicine. Special attention is paid to the questions of in vivo biocompatibility and corrosion behavior of Pt implants. In conclusion, we summarize the benefits of Pt usage for future medicine and diagnostics and indicate the problems to be solved to give the green light for the Pt-based new products to get entry in medical market.

Keywords Platinum · Biomedicine · Medical devices · Biocompatibility
Corrosion · Cancer therapy

O. Sinitsyna (✉)
Laboratory for Physical Chemistry of Polymers, A.N. Nesmeyanov
Institute of Organoelement Compounds of Russian Academy of Sciences,
Vavilova St. 28, 119991 Moscow, Russia
e-mail: sinitsyna@gmail.com

O. Sinitsyna
Department of Chemistry, Moscow State University, 119991 Moscow, Russia

P. Paralikar · R. Pandit · M. Rai
Nanobiotechnology Lab, Department of Biotechnology,
SGB Amravati University, Amravati 444602, Maharashtra, India

M. Rai et al. (eds.), *Biomedical Applications of Metals*,
https://doi.org/10.1007/978-3-319-74814-6_7

7.1 Introduction

Platinum (Pt) is a very expensive metal, and hence, it is used only in those applications where significant benefits are obtained. Pt demand in medical and biomedical sectors has been growing and has reached 8,227 000 oz [ounces troy, 1 kg is equal to 32.15075 oz (NIST 2017)] or about 255,888 kg in 2016, which is about 2.6% of total gross demand (PGM market report 2017). A great interest in Pt for biomedical applications is due to its outstanding mechanical and physico-chemical properties combined with biocompatibility. Pt^{2+} coordination compounds are of extreme importance due to their anticancer activity. In Fig. 7.1, the traditional applications of Pt in medicine are shown.

In the chapter, the main applications of Pt and Pt-containing materials in biomedicine are reported. In each case, an attempt is made to identify the reason why Pt is the best choice. For more details on the Pt application in biomedicine, the reader should consider the following sources. It is worth noting the modern and comprehensive review (Pedone et al. 2017) devoted to the applications of PtNPs in nanobiomedicine and a very informative review on nanoformulations of Pt-based anticancer drugs (Cheng and Liu 2017). The book (Woodward 2014) about the biomedical application of precious metals is highly recommended.

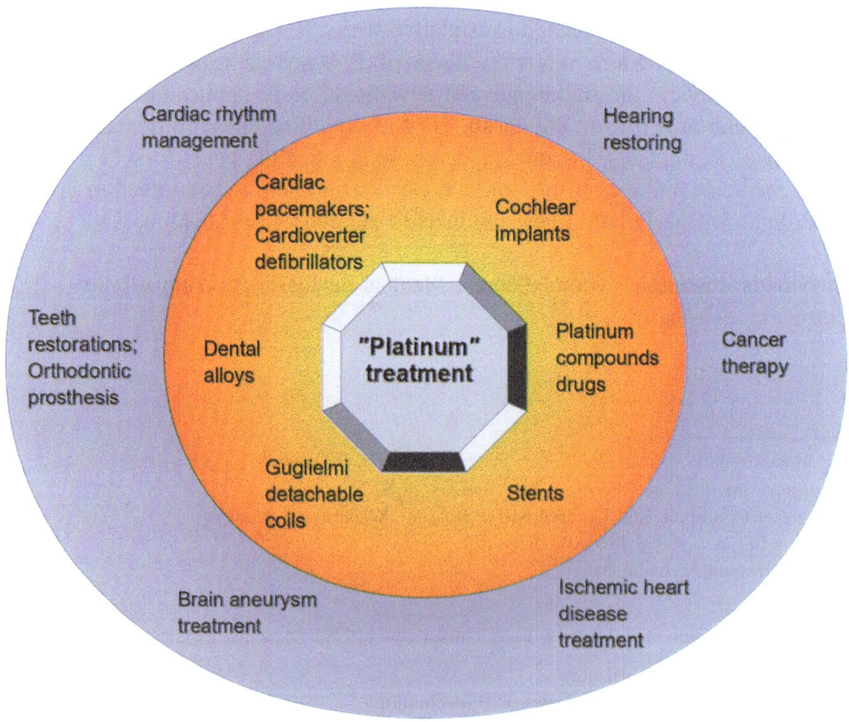

Fig. 7.1 Pt-contained medical devices and drugs

7.2 Pt in Implanted Medical Devices

Due to the outstanding properties of Pt, namely, biocompatibility, inertness, high melting point, excellent workability, electrical conductivity, and radiopacity, it is widely used to manufacture the essential components of permanently implantable medical devices. According to the World Health Organization (WHO) data for 2015, ischemic heart disease was the leading cause of death worldwide (WHO 2017). One of the mainstays of its treatment is coronary stenting. Stents are placed in the coronary arteries to keep them open using the procedure of balloon angioplasty. Owing to Pt high strength, corrosion resistance, chemical stability, and biocompatibility, Pt-containing stents have become an improved alternative to base metals stents (Fig. 7.2). They consist of Pt (33%), Cr (18%), Fe (37%), Ni (9%), Mo (3%), and a trace of Manganese (Mn) (Jorge and Dubois 2015). Greater strength of the Pt-contained alloy allows manufacturers to reduce strut thickness without compromising mechanical properties and radiopacity (providing enhanced X-ray visualization). Small strut thickness tends to improve the stent deliverability and contribute to better procedural outcome. Pt-contained stents have shown a similar clinical safety profile as stainless steel and CoCr (cobalt-chromium) stents during assessment in a non-diseased swine model (Menown et al. 2010).

Another impressive application of Pt wire is the endovascular management of brain aneurysms, especially inoperable ones (Woodward 2014). An aneurysm is filled with the coils (Guglielmi detachable coils), and after blood coagulation, a permanent seal forms.

Dentistry is another field where new Pt-contained products have entered the market. Noble alloys despite their cost continue to be used because of their excellent biocompatibility and corrosion resistance. Noble alloys can become the

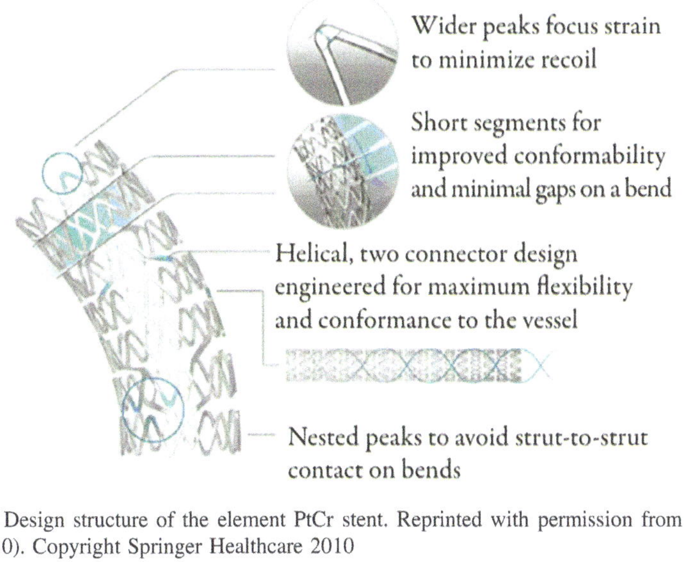

Fig. 7.2 Design structure of the element PtCr stent. Reprinted with permission from (Menown et al. 2010). Copyright Springer Healthcare 2010

only option for patients with contact allergy. Base metal alloys can develop corrosion couples with Ti-based implant fixtures; therefore, noble alloys are recommended for implant restorations. Traditionally, most dental high noble alloys contain at least 70% of gold, Pt, and palladium. Gold is the main component. The addition of Pt increases the melting point of the alloys and reduces their thermal expansion, which is necessary for dental porcelain bonding (Givan 2014). Noble dental alloys are being pushed out of the market, on the one hand, by cheaper base metals alloys (Co–Cr, Ni–Cr, and Ni–Cr–Be), on the other hand, by ceramics and titanium processed by CAD/CAM technologies (Givan 2014). Despite this, a new application of precious alloys was proposed in ceramo-metal teeth restorations known as Captek™ (Argen Corp., San Diego). Traditional noble alloys need thin surface oxide layer for porcelain bonding. In Captek™ gold lattice, strengthened with palladium and Pt, and porcelain interlock micromechanically (Vasani et al. 2009; McArdle 2011). Captek™ crown can be thinner than conventional metals, and they do not contain oxides capable to penetrate the surrounding gingiva.

Pt is an ideal electrode material for cardiac pacemakers, implantable defibrillators, cochlear implants, and other neuromodulation devices (Woodward 2014). Brain–computer interfaces, utilizing intracortical microelectrode arrays (MEAs), are perspective for the restoration of neurological function (Hochberg and Donoghue 2006). The arrays record neural activity. The obtained data can be used to control an artificial arm or a computer cursor.

7.3 Biocompatibility and Corrosion Behavior of Pt Implants

Few cases of contact allergy to Pt contained in jewelry were reported, but most likely, the allergy was related to other components of the alloys (Gedde and Roeder 2003). The presence of intermetallic compounds, such as $AuZn_3$ and Pt_3Zn, in high noble dental alloys can lead to their lower corrosion stability and biocompatibility (Colic et al. 2009). Pt shows no dissolution of artificial saliva (Knosp et al. 2003). Scanning electron microscopic evaluation of Pt scala tympani electrodes from auditory prostheses did not reveal any signs of corrosion after periods of implantation of up to 1000 days (Shepherd and Clark 1991). The corrosion resistance of the Pt stimulating electrode used as a cortical visual prosthetic in human was reported (Donaldson et al. 1985). But in more recent studies, fine particles of Pt were found in tissue surrounding cochlear implant electrodes after long-term implantation in human body, which could be a consequence of the electrodes corrosion (Nadol et al. 2014; Spiers et al. 2016; O'Malley et al. 2017). The pitting of Pt electrode operated in vivo for 4 years was revealed by scanning electron microscopy (Nadol et al. 2014). In another study, long-term impedance drops of chronically implanted MEAs in nonhuman primates were related to the corrosion of Pt (Barrese et al. 2016). In comparison with other studies, the sputtered Pt layers in the MEAs had a very low thickness of about 500 nm. The authors suggested that the corrosion was promoted by mechanical shearing effect caused by the device migration and long-term exposure to the reactive oxygen species (ROS), produced by immune cells during the foreign body reaction. The addition of iridium can improve the corrosive resistance of Pt-contained components. According to (Takmakov 2017), the corrosion of Pt electrodes can be ignored if their size is large, or they are implanted for a short period of time.

Although Pt is a biocompatible material, its implantation leads to tissue reactions. Multinuclear foreign body giant cells were frequently observed near the surface of Pt implants (Killer et al. 2010; Nadol et al. 2014). First, the body tries to dissolve the foreign body, secreting ROS, and then encapsulates it by the fibrous tissue. These effects increase the threshold for stimulation and reduce the signal amplitude from recording electrodes (Gedde and Roeder 2003). For example, in cardiac pacemakers, the pulse generator output is doubled to compensate the increase in threshold current caused by the electrode encapsulation. Anti-inflammatory drug-eluting devices are developed to reduce the thickness of the capsule (Stokes et al. 1983; Radovsky and Van-Vlect 1989; Bennett and Dubois 2013). Also, a reduction in an implant size is associated with smaller thickness of the capsule (Campbell et al. 1991). It is worth noting the importance of noninvasive implantation to the reduction of inflammation response and scar tissue formation (Young et al. 2017).

7.3.1 The Advantages of Nanostructured Pt Electrodes

Roughening of the electrode surface results in a large surface area without increasing the electrode geometric size. Thus, nanostructured electrodes should substantially decrease the impedance between the electrode and the surrounding tissue and increase the signal-to-noise ratios (Young et al. 2017). Nanoclusters and NPs coatings decrease the impedance and provide more stable measurements (Shah et al. 2013; Angelov et al. 2016). PtNP-coated electrodes caused a reduced inflammatory response (Angelov et al. 2016). Electrodes with Au–Pt nanoporous NPs coating showed very low impedance and high signal-to-noise ratios. Initially, the NPs consisted of Au–Pt–Cu alloy. The nanoporous were produced by Cu dissolution (Zhao et al. 2016). Electrodes, consisting of nanoparticles, can match the mechanical properties of a tissue better than electrodes consisting of bulk metal (Vitale et al. 2015).

It is impossible to implant electrodes in the deep regions of the brain, but NPs can be delivered there and act as remote neural interfaces. There are many methods of their remote activation, for example, by light, magnetic field, or ultrasound (Colombo et al. 2016).

The biosafety of nanostructured Pt electrodes should be carefully investigated, since PtNPs can potentially catalyze undesirable chemical reactions in physiological media. It was found that Pt black produced a denser capsule than Pt without a coating (Dimond et al. 1970). Pt black can be attributed to nanostructured Pt, since scanning electron microscopy and X-ray diffraction analysis revealed a porous network of Pt nanocrystals with the size of about 10 nm (Stanca et al. 2017).

Pt electrodes are of considerable interest for sensors of important biological molecules. It is known that diabetes mellitus, an endocrine disorder of carbohydrate metabolism, is a leading cause of morbidity and mortality; therefore, sensors for the determination of glucose level are in most demand. Enzymatic amperometric glucose biosensors are the most common devices (Yoo and Lee 2010). Immobilized glucose oxidase (GOx) is utilized to catalyze the oxidation of β-D-glucose by molecular oxygen with gluconic acid and hydrogen peroxide production. The amount of hydrogen peroxide molecules is proportional to glucose concentration in blood. Catalytic anode is required to oxidize hydrogen peroxide. The first commercially successful glucose biosensor was very expensive because of Pt electrode usage (Yoo and Lee 2010). Very thin Pt-containing nanostructured coatings may significantly reduce the cost of the sensors and improve their characteristics. PtNPs-contained sensors were developed to detect glucose, L-lactate, troponin, and cholesterol (Pareek et al. 2017).

7.4 Pt-Based Drugs for Cancer Therapy

Pt-based drugs have strengthened cancer therapy, as approximately half of the patients undertaking chemotherapeutic treatment receive Pt drugs. In the mid of nineteenth century, Peyrone for the first time prepared coordination complex with the formula *cis*-$[Pt(NH_3)_2Cl_2]$ and named the compound as Peyrone's chloride (Kang et al. 2015). The discovery of the antineoplastic properties of this complex by Barnett Rosenberg began the use of Pt-based compounds. Later, Rosenberg proposed that Pt complex could inhibit bacterial cell division, so it can be used to stop the uncontrolled growth of cell, which is a characteristic feature of cancer cell. In 1969, Rosenberg published his results that *cis*-$[Pt(NH_3)_2Cl_2]$ was effective in treating sarcoma 180 and leukemia L1210 in mice (Rosenberg et al. 1969). After 9 years of the initial publication, i.e., in 1978, Rosenberg described the anti-cancerous activity of this compound and later it was known as cisplatin (Rosenberg 1999). US Food and Drug Administration approved that cisplatin was approved by US Food and Drug Administration in the clinical treatment of genitourinary tumors (Smith 1979; Hoeschele 2009). Platinum-based anticancer agents are widely used as first-line drugs in chemotherapy. It can be used in the treatment of various solid tumors such as bladder cancer, ovarian cancer, melanoma, small cell lung cancer, and lymphomas. The disadvantages of Pt-based drugs are not a single drug is capable of treating all types of cancer, and Pt-based drugs can be inherently resistant to cancer cells (Shaili 2014). The use of cisplatin is limited, because of its side effects such as neurotoxicity, nephrotoxicity, ototoxicity, myelosuppression, intrinsic, and acquired resistance developed by various cancers (McWhinney et al. 2009). Carboplatin, nedaplatin, heptaplatin, and lobaplatin are similar to cisplatin and clinically used as anticancer drugs (Wheate et al. 2010; Johnstone et al. 2014a) (Table 7.1).

Table 7.1 Various platinum-based drugs

Platinum drugs	Treatment of platinum drug in different types of cancer
Cisplatin	Anal, bladder, esophageal, head and neck cancer, cervical cancer
Carboplatin	Ovarian, testicular, soft tissue carcinoma
Oxaliplatin	Colorectal cancer, esophagus, gastric cancer

After the initial work on the anticancer activity of cisplatin, inorganic chemists started preparing a variety of Pt complexes with different ligands and evaluated the antineoplastic effect of Pt-based complexes. It was found that the Pt complex has square planar geometry, neutral charge, and also contains two cis ammine ligands and two cis anionic ligands. Following the initial reports of the anticancer activity of cisplatin, inorganic chemists began preparing a variety of Pt complexes with different ligands and testing their antineoplastic effects. The anionic ligands could not bind Pt too tightly and hence, the activity would be decreased. If the ligands were labile, then compounds exhibited high level of toxicity (Wheate et al. 2010). Instead of using two amine ligands or two cationic ligands, researchers started using chelating diamine or chelating dicarboxylate. Extensive drug studies demonstrated the discovery of two more platinum-based agents, *cis*-diammine cyclobutane-dicarboxylato platinum (II) and *R*,*R*-cyclohexane-1,2-diamine oxalate platinum (II). In the United States, both the platinum-based agents were approved for clinical use by US Food and Drug Administration. The former compound platinum complex is referred to as carboplatin and the latter as oxaliplatin (Wheate et al. 2010; Johnstone et al. 2014b). To solve this problem, novel strategies need to be adopted for Pt-based chemotherapy. As compared with single-drug therapy, combined therapy is capable of reducing drug resistance by targeting different signal pathways. Combinational therapy provides higher therapeutic efficacy through synergistic effect as compared to single-drug therapy. Sometimes, some side effects can be observed as it is the combination of different drugs, which may vary in solubility, biodistribution, and pharmacodynamics. Combination of paclitaxel, docetaxel, and doxorubicin along with Pt-based drugs oxaliplatin, cisplatin, or carboplatin can improve the efficacy of anticancer therapy (Kang et al. 2015).

The second strategy is the use of nanotechnology. Modern nanotechnology has been employed in the delivery of therapeutics and diagnostics, which provide the possibility of targeted delivery of anticancer drugs. Nanoparticle-based delivery system can improve the solubility of drugs, reduce systemic toxicity, increase cell uptake, increase blood circulation time, and provide control release of drug. Nanoparticles can be used in the combination therapy, and nanoparticles can conjugate or encapsulate one or more drugs (Balducci et al. 2010). Combined drugs can be delivered to the target with minimum leakage as nanoparticles protect the drugs. Hence, research community all over the world is interested in nanoparticles-based drug delivery system for combination chemotherapy. Polymeric nanoparticles, solid lipid nanoparticles, and inorganic nanoparticles are developed for the delivery of Pt drugs. Polymer–Pt(II) conjugates such as AP5346 (oxaliplatin) and AP5280 (cisplatin) are being used in clinical study as both the drugs entered into phase II clinical study (Hu et al. 2010; Kang et al. 2015). Kataoka developed NC-6004, the polyglutamic acid Pt (II) drugs. In Japan, NC-6004 drug is used in phase II clinical studies whereas it is used as phase III clinical studies in the USA. One more example of Pt-based drug which is used as phase III drug is lioplatin. Lipoplatin can be used in the treatment of non-small cell lung cancer. As compared with combinational therapy, single-drug therapy is more successful (Plummer et al. 2011).

7.5 Nanoparticle Formulations of Pt Drugs

As mentioned earlier, cisplatin is drug of choice for treatment of different types of cancer, and most types of cancers are sensitive to Pt-based drug treatment. Cisplatin is a Pt-based drug used to treat the cancer of bones, muscles, soft tissues, blood vessels, etc. (Dasari and Tchounwou 2014). Different formulations were developed by cisplatin encapsulation in liposome with differences that consist in the Pt content, composition of lipid bilayer, and drug release profile. This type of formulation results in low lipid ratio with unstable system because of low hydrophilicity and lipophilicity of cisplatin-liposomal formulations, especially in bloodstream (Johnstone et al. 2016; Wani et al. 2016; Duan et al. 2016; Cheng and Liu 2017). Many nanocarriers are designed such as polymeric NPs, micelles, nanocapsules, and hydrogel for the cisplatin delivery (Callaria et al. 2014; Duan et al. 2016). Likewise, different formulations were prepared using polymeric NPs and Pt-based drugs for the treatment of various diseases. The formulations, namely, lipoplatin, SPI-077, Lipoxal, etc., are PEGlayted liposomal formulations used to carry cisplatin and oxaliplatin for treatment of ovarian cancer, gastrointestinal cancer, cervical cancer, etc. (Cheng and Liu 2017).

Moreover, formulation of cisplatin and DACHPt (Pt complex) encapsulated with PGlu-based micelle, namely, NC-6004 and NC-4016, was recommended for treatment of metastatic pancreatic cancer and various other tumors (Min et al. 2015; Cheng and Liu 2017). The other examples of micellar formulations approved for cancer therapy are Genexol-PM (Kim et al. 2007; Lee et al. 2008), NK105 (Hamaguchi et al. 2007), NK911 (Tsukioka et al. 2002; Matsumura et al. 2004), and nanoplatin-NC6004 (Uchino et al. 2005). Among these, Genexol-PM is first non-targeted micellar formulation approved for cancer therapy by Korea in 2006 for metastatic breast and NSCL cancer treatment as a first-line therapy (Kim et al. 2007).

Carboplatin-based formulations were developed especially for treatment of multidrug-resistant cancer cell lines. Carboplatin was incorporated in hybrid nanomaterial or in polymeric NPs via non-covalent interactions (Uivarosi et al. 2017). Carboplatin-polymeric formulations were developed by encapsulating the carboplatin with PLGA [poly(D-L-lactide-co-glycolide)] polymer. Sadhukha and Prabha in (2014) reported that carboplatin encapsulated polymeric nanocarriers exhibit anticancer activity against A549 (lung) and MA148 (ovarian) tumor cells.

The study revealed that nanocarriers enhanced the cellular uptake of carboplatin and improved therapeutic efficacy with minimum toxicity. Karanam et al. (2015) reported that poly (ε-caprolactone) NPs of carboplatin significantly showed cytotoxicity in human glioma cell lines. Khan et al. (2017) demonstrated the enhanced antiproliferative effect of chitosan-based formulations against MCF-7 breast cancer cell line. Moreover, Ahmeda et al. (2014) revealed that carboplatin loaded protein NPs exhibit significant cellular uptake with high encapsulation efficacy in retinoblastoma cells with sustained drug retention. The nanohybrid materials were also widely studied to improve the pharmacological profile of carboplatin. Balas et al. (2016) functionalized MWCNT (multiple functionalization of multiwalled carbon nanotubes) with amino group and antitumor drug carboplatin for treatment of human mammary adenocarcinoma-derived epithelial cell line MDA-MB-231. The resultant hybrid showed the considerable decrease of MDA-MB-231 cell viability with inhibition in protein expression. Similarly, another nanohybrid formulation by carboplatin loaded nanographene oxide–gelatin material also exhibits significant efficacy against human neuroblastoma cell line IMR-32 (Makharza et al. 2015).

Formulation of Pt drugs NPs has made a profound impact on management of cancer. The interaction between Pt drug and nanocarriers is a central strength of their performance. The use of such formulations will ensure the effective targeted drug release to tumor cells, and it will also help to deliver Pt resistant modulators. So, there are huge opportunities for research in this field and in future, and this nanoformulation technology may appear promising.

7.6 PtNPs for Biomedical Applications

High catalytic activity of PtNPs encourages to use them as artificial enzymes (nanozymes). Their main advantages are efficiency, selectivity, and insensitivity to the environment. PtNPs can mimic enzymes devoted to the control of ROS homeostasis, specifically catalase (CAT), glutathione peroxidase, and superoxide dismutase (SOD) (Hirakawa and Sano 2009; Li et al. 2016; Moglianetti et al. 2016; Ye et al. 2017). Thus, PtNPs are able to quench hydrogen peroxide (H_2O_2) and superoxide anions (O^{2-}). The mixture of Pt and palladium nanocolloid PAPLAL has been used in Japan over the past 60 years for treatment of conditions related to excessive reactive oxygen. The SOD and CAT activity of the Pt nanoparticles is significantly reduced due to oxidation in air and palladium NPs prevent this oxidative deterioration (Shibuya et al. 2014).

PtNPs show great potential for application in nanomedicine. Polyvinylpyrrolidone (PVP) coated PtNPs with dimensions of about 1–2 nm prolonged the life span of mutant nematode *Caenorhabditis elegans* with high level of oxidative stress (Kim et al. 2010; Sakaue et al. 2010). PtNPs (2 nm) with polyacrylic acid (PAA) coating were successfully used as therapeutic agents for cigarette smoking-related inflammatory lung diseases (Onizawa et al. 2009). A study in mice demonstrated that

PtNP-contained gel protected against UV-induced skin damage (Yoshihisa et al. 2010). Phytochemical-coated PtNPs showed antioxidant and neurorescue activities on the zebrafish model of Parkinson's diseases (Nellore et al. 2013).

Anticancer effect of PtNPs was found in several studies. Biosynthesized PtNPs showed anti-ovarian cancer activity without affecting the normal cells (Bendale et al. 2017). The type of capping agent is crucial for antitumor activity. High cytotoxicity of PtNPs with folic acid on MCF7 breast cancer cells was related to the increase in receptor-mediated endocytosis (Teow and Valiyaveettil 2010). Further studies are required to clarify the molecular mechanism of PtNPs antitumor effect. PtNPs were used to successful photothermal treatment of Neuro 2A cancer cells (Manikandan et al. 2013).

Much efforts are being made to find new antimicrobial agents, taking into account the increasing prevalence of bacteria with antibiotic resistance. Bacteriotoxic properties of PVP-coated PtNPs on *P. aeruginosa* were found in Gopal et al. (2013). It was shown that only small particles with the size less than 5 nm entered the bacteria. Another key parameter is zeta potential of the NPs. NPs with more negative zeta potential than the membrane potential of bacterial cells caused the rupture of the membrane and cell walls (Chwalibog et al. 2010). The bacteriotoxicity of PtNPs was demonstrated against Gram-negative *E. coli, P. aeruginosa* (Gopal et al. 2013; Konieczny et al. 2013; Ahmed et al. 2016), and Gram-positive *S. aureus* bacteria (Chwalibog et al. 2010). The mechanism of AuPtNPs antibacterial activity against *E. coli* was studied by Zhao et al. (2014). The authors suggest that bacteriotoxic effect of the NPs is caused by intracellular hyperproduction of adenosine triphosphate (ATP) and the reduction of cell membrane potential accompanied by the membrane disruption and the cell lysis.

The biosafety of PtNPs is still an open question. A number of studies reveal almost no cytotoxic effects of PtNPs (Elder et al. 2007; Hamasaki et al. 2008; Horie et al. 2011; Moglianetti et al. 2016). In other studies, PtNPs were found to be toxic (Asharani et al. 2010; Park et al. 2010; Teow and Valiyaveettil 2010; Manikandan et al. 2013; Yamagishi et al. 2013). The possible mechanism of toxicity is DNA damage by Pt^{2+} ions released from NPs (Pelka et al. 2009; Asharani et al. 2010; Gehrke et al. 2011). The presence of contaminants in PtNP solutions such as reaction by-products and Pt ions may be responsible for the toxic effects (Pedone et al. 2017).

7.7 Conclusions

The overview of modern applications of Pt-contained materials in biomedicine shows that new Pt-contained products continue to enter the market. It is believed that new highly effective drugs that exploit the antioxidant properties of PtNPs and anticancer activity of Pt compounds will be approved for use in near future. However, additional data are required on the mechanisms of PtNPs interaction with human body and biosafety of Pt nanomaterials. The long-term corrosion resistance of Pt components should be carefully evaluated.

References

Ahmed KBA, Raman T, Anbazhagan V (2016) Platinum nanoparticles inhibit bacteria proliferation and rescue zebrafish from bacterial infection. RSC Adv 6:44415–44424

Ahmeda F, Alib MJ, Kondapi AK (2014) Carboplatin loaded protein nanoparticles exhibit improve anti-proliferative activity in retinoblastoma cells. Int J Biol Macromol 70:572–582

Angelov SD, Koenen S, Jakobi J, Heissler HE, Alam M, Schwabe K, Barcikowski S, Krauss JK (2016) Electrophoretic deposition of ligand-free platinum nanoparticles on neural electrodes affects their impedance in vitro and in vivo with no negative effect on reactive gliosis. J Nanobiotechnol 14:3

Asharani PV, Xinyi N, Hande MP, Valiyaveettil S (2010) DNA damage and p53-mediated growth arrest in human cells treated with platinum nanoparticles. Nanomedicine 5:51–64

Balas M, Constanda S, Duma-Voiculet A, Prodana M, Hermenean A, Pop S, Demetrescu I, Dinischiotu A (2016) Fabrication and toxicity characterization of a hybrid material based on oxidized and aminated MWCNT loaded with carboplatin. Toxicol In Vitro 37:189–200

Balducci A, Wen Y, Zhang Y, Helfer BM, Hitchens TK, Meng WS, Wesa AK, Janjic JM (2010) Combination therapies for effective cancer treatment. Ther Deliv 1:323–334

Barrese JC, Aceros J, Donoghue JP (2016) Scanning electron microscopy of chronically implanted intracortical microelectrode arrays in non-human primates. J Neural Eng 13:026003

Bendale Y, Bendale V, Paul S (2017) Evaluation of cytotoxic activity of platinum nanoparticles against normal and cancer cells and its anticancer potential through induction of apoptosis. Integr Med Res 6(2):141–148

Bennett J, Dubois C (2013) A novel platinum chromium everolimus-eluting stent for the treatment of coronary artery disease. Biologics 7(1):149–159

Callaria M, Aldrich-Wright JR, de Souza PL, Stenzel MH (2014) Polymers with platinum drugs and other macromolecular metal complexes for cancer treatment. Prog Polym Sci 39:1614–1643

Campbell PK, Jones KF, Huber RJ, Horch KW, Normann RA (1991) A silicon-based, three-dimensional neural interface. IEEE Trans Biomed Eng 38:758–768

Cheng Q, Liu Y (2017) Multifunctional platinum-based nanoparticles for biomedical applications. WIREs Nanomed Nanobiotechnol 9. https://doi.org/10.1002/wnan.1410

Chwalibog A, Sawosz E, Hotowy A, Szeliga J, Mitura S, Mitura K, Grodzik M, Orlowski P, Sokolowska A (2010) Visualization of interaction between inorganic nanoparticles and bacteria or fungi. Int J Nanomed 5:1085–1094

Colombo E, Feyen P, Antognazza MR, Lanzani G, Benfenati F (2016) Nanoparticles: a challenging vehicle for neural stimulation. Front Neurosci 10:105

Colic M, Stamenkovic D, Anzel I, Lojen G, Rudolf R (2009) The influence of the microstructure of high noble gold-platinum dental alloys on their corrosion and biocompatibility in vitro. Gold Bull 42(1):34–47

Dasari S, Tchounwou PB (2014) Cisplatin in cancer therapy: molecular mechanisms of action. Eur J Pharmacol 740:364–378

Dimond AM, Kaechele LE, Jurist JM, Crandall PH (1970) Brain tissue reaction to some chronically implanted metals. J Neurosurg 33:574–580

Donaldson PE, Donaldson ND, Brindley GS (1985) Life of Pt and Pt–Ir stimulating electrodes in neurological prostheses. Med Biol Eng Comput 23:84–86

Duan X, He C, Kron SJ, Lin W (2016) Nanoparticle formulations of cisplatin for cancer therapy. WIREs Nanomed Nanobiotechnol 8(5):776–791

Elder A, Yang H, Gwiazda R, Teng X, Thurston S, He H, Oberdörster G (2007) Testing nanomaterials of unknown toxicity: an example based on platinum nanoparticles of different shapes. Adv Mater 19:3124–3129
Gedde LA, Roeder R (2003) Criteria for the selection of materials for implanted electrodes. Ann Biomed Eng 33:879–890
Gehrke H, Pelka J, Hartinger C, Blank H, Bleimund F, Schneider R, Gerthsen D, Bräse S, Crone M, Türk M, Marko D (2011) Platinum nanoparticles and their cellular uptake and DNA platination at non-cytotoxic concentrations. Arch Toxicol 85:799–812
Givan DA (2014) Precious metal alloys for dental applications. In: Baltzer N, Copponnex T (eds) Precious metals for biomedical applications. Woodhead Publishing is an imprint of Elsevier, Cambridge, UK, pp 109–129
Gopal J, Hasan N, Manikandan M, Wu HF (2013) Bacterial toxicity/compatibility of platinum nanospheres, nanocuboids and nanoflowers. Sci Rep 3:1260
Hamaguchi T, Kato K, Yasui H, Morizane C, Ikeda M, Ueno H, Muro K, Yamada Y, Okusaka T, Shirao K, Shimada Y, Nakahama H, Matsumura Y (2007) A phase I and pharmacokinetic study of NK105, a paclitaxel-incorporating micellar nanoparticle formulation. Br J Cancer 97:170–176
Hamasaki T, Kashiwagi T, Imada T, Nakamichi N, Aramaki S, Toh K, Morisawa S, Shimakoshi H, Hisaeda Y, Shirahata S (2008) Kinetic analysis of superoxide anion radical-scavenging and hydroxyl radical-scavenging activities of platinum nanoparticles. Langmuir 24:7354–7364
Hirakawa K, Sano S (2009) Platinum nanoparticle catalyst scavenges hydrogen peroxide generated from hydroquinone. Bull Chem Soc Jpn 82:1299–1303
Hochberg LR, Donoghue JP (2006) Sensors for brain–computer interfaces. IEEE Eng Med Biol Mag 25:32–38
Hoeschele JD (2009) In remembrance of Barnett Rosenberg. Dalton Trans 0:10648–10650
Horie M, Kato H, Endoh S, Fujita K, Nishio K, Komaba LK, Fukui H, Nakamura A, Miyauchi A, Nakazato T, Kinugasa S, Yoshida Y, Hagihara Y, Morimoto Y, Iwahashi H (2011) Evaluation of cellular influences of platinum nanoparticles by stable medium dispersion. Metallomics 3:1244–1252
Hu CM, Aryal S, Zhang L (2010) Nanoparticle-assisted combination therapies for effective cancer treatment. Ther Deliv 1:323–334
Johnstone TC, Alexender SM, Lin W, Lippard SJ (2014a) Effects of monofunctional platinum agents on bacterial growth—a retrospective study. J Am Chem Soc 136(1):116–118
Johnstone TC, Oark GY, Lippard S (2014b) Understanding and improving platinum anticancer drugs phenanthriplatin. Anticancer Res 34(1):471–476
Johnstone TC, Suntharalingam K, Lippard SJ (2016) The next generation of platinum drugs: targeted Pt(II) agents, nanoparticle delivery, and Pt(IV) prodrugs. Chem Rev 116:3436–3486
Jorge C, Dubois C (2015) Clinical utility of platinum chromium bare-metal stents in coronary heart disease. Med Devices: Evid Res 8:359–367
Kang X, Xiao HH, Song HQ, Jing XB, Yan LS, Qi RG (2015) Advances in drug delivery system for platinum agents based combination therapy. Cancer Biol Med 12:362–374
Karanam V, Marslin G, Krishnamoorthy B, Chellan V, Siram K, Natarajan T, Bhaskar B, Franklin G (2015) Poly(ε-caprolactone) nanoparticles of carboplatin: preparation, characterization and in vitro cytotoxicity evaluation in U-87 MG cell lines. Colloids Surf B 130:48–52
Khan MA, Zafaryab M, Mehdi SH, Quadri J, Rizvi MM (2017) Characterization and carboplatin loaded chitosan nanoparticles for the chemotherapy against breast cancer in vitro studies. Int J Biol Macromol 97:115–122
Killer M, Arthur AS, Barr JD, Richling B, Cruise GM (2010) Histomorphology of thrombus organization, neointima formation, and foreign body response in retrieved human aneurysms treated with hydrocoil devices. J Biomed Mater Res Part B: Appl Biomater 94B:486–492

Kim DW, Kim SY, Kim HK, Kim SW, Shin SW, Kim JS, Park K, Lee MY, Heo DS (2007) Multicenter phase II trial of Genexol-PM, a novel Cremophor-free, polymeric micelle formulation of paclitaxel, with cisplatin in patients with advanced non-small-cell lung cancer. Ann Oncol 18:2009–2014

Kim J, Shirasawa T, Miyamoto Y (2010) The effect of TAT conjugated platinum nanoparticles on lifespan in a nematode *Caenorhabditis elegans* model. Biomaterials 31:5849–5854

Knosp H, Holliday RJ, Corti CW (2003) Gold in dentistry: alloys, uses and performance. Gold Bull 36(3):93–102

Konieczny P, Goralczyk AG, Szmyd R, Skalniak L, Koziel J, Filon FL, Crosera M, Cierniak A, Zuba-Surma EK, Borowczyk J, Laczna E, Drukala J, Pyza E, Semik D, Woznicka O, Klein A, Jura J (2013) Effects triggered by platinum nanoparticles on primary keratinocytes. Int J Nanomed 8:3963–3975

Lee KS, Chung HC, Im SA, Park YH, Kim CS, Kim SB, Rha SY, Lee MY, Ro J (2008) Multicenter phase II trial of Genexol-PM, a Cremophor-free, polymeric micelle formulation of paclitaxel, in patients with metastatic breast cancer. Breast Cancer Res Treat 108:241–250

Li J, Lv L, Zhang G, Zhou X, Shen A, Hu J (2016) Core shell Fructus *Broussonetia*-like Au@ Ag@ Pt nanoparticles as highly efficient peroxidase mimetics for supersensitive resonance-enhanced Raman sensing. Anal Methods 8:2097–2105

Makharza S, Vittorio O, Cirillo G, Oswald S, Hinde E, Kavallaris M, Büchner B, Mertig M, Hampel S (2015) Graphene oxide–Gelatin nanohybrids as functional tools for enhanced carboplatin activity in neuroblastoma cells. Pharm Res 32:2132–2143

Manikandan M, Hasan N, Wu HF (2013) Platinum nanoparticles for the photothermal treatment of Neuro 2A cancer cells. Biomaterials 34:5833–5842

Matsumura Y, Hamaguchi T, Ura T, Muro K, Yamada Y, Shimada Y, Shirao K, Okusaka T, Ueno H, Ikeda M, Watanabe N (2004) Phase I clinical trial and pharmacokinetic evaluation of NK911, a micelle-encapsulated doxorubicin. Br J Cancer 91:1775–1781

McArdle BF (2011) Clinical indications for a composite-metal PFM restorative. Cosmet Dent 1:16–20

McWhinney SR, Goldberg RM, McLeod HL (2009) Platinum neurotoxicity pharmacogenetics. Mol Cancer Ther 8:10–16

Menown IBA, Noad R, Garcia EJ, Meredith I (2010) The platinum chromium element stent platform: from alloy, to design, to clinical practice. Adv Ther 27(3):29–141

Min Y, Caster JM, Eblan MJ, Wang AZ (2015) Clinical translation of nanomedicine. Chem Rev 115:11147–11190

Moglianetti M, De Luca E, Pedone D, Marotta R, Catelani T, Sartori B, Amenitsch H, Retta SF, Pompa PP (2016) Platinum nanozymes recover cellular ROS homeostasis in an oxidative stress-mediated disease model. Nanoscale 8:3739–3752

Nadol JB Jr, O'Malley JT, Burgess BJ, Galler D (2014) Cellular immunologic responses to cochlear implantation in the human. Hear Res 318:11–17

Nellore J, Pauline C, Amarnath K (2013) *Bacopa monnieri* phytochemicals mediated synthesis of platinum nanoparticles and its neurorescue effect on 1-methyl 4-phenyl 1,2,3,6 tetrahydropyridine-induced experimental Parkinsonism in zebrafish. J Neurodegener Dis 2013:972391

NIST (2017) Handbook 44. Appendix C. General tables of units of measurement. Available from: https://www.nist.gov/file/330151pdf

O'Malley JT, Burgess BJ, Galler D, Nadol JB (2017) Foreign body response to silicone in cochlear implant electrodes in the human. Otol Neurotol 38(7):970–977

Onizawa S, Aoshiba K, Kajita M, Miyamoto Y, Nagai A (2009) Platinum nanoparticle antioxidants inhibit pulmonary inflammation in mice exposed to cigarette smoke. Pulm Pharmacol Ther 22:340–349

Pareek V, Bhargava A, Gupta R, Jain N, Panwar J (2017) Synthesis and applications of noble metal nanoparticles: a review. Adv Sci Eng Med 9(7):527–544

Park EJ, Kim H, Kim Y, Park K (2010) Intratracheal instillation of platinum nanoparticles may induce inflammatory responses in mice. Arch Pharmacol Res 33:727–735

Pedone D, Moglianetti M, De Luca E, Bardi G, Pompa PP (2017) Platinum nanoparticles in nanobiomedicine. Chem Soc Rev 46:4951–4975

Pelka J, Gehrke H, Esselen M, Türk M, Crone M, Bräse S, Muller T, Blank H, Send W, Zibat V, Brenner P, Schneider R, Gerthsen D, Marko D (2009) Cellular uptake of platinum nanoparticles in human colon carcinoma cells and their impact on cellular redox systems and DNA integrity. Chem Res Toxicol 22:649–659

PGM market report (2017) May (2017). Johnson Matthey

Plummer R, Wilson RH, Calvert H, Boddy AV, Griffin M, Sludden J, Tidy MJ, Eatock M, Pearson DG, Ottley CJ, Matsumura Y, Kataoka K, Nishiya T (2011) A phase I clinical study of cisplatin-incorporated polymeric micelles (NC-6004) in patients with solid tumours. Br J Cancer 104:593–598

Radovsky AS, Van-Vlect JS (1989) Effects of dexamethasone elution on tissue reaction around stimulating electrodes of endocardial pacing leads in dogs. Am Heart J 117:1288–1298

Rosenberg B, VanCamp L, Trosko JE, Mansour VH (1969) Platinum compounds: a new class of potent antitumour agents. Nature 222:385–386

Rosenberg B (1999) In: Lippert B (ed) Cisplatin: chemistry and biochemistry of a leading anticancer drug. Verlag Helvetica Chimica Acta, Zürich, pp 1–27

Sadhukha T, Prabha S (2014) Encapsulation in nanoparticles improves anti-cancer efficacy of carboplatin. AAPS Pharm Sci Technol 5:1029–1038

Sakaue Y, Kim J, Miyamoto Y (2010) Effects of TAT-conjugated platinum nanoparticles on lifespan of mitochondrial electron transport complex I-deficient *Caenorhabditis elegans, nuo-1*. Int J Nanomed 5:687–695

Shah KG, Tolosa VM, Tooker AC, Felix SH and Pannu SS (2013) Improved chronic neural stimulation using high surface area platinum electrodes. In: 2013 35th annual international conference of the IEEE engineering in medicine and biology society (EMBC), Osaka, 2013, pp 1546–1549

Shaili E (2014) Platinum anticancer drugs and photochemotherapeutic agents: recent advances and future developments. Sci Prog 97:20–40

Shepherd BK, Clark GM (1991) Scanning electron microscopy of platinum scala tympani electrodes following chronic stimulation in patients. Biomaterials 12(4):417–423

Shibuya S, Ozawa Y, Watanabe K, Izuo N, Toda T, Yokote K et al (2014) Palladium and platinum nanoparticles attenuate aging-like skin atrophy via antioxidant activity in mice. PLoS ONE 9 (10):e109288

Smith GH (1979) New drugs released in 1978. Nurse Pract 4:35–41

Spiers K, Cardamone T, Furness JB, Clark JCM, Patrick JF, Clark GM (2016) An X-ray fluorescence microscopic analysis of the tissue surrounding the multi-channel cochlear implant electrode array. Cochlear Implants Int Interdisc J 17(3):129–131

Stanca SE, Hänschke F, Ihring A, Zieger G, Dellith J, Kessler E, Meyer HG (2017) Chemical and electrochemical synthesis of platinum black. Sci Rep 7:1074

Stokes KB, Bornzin GA, Weabusch WA (1983) A steroid-electing, low-threshold, low polarizing electrode. In: Steinkoff D (ed) Cardiac Pacing. Verlag, Darnstadt, p 369

Takmakov PA (2017) Electrochemistry of a robust neural interface. Electrochem Soc Interface 26 (3):49–51

Teow Y, Valiyaveettil S (2010) Active targeting of cancer cells using folic acid-conjugated platinum nanoparticles. Nanoscale 2:2607–2613

Tsukioka Y, Matsumura Y, Hamaguchi T, Koike H, Moriyasu F, Kakizoe T (2002) Pharmaceutical and biomedical differences between micellar doxorubicin (NK911) and liposomal doxorubicin (Doxil). Jpn J Cancer Res 93:1145–1153

Uchino H, Matsumura Y, Negishi T, Koizumi F, Hayashi T, Honda T, Nishiyama N, Kataoka K, Naito S, Kakizoe T (2005) Cisplatin-incorporating polymeric micelles (NC-6004) can reduce nephrotoxicity and neurotoxicity of cisplatin in rats. Br J Cancer 93:678–687

Uivarosi V, Olar R and Badea M (2017) Nanoformulation as a tool for improve the pharmacological profile of platinum and ruthenium anticancer drugs. In: Akitsu T (ed) Descriptive inorganic chemistry researches of metal compounds. ISBN 978-953-51-3398-8, Print ISBN 978-953-51-3397-1, Published: 23 Aug 2017 under CC BY 3.0 license. © The Author(s)

Vasani R, Kawashima I, Ziebert GJ, Berzins DW (2009) Metal-ceramic interface evaluation of a gold-infiltrated alloy. J Prosthodont 18:560–565

Vitale F, Summerson SR, Aazhang B, Kemere C, Pasquali M (2015) Neural stimulation and recording with bidirectional, soft carbon nanotube fiber microelectrodes. ACS Nano 9:4465

Wani WA, Prashar S, Shreaz S, Gómez-Ruiz S (2016) Nanostructured materials functionalized with metal complexes: in search of alternatives for administering anticancer metallodrugs. Coord Chem Rev 312:67–98

Wheate NJ, Walker S, Craig GE, Oun R (2010) The status of platinum anticancer drugs in the clinic and in clinical trials. Dalton Trans 39:J8113–J8127

WHO (2017) The top 10 causes of death. Fact sheet Available from: http://www.who.int/mediacentre/factsheets/fs310/en/

Woodward BK (2014) Platinum group metals (PGMs) for permanent implantable electronic devices. In: Baltzer N, Copponnex T (eds) Precious metals for biomedical applications. Woodhead Publishing is an imprint of Elsevier, Cambridge, UK, pp 130–147

Yamagishi Y, Watari A, Hayata Y, Li X, Kondoh M, Tsutsumi Y, Yagi K (2013) Hepatotoxicity of sub-nanosized platinum particles in mice. Die Pharmazie-Int J Pharm Sci 68:178–182

Ye H, Liu Y, Chhabra A, Lilla E, Xia X (2017) Polyvinylpyrrolidone (PVP)-capped Pt nanocubes with superior peroxidase-like activity. Chem Nano Mat 3:33–38

Yoshihisa Y, Honda A, Zhao QL, Makino T, Abe R, Matsui K, Shimizu H, Miyamoto Y, Kondo T, Shimizu T (2010) Protective effects of platinum nanoparticles against UV-light-induced epidermal inflammation. Exp Dermatol 19:1000–1006

Yoo EH, Lee SY (2010) Glucose biosensors: an overview of use in clinical practice. Sensors 10:4558–4576

Young AT, Cornwell N, Daniele MA (2017) Neuro-nano interfaces: utilizing Nano-coatings and nanoparticles to enable next-generation electrophysiological recording, neural stimulation, and biochemical modulation. Adv Funct Mater 2017:1700239

Zhao Y, Ye C, Liu W, Chen R, Jiang X (2014) Tuning the composition of AuPt bimetallic nanoparticles for antibacterial application. Angew Chem Int Ed 53:8127–8131

Zhao Z, Gong R, Zheng L, Wang J (2016) In vivo neural recording and electrochemical performance of microelectrode arrays modified by rough-surfaced AuPt alloy nanoparticles with nanoporosity. Sensors 16:1851

Chapter 8
Metal-Based Drugs for Treatment of Malaria

Paulo Ricardo Franco Marcelino, Mariete Barbosa Moreira, Talita Martins Lacerda and Silvio Silvério da Silva

Abstract Despite the incessant efforts to decrease exorbitant number of daily deaths, malaria remains a major threat to the public health in many countries. Transmitted by *Anopheles* mosquitoes, it is caused by infection with *Plasmodium* parasites that have become resistant to many antimalarial drugs. In this context, series of metal-based compounds have been screened for optimal activity against different *Plasmodium* species and strains. This chapter briefly reviews current and potential uses of metal complexes (such as iron, cobalt, nickel, gallium, copper, gold, and silver), metal chelators, and organometallic compounds, as interesting medicinal agents that greatly benefits the fight against malaria.

Keywords Malaria · Plasmodium · Anopheles · Metals · Drug

8.1 Introduction

Malaria is a neglected tropical disease caused by the protozoan of the genus *Plasmodium* and transmitted by the female *Anopheles* (*Culicidae*) mosquitoes (França et al. 2008). Probably originated in Africa, malaria has been plaguing the humanity for millennia, which can be inferred from documents of ancient civilizations that preceded the Christian era (Egyptians, Chinese, Mesopotamian, Hindus, Greeks, and Romans). Important figures in the human history, such as Pharaoh Tutankhamun and his family (1324 BC), Saint Augustine (579 BC), Dante Alighieri (1321 AD), and Charles V of the Holy Roman Germanic Empire (1558 AD), were affected by severe intermittent fevers (Celli 1925; Bruce-Chwatt 1988; Hawass et al. 2010; Fiocruz 2017).

P. R. F. Marcelino (✉) · M. B. Moreira · T. M. Lacerda · S. S. da Silva (✉)
Department of Biotechnology, Engineering School of Lorena,
São Paulo University, CEP 12602-810, Lorena, Brazil
e-mail: paulorfm1@hotmail.com

S. S. da Silva
e-mail: ssilverio@gmail.com

M. Rai et al. (eds.), *Biomedical Applications of Metals*,
https://doi.org/10.1007/978-3-319-74814-6_8

The great navigations and the consequent territorial conquests were the perfect opportunity for malaria to spread to other regions of the planet, being considered one of the most devastating diseases of North American colonies between the XVI and the XVIII centuries (Duffy 1953; Ackerknecht 1966; Russell 1968). At the XVIII century, Italians thought that the symptoms of intermittent fever were due to unhealthy air—"*mal aire*"—and that expression gave rise to the current name of the disease, malaria. In South America, this disease arrived through the ships that brought the slaves to work mainly in Brazil (Yalcindag et al. 2012). At the XVII century, as the mortality increased, South American, Indians, and Jesuit priests started using teas and beverages prepared with *Cinchona* sp. as treatment (Lee 2002; Ockenhouse et al. 2005). In 1820, Pierre Pelletier and Joseph Caventau isolated quinine from *Cinchona* sp., proved its antimalarial effect, and in the next year, quinine and quinine sulfate were commercially available as the first anti-malarial drugs (Cunico et al. 2008). Despite the discovery of an effective active principle, it took some decades to elucidate the causes of malaria. It was in 1880 that the French physician Charles Alphonse Laveran observed the malaria-causing protozoa in red blood cells of one of his patients. Between 1897 and 1899, Italian researchers Amico Bignami, Giuseppe Bastianelli, Battista Grassi, and the English physician Ronald Ross identified the female of the *Anopheles* mosquito as the transmitter of *Plasmodium* protozoan to the mammals and defined its life cycle, for which he was awarded Nobel Prizes in 1902 and 1907 (Keeble 1997; Despomnier et al. 2006; FioCruz 2017).

Up to the I World War, quinine was the only drug used to treat malaria. The difficulty to obtain the bark of *Cinchona* motivated the Germans to develop, in 1920, a synthetic molecule, 9-aminoacridine, that has been marketed since 1930 by the trade name Atabrine (Wallace 1989). Despite the advances, the countries involved in the I World War reported large decrease in their populations due to malaria. In the XI Pan American Sanitary Conference in 1942, malaria was identified as the continent's most devastating disease (Rocha et al. 2006).

In the II World War, also driven by the inherent difficulties for the extraction of quinine from the bark of *Cinchona*, the United States started working in 1942 on an alternative synthetic drug, Atabrine (Curico et al. 2008). A couple of years later, american researchers in collaboration with pharmaceutical industries attempted to produce a synthetic quinine, but technical drawbacks and the large-scale production costs made this attempt impossible (Lee 2002).

The failures in the laboratory synthesis of quinine greatly motivated researches for the prospection of new antimalarial drugs such as Amodiaquine, Primaquine, Proguanil, Pyrimethamine, and Chloroquine (Boss et al. 2003; Ockenhouse et al. 2005; Silva et al. 2005). Chloroquine has been highlighted among these drugs due to its efficiency, low production costs, low toxicity, and the possibility of being consumed by pregnant women. These advantages made chloroquine the first choice in the treatment of malaria (Robert et al. 2001; Silva et al. 2005).

During the Korean (1950–1953) and Vietnam (1950–1957) wars, the US Army observed that some malaria patients did not respond to chloroquine. Again, a new drug prospection program was conducted, in which Dapsone, Pyrimethamine,

Sulfadoxine, Sulfalene, Mefloquine, and Halofantrine were developed (Boss et al. 2003; Foley et al. 2005; Ockenhouse et al. 2005; Nzila et al. 2006).

More recently, it was observed that the number of *Plasmodium* strains resistant to the drugs available on the market has increased dramatically, and researches for the discovery of new antimalarial drugs have become increasingly necessary. Some emerging countries like Brazil, India, and China have invested extensively in researches for the treatment of neglected tropical diseases, especially malaria. In the 1970s, Chinese researchers presented artemisinin and its semisynthetic derivatives (Artemether, Arteether, Artesunate, Artemisinic acid, and Dihydroartemisin) as potential antimalarial drugs (Li et al. 1998; Prince 2000; Haynes 2001). The success of these drugs in the treatment of malaria is due to the fact that the *Plasmodium* strains have still little or no resistance to them.

Currently, statistics related to the number of malaria deaths are lower than in previous decades, with a decrease of approximately 52% in the last 15 years (Fig. 8.1). However, malaria is still present in 108 countries, and in 2015, it was estimated that 212 million people were affected by the disease, with most of the cases concentrated in Southeast Asia, sub-Saharan Africa, and Amazon due to their tropical or subtropical climates that favor the survival and reproduction of *Anopheles* mosquitoes. Also, countries with the highest number of malaria cases are in regions with poor sanitary conditions that also favor the reproduction and development of the malaria vector.

Projects such as the "Roll Back Malaria Partnership" (RBM) must invest approximately 93 billion euros until 2030 (www.rollbackmalaria.org) for the treatment and total eradication of malaria. However, the success of such initiatives can be compromised once again by problems caused by the resistance of *Plasmodium* lineages. For this reason, research for the development of new antimalarial drugs must be constant. Recently, metal-based drugs have been actively explored for the treatment of a variety of parasites, with an important effect in the treatment of malaria. The following paragraphs aim to present the state-of-the-art of such strategy.

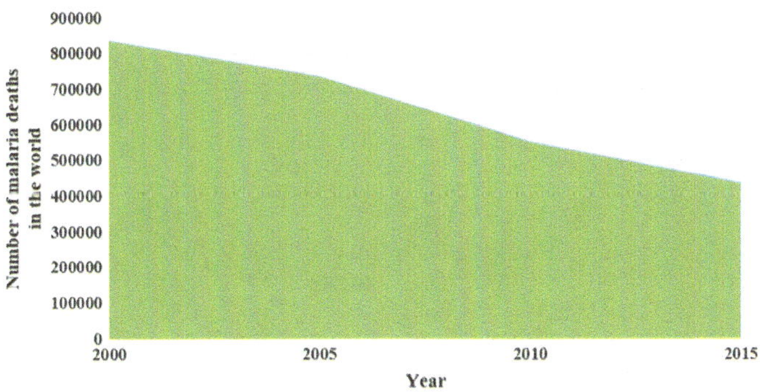

Fig. 8.1 Number of malaria deaths in the world in the last 15 years (*Source* World Health Organization 2017)

8.2 General Aspects of Malaria: The Mechanisms of Action of Classic Drugs and the Resistance of the Protozoan

Malaria is a protozoan infection caused by *Plasmodium* (*P. falciparum, P. vivax, P. ovale* and *P. malariae*), with *P. falciparum* being the most dangerous form of the disease due to the related highest rates of complications and mortality. The main vector to humans and other mammals is mosquitoes of the genus *Anopheles*, which comprises more than 400 species, with only a few epidemiologically important. These mosquitoes have nocturnal habits, and only females feed on blood and are responsible for the transmission of the *Plasmodium* (Rabinovitch et al.1998; FioCruz 2017).

The life cycle of the protozoan is divided between a host and an insect vector, as briefly described below and illustrated schematically in Fig. 8.2. (**I**) By stinging the host, the sporozoite form of *Plasmodium*, lodged in the mosquito's salivary glands, is injected into the bloodstream until it reaches the liver. (**II**) In hepatic cells, the sporozoites reproduce asexually generating other cells called merozoite (not all merozoites reproduce asexually, some develop sexually). (**III**) The merozoites destroy the erythrocytes, causing anemia in the host and initiating a series of reproductive cycles. (**IV**) Some merozoites will become immature gametocytes, precursors of male and female gametes. (**V**) By re-stinging the host, the

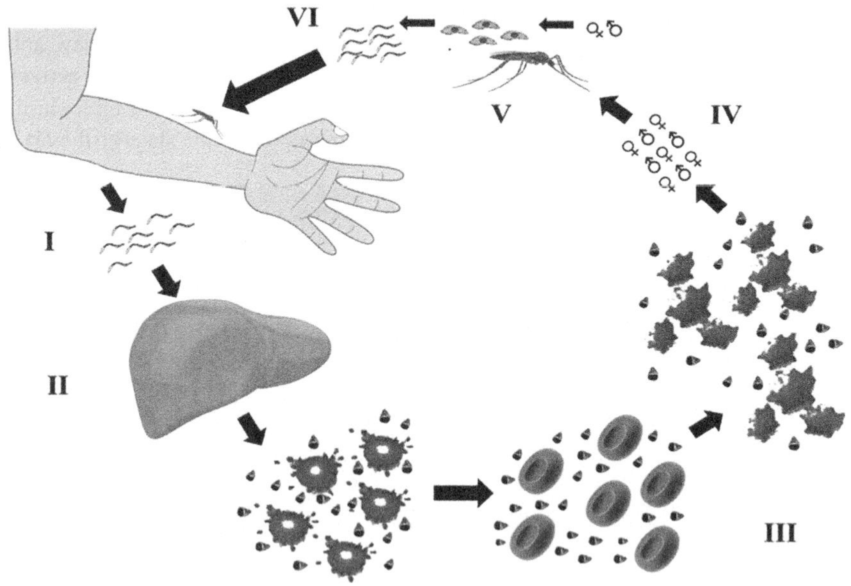

Fig. 8.2 *Plasmodium* life cycle. The stages **I–IV** occur in the host cells and stages **V** and **VI** occur in the *Anopheles* mosquito

gametocytes will be collected and matured in the mosquito's digestive system. **(VI)** The fusion of gametocytes will result in zygotes (also named as ookinetes) that will subsequently be converted into sporozoites, which migrate to the salivary glands of the mosquito, thus initiating a new infectious cycle (Rabinovitch et al. 1998; Cunico et al. 2008; FioCruz 2017).

The knowledge of the *Plasmodium* life cycle is of fundamental interest in the selection and administration of drugs for the treatment of the infected host. According to Korolkovas and Burckhalter (1982), the antimalarials commonly used act on the evolutionary stage of the parasite and can be classified as follows:

(I) Blood schizonticides or suppressive agents: drugs that act on the asexual forms of the parasite found in the bloodstream;
(II) Tissue schizonticides: drugs that act on the asexual forms of the parasite found in the tissues;
(III) Gametocytes: drugs that act on the sexual forms of the parasites;
(IV) Sporonticides: drugs that act indirectly on the vegetative forms found in the mosquito vector through gametocytes;
(V) Sporozoiticides: drugs that act on the forms of the parasite infecting the host.

The effects of the above antimalarial drugs on parasite cells are variable according to the infecting species; however, these drugs may act as hemozoin production inhibitors, folic acid synthesis inhibitors, transcription inhibitors or inhibitors of the mitochondrial respiratory chain, transport proteins inhibitors, and genetic material modifiers (Cunico et al. 2008; Rai et al. 2017). Table 8.1 shows the main classes of antimalarial used, their molecular structures, and their effects on the parasite.

The importance of drugs with the quinoline group (highlighted in bold in the structural formulas of Table 8.1) is highlighted in several drugs, especially synthetic quinine derivatives that in the last century have achieved significant space in the pharmaceutical market. In addition to the antimalarial effect, recent studies have shown that the active ingredients quinolinics and derivatives presented antiviral activity (antiviral) (Achan et al. 2011; www.cureffi.org).

Despite a variety of drugs used in the treatment of malaria, *Plasmodium* species have become resistant to many compounds. Sibley and Ringwald (2007) reported that the emergence of resistance to antimalarial drugs is directly related to an enormous amount of pathogenic populations and the short time of reproduction of the parasite. In addition, the indiscriminate and extensive use of antimalarial drugs also contributes to the process of resistance.

Trying to solve this issue, the World Health Organization (WHO) recommends the use of combinations of antimalaria drugs instead of monotherapy, mainly Artemether/Lumefantrine, Artesunate/Amodiaquine, Artesunate/Mefloquine, Artesunate/Sulfadoxine, and Artesunate/Pyrimethamine (WHO 2007; Cunico et al. 2008). Some in vitro studies demonstrated that the compounds verapamil, desipramine, and promethazine may reverse the resistance of *P. falciparum* to

Table 8.1 Main classes of antimalarial drugs used in the treatment and their effects on the parasite

Classes of antimalarial drugs and effects on the parasite	Main Drugs used on treatment	
Aryl-alcohols: hemozoin production inhibitors	**Quinine**	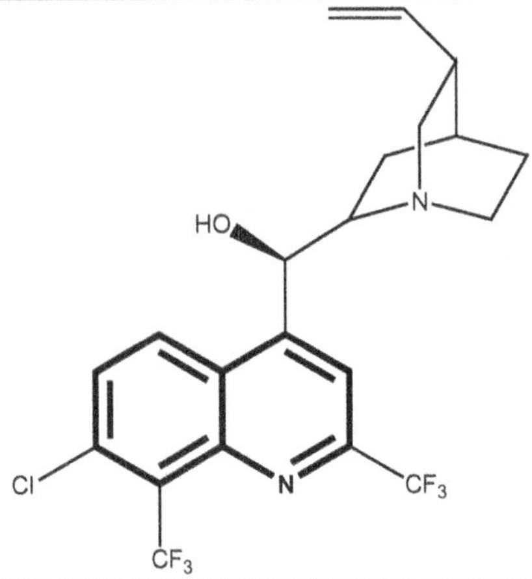
	Mefloquine	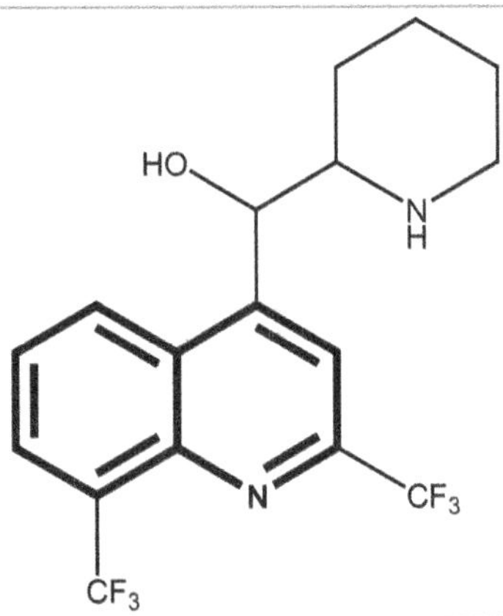
	Halo-fantrine	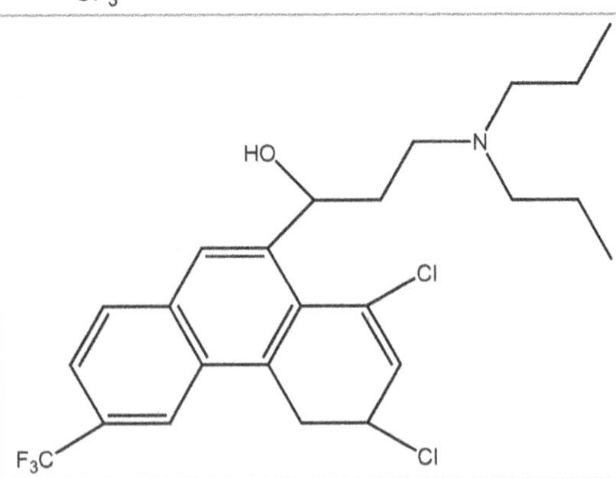

(continued)

Table 8.1 (continued)

Classes of antimalarial drugs and effects on the parasite	Main Drugs used on treatment	
	Pyronar-idine	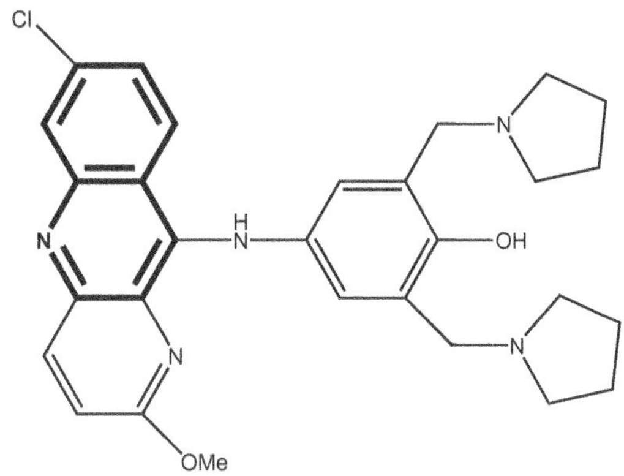
	Lume-fantrine	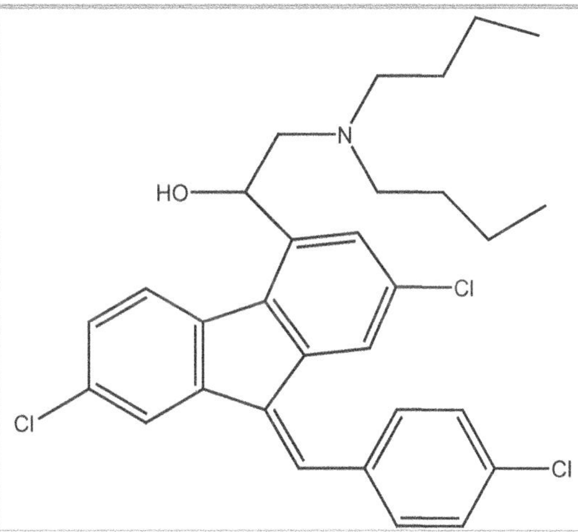
Artemisinin and derivatives: hemozoin production inhibitors, mitochondrial respiratory chain inhibitors, and transport proteins	**Artemisin**	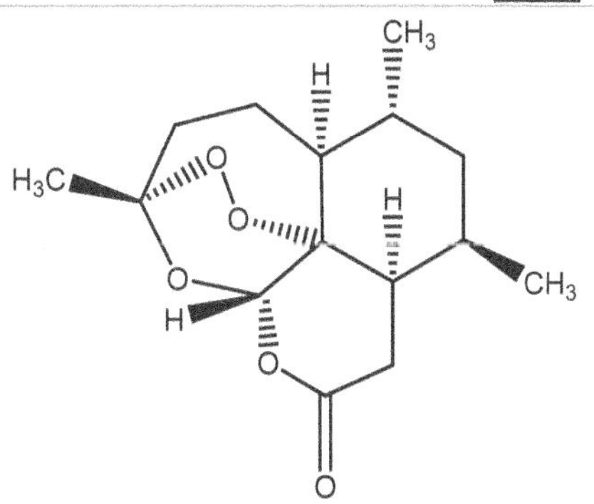

(continued)

Table 8.1 (continued)

Classes of antimalarial drugs and effects on the parasite	Main Drugs used on treatment	
	Artemether	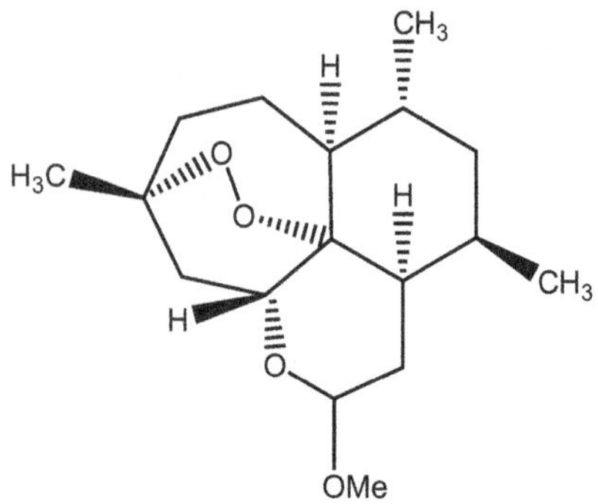
	Arteether	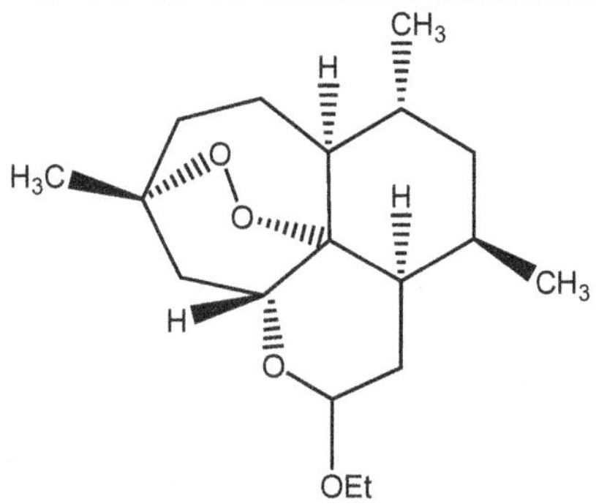
	Artesunate	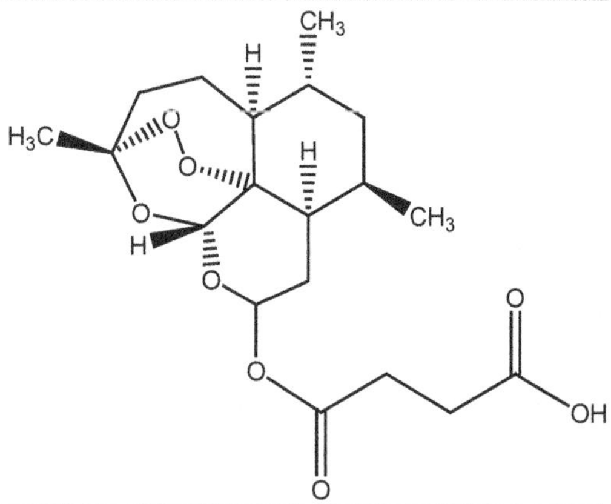

(continued)

Table 8.1 (continued)

Classes of antimalarial drugs and effects on the parasite	Main Drugs used on treatment	
	Artenilic acid	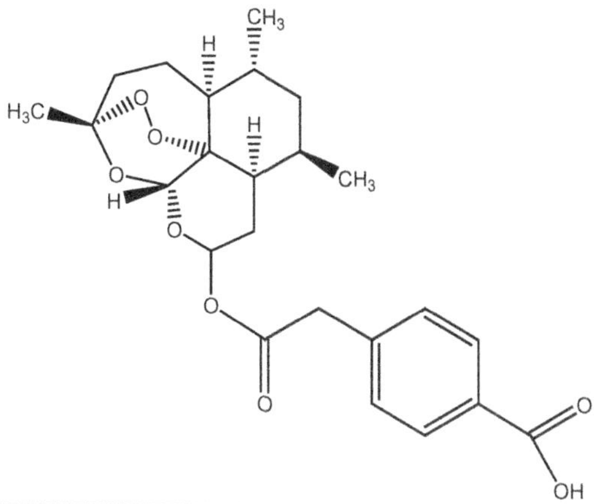
	Dihydroartemisin	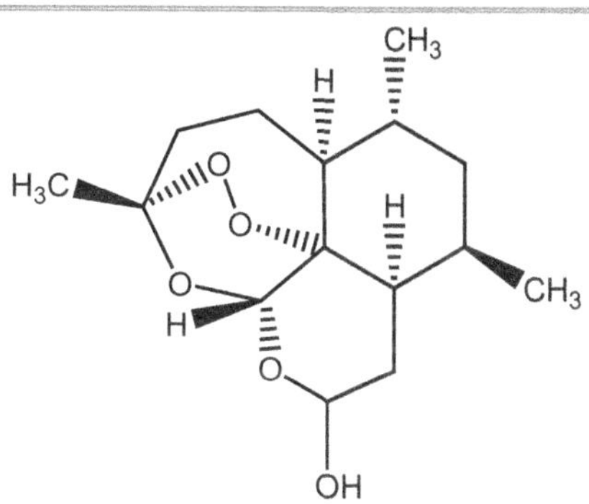
Biguanides and derivatives: folic acid synthesis inhibitors	**Chloro-proguanil**	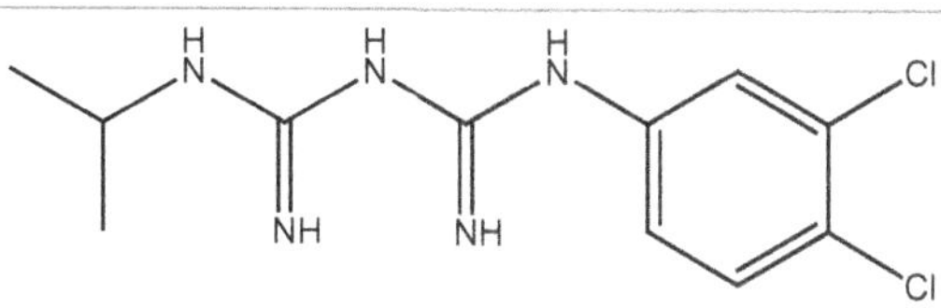
	Cyclo-chloro-proguanil	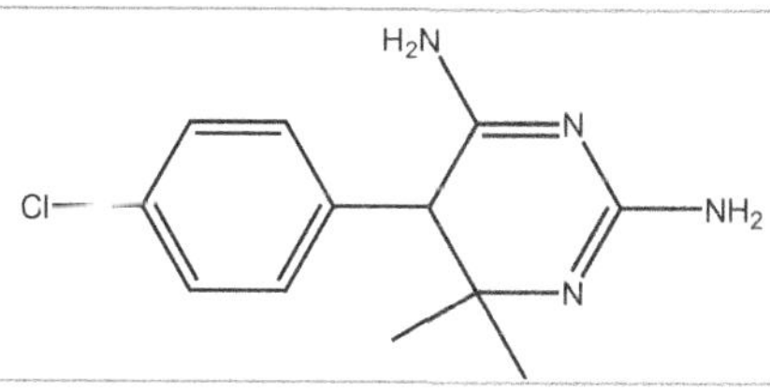

(continued)

Table 8.1 (continued)

Classes of antimalarial drugs and effects on the parasite	Main Drugs used on treatment	
Naphthoquinones: mitochondrial respiratory chain inhibitors	**Atovaquone**	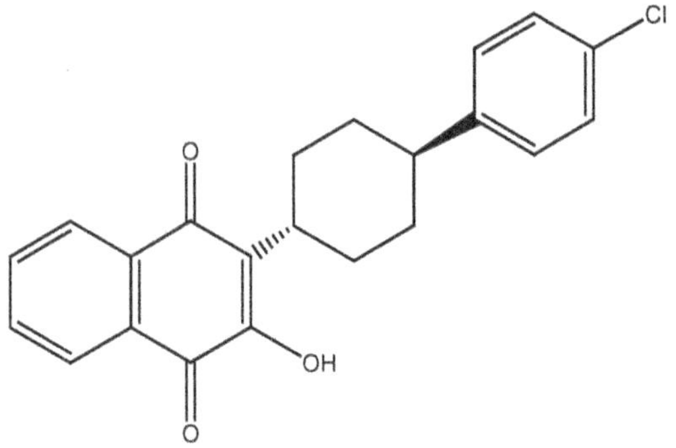
	Ubiquinone	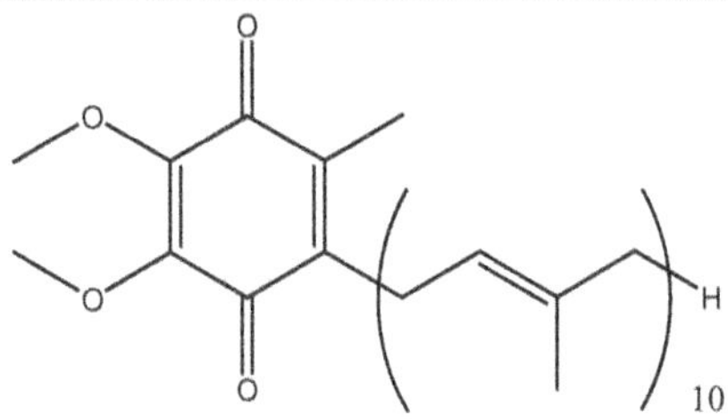
Quinolines: hemozoin production inhibitors and genetic material (DNA) modifiers	**Amodiaquine**	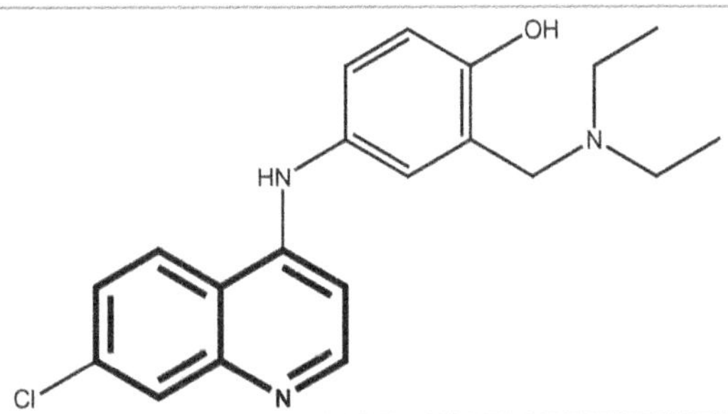
	Primaquine	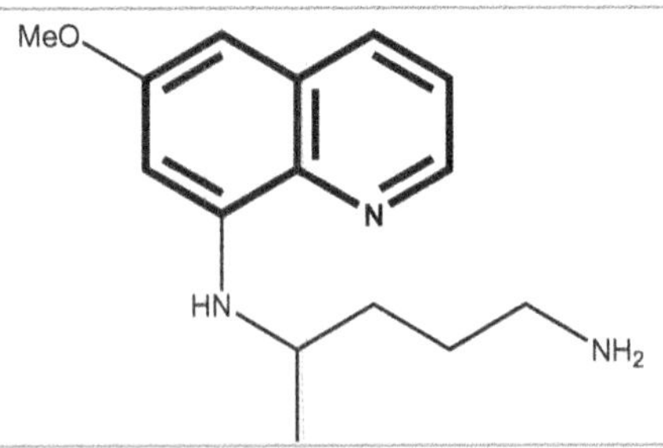

(continued)

Table 8.1 (continued)

Classes of antimalarial drugs and effects on the parasite	Main Drugs used on treatment	
	Chloroquine	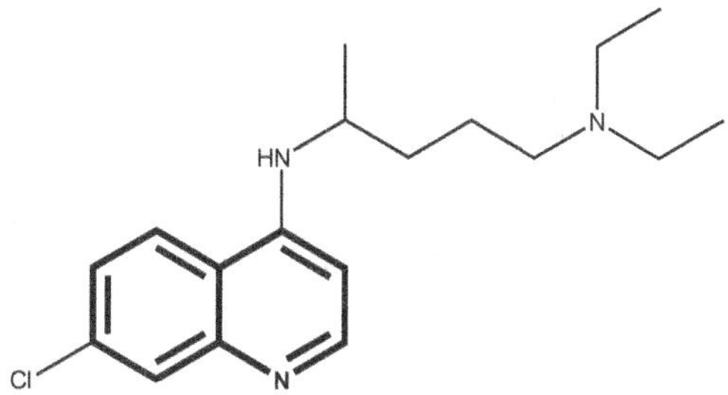
	Etaquine	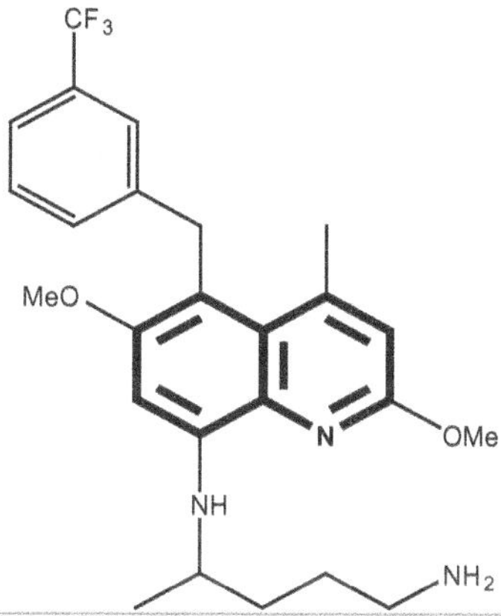
	Hydroxychloroquine	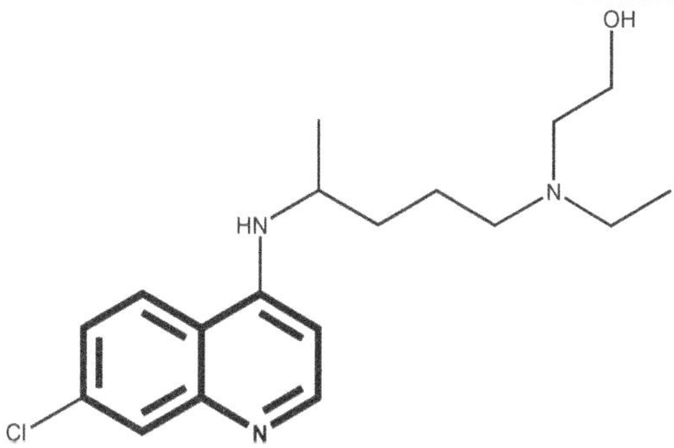
	Plasmoquine	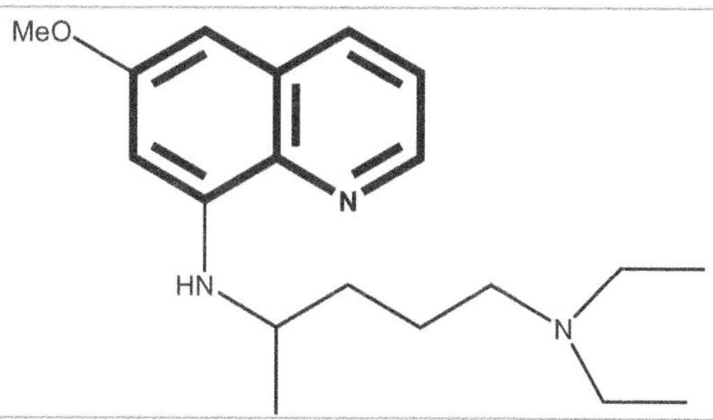

(continued)

Table 8.1 (continued)

Classes of antimalarial drugs and effects on the parasite	Main Drugs used on treatment	
Sulfones: inhibitors of folic acid synthesis	**Dapsone**	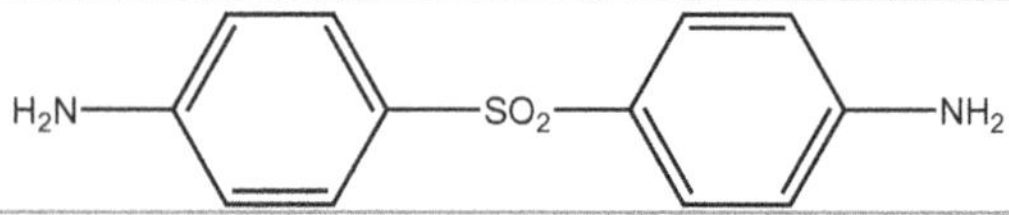
	Sulfa-doxine	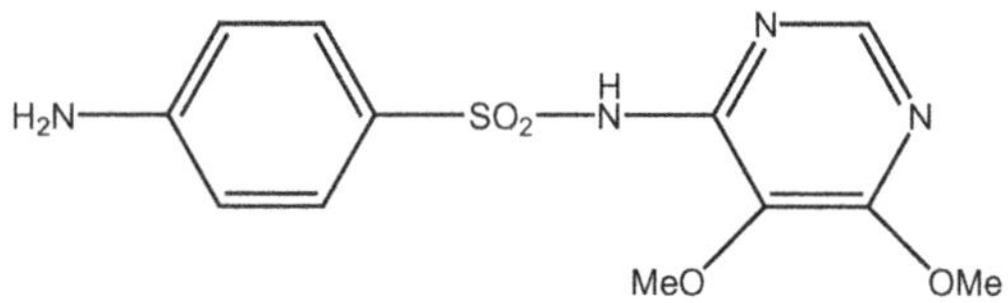
	Sulfalene	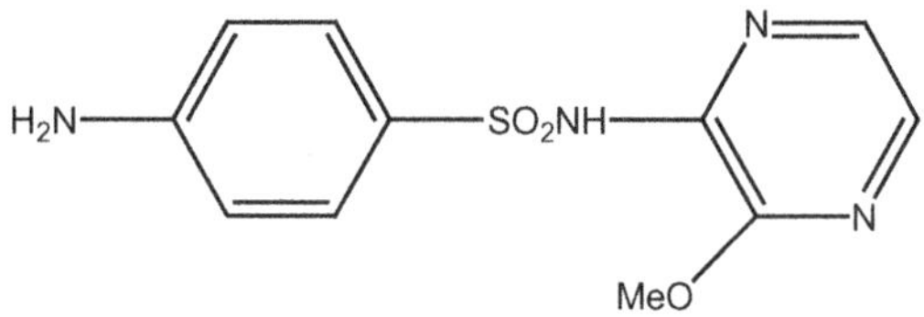

chloroquine; however, the mechanisms of this reversal are not yet known (Van Schalkuyk et al. 2001; Ridley 2002; Cunico et al. 2008).

The resistance of the parasites to the classic antimalarial drugs has enormously motivated the prospection of new drugs, and metal-based compounds play an important role in this context. Strategies for the discovery and development of metal-based drugs are driven by the elucidation of the biological profile of the parasite and by the identification of therapeutic targets. Metalloantimalarials are considered very attractive new antimalaria agents as we will see in the following topics.

8.3 Metalloantimalarials

8.3.1 Metal Complexes

The use of metals for therapeutic purposes has following advantages: the possibility of preparing stable complexes with predictable structures, the selective choice of ligands according to their affinity, and the increasing know-how on the metal complexes behavior in biological environments (Allesio 2011). The antimalarial activities of several metal complexes were already demonstrated, proving their high potential as alternative treatment against resistant *Plasmodium* species (Biot et al. 2012; Salas et al. 2013; Wani et al. 2015).

8.3.2 Metal Complexes of Quinoline

The attachment of a metal atom to an already existent antimalarial drug is an interesting strategy used to enhance its efficacy (Navarro 2009). Quinoline-containing antimalarial drugs are widely used in malaria therapy, as mentioned in Table 8.1 (Salas et al. 2013).

Chloroquine (CQ) and aminoquinoline were extensively used for many years (Sharma 2005; Navarro et al. 2010). Ruthenium complexes, widely investigated for many applications in medicine, exhibit anticancer, anti-allergic, and antiparasitic potential, as they correspond to nitric oxide donors for vascular relaxation induction (Donnici et al. 2009; Levina et al. 2009; Gambino and Otero 2012; Lima et al. 2014; Seuanes et al. 2015; Correa et al. 2016; Furrer et al. 2016; Mazuryk et al. 2016; Zhang et al. 2016). The synthesis of ruthenium complexes containing CQ as ligands is an interesting strategy to improve the effectiveness of antimalarial drugs (Sanchez-Delgado et al. 1996; Biot et al. 2011; Martínez et al. 2011).

Historically, ruthenium CQ complexes were the first class of compounds investigated for this purpose. According to the literature, the binuclear complex of Ru(II) chloroquine $[RuCQCl_2]_2$ (**complex 1**, Fig. 8.3) was five times more potent than standard chloroquine against *P. berghei* and *P. falciparum* strains. The mechanism of action of **complex 1** was described as the posthydrolytic binding to hematin in solution inhibiting its aggregation to β-hematin. Results show that the presence of the metal resulted in significantly enhanced activity against CQ-resistant strains (Sanchez-Delgado et al. 1996; Martínez et al. 2008; Salas et al. 2013).

Sanches-Delgado et al. (1996) synthesized the first class of ruthenium complexes containing CQ as ligand. In vitro experiments showed that arena ruthenium complexes were more effective than CQ against resistant strains of *P. falciparum.* Arene-Ru(II)-chloroquine (**complexes 2–4**, Fig. 8.3) demonstrated appreciable antimalarial activity. Additionally, the interaction between these ruthenium derivatives and target biomolecules was investigated (Martínez et al. 2011).

Another promising class of chloroquine complexes for the development of therapeutic agents are gold complexes (Navarro 2009; Navarro et al. 2010). These compounds exhibit antiparasitic potential for the treatment of leishmaniasis, trypanosomiasis, schistosomiasis, and malaria (Fricker et al. 2008; Navarro 2009; Vieites et al. 2009; Navarro et al. 2010; Biot et al. 2012).

The antiplasmodial potential of gold complexes was investigated, with a high number of possible ligands that can be coordinated to CQ or chloroquine diphosphate (CQDP), allowing the investigation of antimalarial properties of the several complexes (Navarro 2009).

In vitro tests showed that the gold complex $[Au(PPh_3)(CQ)]PF_6$ (**complex 5**, Fig. 8.3) caused inhibition of two resistant strains of *P. falciparum*, with IC_{50} values of 5 and 23 nM, and against a *P. berghei* strain. Studies on the elucidation of the possible mechanism of action of this complex include two targets, i.e., the inhibition of hemozoin (malarial pigment) and DNA interaction. Experiments with mice showed that treatment 1 mg/kg of AuCQ, and parallely with equivalent concentrations of CQDP, induced a reduction in parasite cells of 84 and 44%, respectively, when compared to the untreated control. These results suggest that the complexation of gold to CQ increased the in vivo susceptibility of *P. berghei* to CQ (Navarro et al. 1997, 2011) and lead to the search for novel gold–CQ complexes, which were synthesized, characterized, and evaluated against CQ-sentitive and CQ-resistant strains of *P. falciparum*. In this perspective, changes in the molecular structure of the $[Au(PPh_3)(CQ)]PF_6$ complex were performed, such as variation in the counter anion (**complex 6**, Fig. 8.3), in the phosphine ligand (**complex 7**, Fig. 8.3), and in gold oxidation state (Au (I) and Au (III)) (Navarro et al. 1997, 2004).

The literature also reported the antimalarial activities of iron, cobalt, and nickel complexes containing chloroquine (CQ) and Mefloquine (Mef) as ligands. The complexes of general formula $[M(II)L_1L_2Cl_2]$ and $[M(III)(Mef)(CQ)Cl_3)]$, where

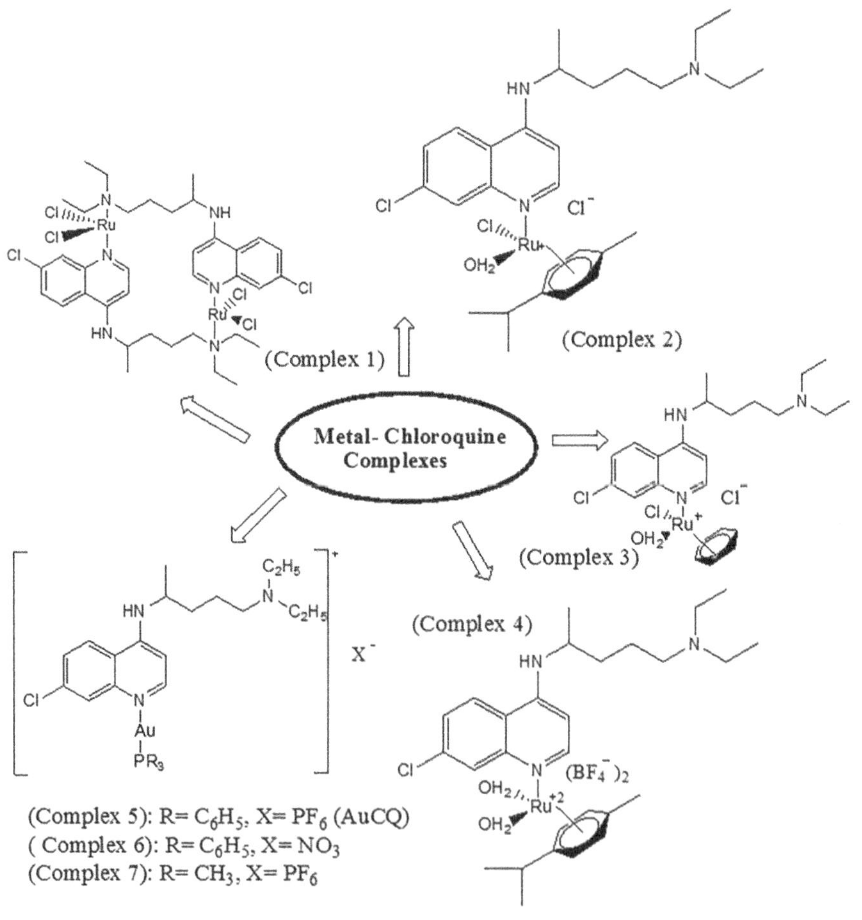

Fig. 8.3 Gold and ruthenium complexes of chloroquine

L_1 = Mefloquine, L_2 = chloroquine, M = Co^{2+}, Ni^{2+}, and Fe^{3+}, were synthesized, characterized, and evaluated. The in vivo tests revealed that the mixed metal complexes of Mefloquine and chloroquine [Co(Mef)(CQ)Cl_2] and [Fe(Mef)(CQ)Cl_3)] exhibited higher antimalarial potential. Furthermore, toxicity studies showed that these complexes demonstrated less toxicity than the Ni(II) analogue (Adediji et al. 2009). Other quinoline derivatives, Amodiaquine and primaquine, were complexed to several metal ions. The complexes of general formula [M^{2+}(Amodiaquine)$(Cl)_2$] and [Mn^+(primaquine)$_2$(X)$_n$(H_2O)$_y$], where M= VO(II), Cr(III), Fe(III), Cu(II), Co(II), Ni(II), Zn(II), Cd(II), Hg(II), Rh(III), Pd(II), Au(III), Ag(I), Mn(II), Sn(II), and Pt(II), were prepared and studied as potential antimalarial agents (Wasi et al. 1987). The antimalarial activity of platinum (II) complexes containing 4-aminoquinoline analogues was also considered (Souza et al. 2011). All these results indicated that metal complexation to traditional antimalarial quinolones represents an attractive alternative to the development of new antimalarials agents.

8.3.3 Metal Complexes of Other Ligands

In a very informative review on gallium(III) complexes as new promising metal-based drug candidates, Lessa et al. (2012) mentioned the complex of general formula [Ga-3-Madd]ClO_4, where H_2-3-Madd = 1,12 bis-(2-hydroxy-3-methoxybenzyl)-1,5,8,12-tetraazododecane, active against chloroquine-resistant FCR-3 and Indo-1 lineages at low micromolar concentrations. The complexes [Fe-3-Eadd]ClO_4 (**complex 8**, Fig. 8.4) and [Ga-3-Eadd]ClO_4 (**complex 9**, Fig. 8.4), where H_2-3-Eadd = 1,12-bis-(2-hydroxy-3-ethyl-benzyl-1,5,8,12-tetraazadodecane, were investigated in respect to their antimalarials activities against HB3 (chloroquine-sensitive) and Dd2 (chloroquine-resistant) *P. falciparum* strains. The results revealed that both complexes were effective against the HB3 chloroquine-resistant strains, but were 10–30 times less potent against Dh2 chloroquine-resistant strains. In the case of HB3 strains, both complexes were good inhibitors of hemozoin formation and modest to Dh2 strain. According to the authors, these results suggested that due to the similar antimalarial activities of the complexes, gallium(III) can replace iron(III) in biological environments.

The structure–activity correlation of some metallic antimalarial complexes was studied. A series of copper (II) complexes containing naphthoquinone ligands were synthesized, characterized, and evaluated. All complexes exhibit enhanced antimalarial activity against 3D7 *P. falciparum* strains. Furthermore, correlations between the antimalarial activity and the metal redox couple indicate the component of the parasitic electron transport chain as a possible target of such compounds (Gokhale et al. 2006). Complexes containing buparvaquone of general formula [M(II)$(L1)_2$(C2H_5OH)$_2$], where M(II) = Cu, Co, Ni, Mn, and Fe and L1 = buparvaquone ({3-trans-(4-tert-butylcyclohexyl) methyl-2-hydroxy-1,4-naphthoquinone}), were studied (Gokhale et al. 2003). The copper complex that

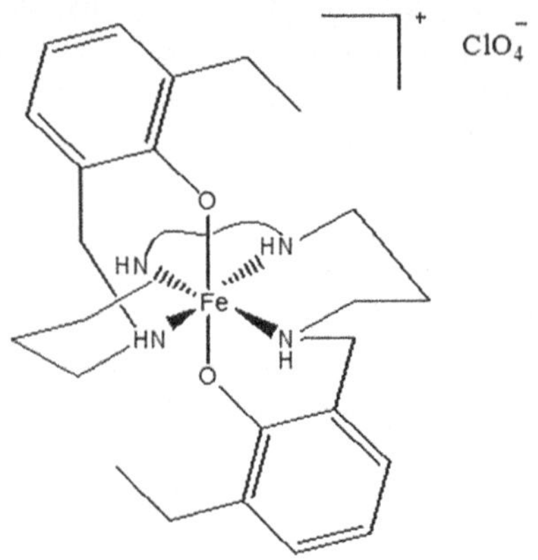

(Complex 8)

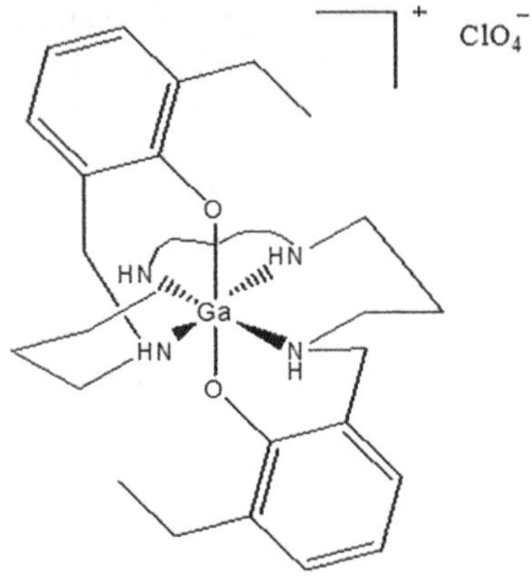

(Complex 9)

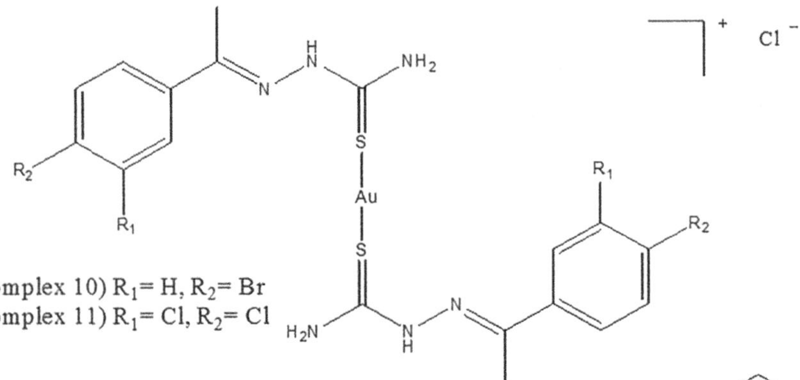

(Complex 10) R_1= H, R_2= Br
(Complex 11) R_1= Cl, R_2= Cl

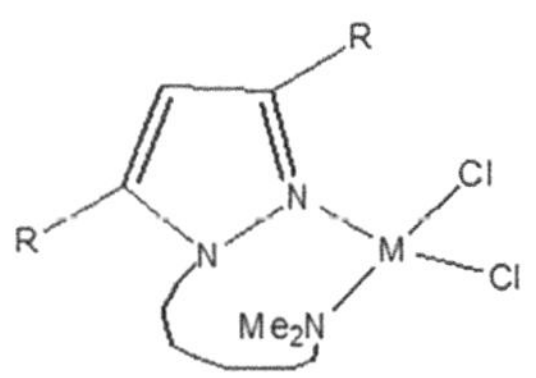

(Complex 12) M= Pt, R= H
(Complex 13) M= Pd, R= H
Me = Methyl

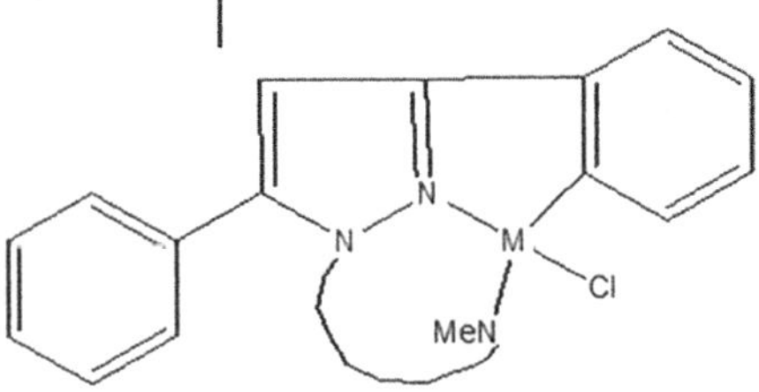

(Complex 14)
M= Pt
(Complex 15)
M= Pd
Me = Methyl

Fig. 8.4 Chemical structure of some metal complexes with antimalarial activity

showed better results demonstrated a thousand-fold enhancement in the antimalarial activity of parent quinone against 3D7 strain. Furthermore, this complex was three times more active against the chloroquine-resistant *P. falciparum* K1 strain when compared to the free ligand. Experiments with this strain cellular showed a 90%

reduction in parasitemia at a dose of 15 mg/kg, which demonstrates the high potential of the copper complex as antimalarial agent (Gokhale et al. 2003). The antimalarial activity of gold(I) thiosemicarbazone complexes (**complexes 10** and **11**, Fig. 8.4) and platinum (II) and palladium(II) complexes with ligands derived from pyrazole (**complexes 12–15**, Fig. 8.4) was also investigated. These complexes exhibited better efficacy in comparison to their free ligands against D10, W2, and 3D7 strains of *P. falciparum* (Khanye et al. 2010; Quirante et al. 2011). Besides the enhancement of the efficacy of organic drugs, the metal complexes correspond to new alternatives for the treatment of malaria, such as the inhibition of the parasite establishment in the vector mosquito.

Recently, Tapanelli et al. (2017) showed that Cu(I), Au(I), and Ag(I) phosphene complexes exhibited notable activity against the *Plasmodium* early sporogonic stages. The results showed that the metal complexes of general formula $[M(L)_4]PF_6$ (M = Cu(I), Ag(I) and $[Au(L)_4]Cl$ with L = Thp (tris(hydroxymethyl) phosphene) or PTA (1,3,5-triaza-7-phosphaadamantane) interfere with the early sporogonic stage of *Plasmodium,* inhibiting the parasite establishment in the vector mosquito.

8.3.4 Metal Chelators

All microorganisms need iron for their growth and replication (Crumbliss 1990). Several metabolic processes of the erythrocytic malaria parasite are dependent on iron, such as heme synthesis, DNA synthesis, proteolysis of hemoglobin, glycolysis pentose phosphate shunt, mitochondrial electron transport, and CO_2 fixation. It is therefore an indication that capturing iron from the parasite may interfere negatively on its metabolism (Sharma 2005).

This strategy corresponds to an interesting alternative for malaria treatment. Common iron-chelating compounds are siderophore, naturally produced by microorganisms to acquire iron from the environment. These compounds can also be administered in the form of free ligands to sequestrate iron, causing the death of the parasite due to deprivation, or in the form of toxic complexes with iron that inhibit parasite growth (Mabeza et al. 1999).

Some characteristics are very important for effective iron-chelating, such as a hydrophilic–hydrophobic balance, the structure of the hex dentate ligand, a selectivity for iron(III), and high affinity for iron and for others cations. The affinity for iron is a main prerequisite for antimalarial activity of an iron-chelating drug, with values of affinity constants iron(III) chelators ranging from 10^{24} to 10^{38}, according to the literature. The classic chelator desferrioxamine (DFO) (**complex 16**, Fig. 8.5), for example, presents an affinity constant value of 10^{31}, forming a stable complex with iron and, therefore, a high antimalarial activity. The chelator must have additional affinity for other metals such as calcium, magnesium, and zinc, as their removal may be detrimental for the parasite (Goodwin and Whitten 1965; Albert 1981; Lytton et al. 1993; Ponka et al. 1994; Cabantchik et al. 1996).

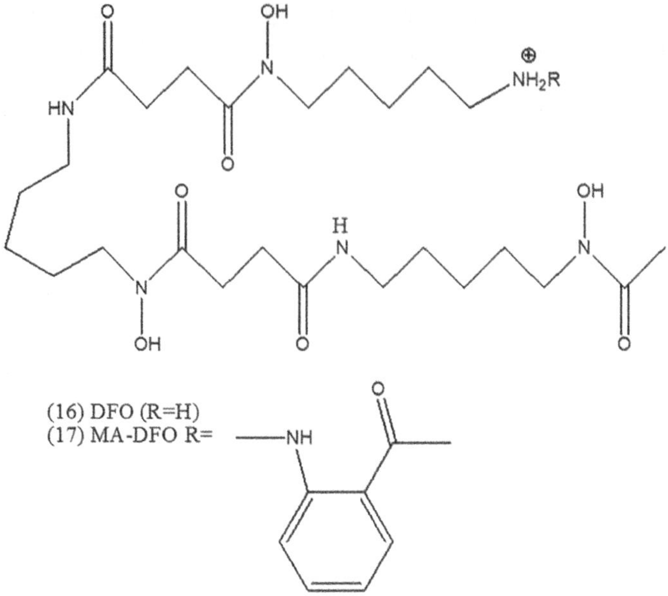

(16) DFO (R=H)
(17) MA-DFO R=

Fig. 8.5 Metal chelators used for malaria

The intensity of the antimalarial activity of iron chelators correlates with their hydrophilic/hydrophobic balance, as they can be capable of permeating cell membranes (Scheibel and Rodriguez 1989). Experimental studies with amino-terminal derivatives of desferrioxamine showed a preserved ability to bind to iron(III) species and a corresponding reduction to bind to iron(II) (Glickstein et al. 1996). Moreover, iron (III) forms stable complexes with coordination number equal six (Mabeza et al. 1999).

Desferrioxamine (DFO) is an important representative of iron-chelator and the first example of metal-based drug used to treat malaria. This siderophore occurs naturally in the form of trihydroxamic acid in *Streptomyces pilosus* and is used to treat hemochromatosis. However, the inherent slow permeation into infected cells and the restriction to advanced stages of *P. falciparum* are examples of drawbacks that limit its application (Modell and Berdoukas 1984; Brittenham 1988), and some structural modifications were conducted to produce more active and lipophilic derivatives, with broader efficiency for different stages of the infected cells.

As example of this strategy, a more lipophilic complex (MA-DFO, **complex 17**, Fig. 8.5) was synthesized by attaching N-methylanthranilic acid to the N-terminus, leading to a higher antimalarial activity. Zinc–desferrioxamine (Zn-DFO) complex exhibited increased permeability and improved antimalarial activity when compared to free DFO. A metal substitution reaction occurs inside the erythrocyte, forming the Fe(III)-DFO complex, which is more stable than the Zn-DFO complex (Loyevsky et al.1993; Chevion et al.1995).

During the last decades, the antimalarial activities of iron-chelating compounds have been investigated and metal chelators such as 1-(N-acetyl-6-aminohexyl)-3-hydroxy-2-methylpyridin-4-one demonstrated notable ability to inhibit the growth of *P. falciparum* in erythrocytes (Pangjit et al. 2015). Therefore, iron chelators correspond to a promising area to explore and obtain effective metal-based drugs for malaria.

8.3.5 Organometallic Compounds

In organometallic compounds, a metal–carbon bond (σ or π) provides special features to classic compounds. Many of these complexes have electronic structures based in 18 valence electrons (Miessler and Tarr 2004) and, due to their use in catalysis and other applications, are considerate potential therapy agents (Chavain and Biot 2010).

The first organometallic compounds for application in medicine, salvarsan (arsphenamine) and neosalvarsan, were based in arsenic and reported by Paul Ehrlich to treat syphilis and trypanosomiasis (Salas et al. 2013). Several organometallic complexes were prepared and valued as potential antimalarial agents, with ferrocene exhibiting the hightest antimalarial activity (Wani et al. 2015). Ferrocenes are highly liposoluble, stable, and nontoxic and have accessible redox potential, which make them very attractive to therapeutic applications (Van-Staveren and Metzler-Nolte 2004; Fouda et al. 2007), including malaria treatment. Inspired in ferrocene, several ferrocene-conjugated analogue structures were synthesized such as Mefloquine, artemisia, mepacrine, quinine, atovaquone, and other molecules (Biot et al. 2000; Blackie et al. 2003; Blackie and Chibale 2008).

Until the present moment, ferrochloroquine or ferroquine (FQ) (**complex 18**, Fig. 8.6) is the most successful metal-based drug for malaria therapy. This compound was described in 1997 as the first chloroquine derivative containing a ferrocene molecule, incorporating the ferrocene to the lateral side chain of chloroquine (Biot et al. 1997). Although there are structural similarities between chloroquine and FQ, the in vitro activities against *P. falciparum* of these compounds are distinct.

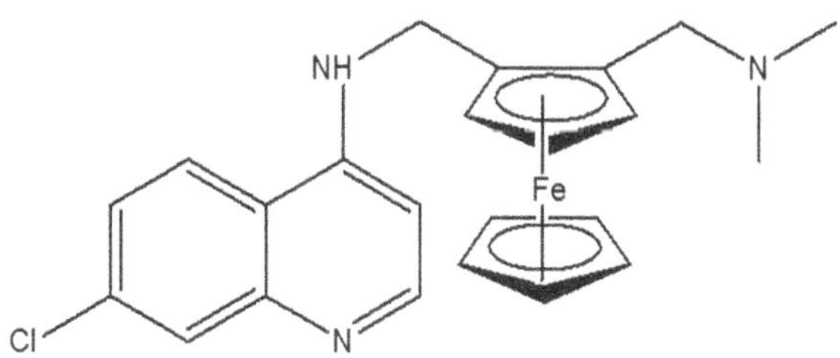

Complex 18 - FQ

Fig. 8.6 Chemical structure of ferroquine (FQ)

FQ has high efficiency against chloroquine-sensitive and chloroquine-resistant *P. falciparum* parasite strains, reaching efficiencies 20 times higher than chloroquine. FQ exhibited high activity in vivo against *P. yoeli, P. vinckei*, and *P. berghei* strains (Biot et al. 1999, 2006).

Some evidences point that the action of FQ seems to be related to inhibition of the hemozoin formation in the food vacuole of the parasite. Despite the similarity in mechanism when compared to CQ, studies indicated that FQ is more efficient than CQ to inhibit the formation of β-hematin. FQ and CQ showed IC50 values of 0.8 and 1.9, respectively (Biot et al. 2005).

The ferroquine compound FQ (SSR97193) is a successful representative of an organometallic drug (Sharma 2005; Biot et al. 2011). Because of its good antimalarial activity, it has been the object of many studies (Barends et al. 2007; Biot et al. 2011; Wani et al. 2015) and is now the only metal-based compound that is in phase II clinical test for malaria therapy. Daher et al. (2006) reported in vitro studies on the metabolism of ferroquine (SSR97193) in animals and humans, indicating potential applications of ferroquine in malaria therapy.

These previous interesting results stimulated the synthesis of several ferroquine derivatives, such as thiosemicarbazones, trioxaferroquines, ferrocene dual conjugates, hydroxyferroquines, and benzothiazoles (Wani et al. 2015; Adams et al. 2017). Thiosemicarbazones (TSCs) correspond to a very important class of compound for medicinal chemistry (Leovac et al. 2007), with interesting biological effects, including antimalarial activity (Bahl et al. 2010).

In vitro tests against *P. falciparum* strains demonstrated that the antiplasmodial activity of FQ conjugates and thiosemicarbazones was higher than for free thiosemicarbazone. Also, FQ-TSCs (**complex 19**, Fig. 8.7) displayed higher

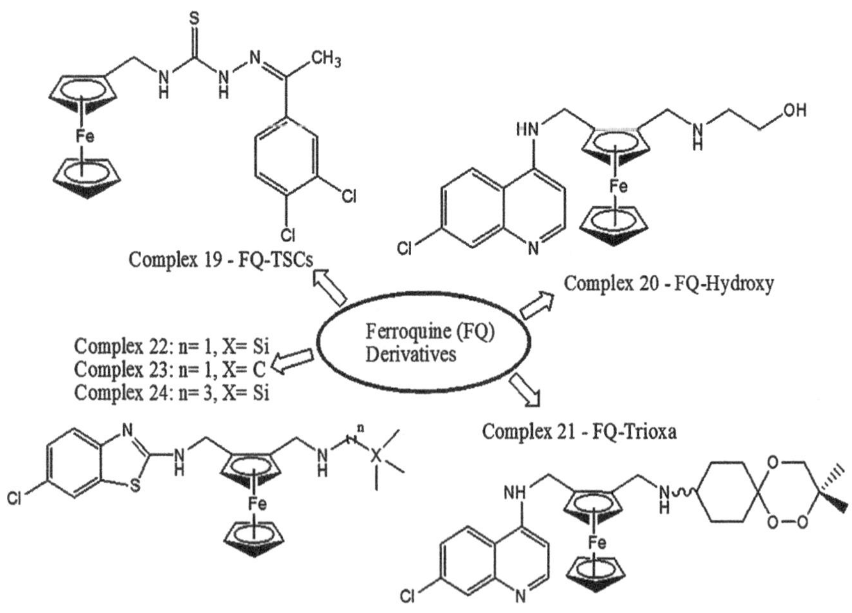

Fig. 8.7 Derivatives of metal complexes of ferroquine

efficiency against four *Plasmodium* strains with IC_{50} values at micromolar range (Biot et al. 2007). Hydroxyferroquine derivatives were also tested, and Wani et al. (2015) observed that they exhibited antiplasmodial activity and antiviral effects against coronavirus severe acute respiratory syndrome. Hydroxyferroquine (FQ-hydroxy) derivatives (**Complex 20**, Fig. 8.7) represent thus an excellent alternative to treat malaria infections caused by coronavirus in some specific geographical regions.

FQ-trioxaquines (FQ-trioxa) (**Complex 21**, Fig. 8.7) are potential antiplasmodial agents. In vitro and in vivo experiments demonstrated that these compounds are highly effective against CQ-resistant strains (Wani et al. 2015).

Benzothiazoles exhibit appreciable biological activity, and recently, Adams et al. (2017) evaluated antimalarial activity of ferrocenyl-containing benzothiazoles (**Complex 22–24**, Fig. 8.7). According to the authors, these compounds presented antiplasmodial activity against CQ-resistant and CQ-sensitive strains. They also observed that ferroquine derivatives were not able to inhibit the formation of β-hematin, indicating that FQ and its derivatives have different mechanisms of action.

The binding of active pharmacophores through covalent linkages is an interesting strategy used for the design of new antimalarial agents, such as ferrocene dual conjugates. The advantage of this strategy is the fact that it causes an increase in the conjugated molecule bioavailability, which diminishes its resistance. Some ferrocene dual conjugates demonstrated good antiplasmodial activities (Meunier 2008).

The development of ferrocene chemistry led to the investigation of ruthenocene analogues as antimalarial agents. Ruthenoquine (RQ) (**complex 25**, Fig. 8.8) and its derivatives (**complexes 26** and **27**, Fig. 8.8) were synthesized and presented good

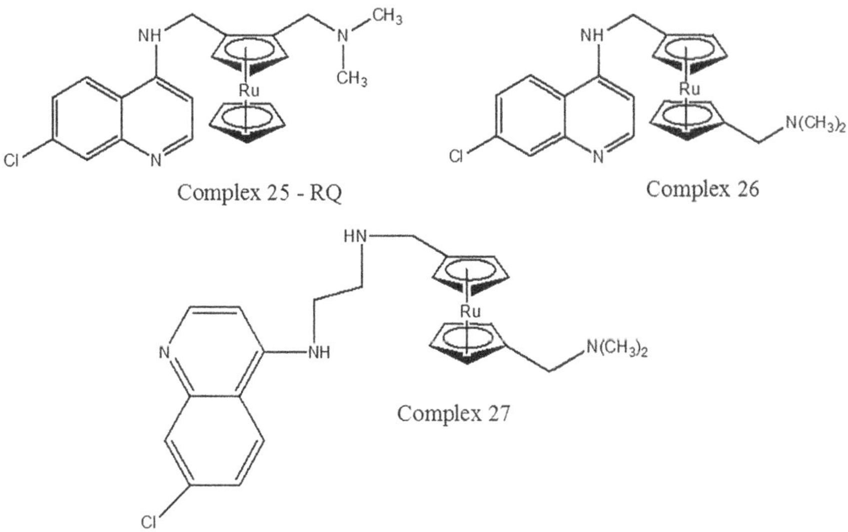

Fig. 8.8 Ruthenoquine and their derivative compounds

inhibition of *P. falciparum* growth, with similar mechanism of action as FQ (Beagley et al. 2002). All the results available up to the present moment point to an enormous potential of ferroquine and its derivatives for the development of antiplasmodial agents.

8.4 Conclusions

The emergence of drug-resistant strains of *Plasmodium* spp. led to an urgent need to develop more effective drugs, and metal-based drugs have been considered a promising strategy against new antiplasmodial agents. In this context, metalloantimalarials based on antimalarial drugs, metal chelators, and organometallic complexes were evaluated. Among all these compounds, ferroquine is the most successful representative, already being tested in phase II clinical trials. Studies on the physiology of the parasite allowed the understanding of the mechanisms of action of new drugs and stimulated the design of new more efficient drugs. With these studies, in the near future, it is expected that metallodrugs with low toxicity and high efficiency will be found for the treatment of neglected tropical diseases such as malaria. In addition, the production costs and the final product are extremely important factors, since this guarantees the accessibility of the population of poor countries affected by these diseases.

Acknowledgments The authors thank FAPESP (process number 15/06238-4) and CNPq (process number 304826/2013-8) for the financial support of research carried out in our laboratories.

References

Achan J, Talisuna AO, Erhart A, Yeka A, Tibenderana JK, Baliraine FN, D'Alessandro U (2011) Quinine, an old anti-malarial drug in a modern world: role in the treatment of malaria. Malaria J 10:144

Ackerknecht EH (1966) Malaria in the Upper Mississipi Valley, 1760-1900. Johns Hopkins Press, Baltimore

Adams M, Kock C, Smith JP, Chibale K, Smith SG (2017) Evaluation of ferrocenyl-containing benzothiazoles as potential antiplasmodial agents. Eur J Inorg Chem 2:242–246

Adediji FJ, Olayinka TE, Adebayo AM, Babatunde O (2009) Antimalarial mixed ligand metal complexes: synthesis, physicochemical and biological activities. Int J Phys Sci 9:529–534

Albert A (1981) Selective toxicity. Chapman and Hill, New York

Alessio E (2011) Bioinorganic medicinal chemistry. Wiley-VCH Velarg & Co, Germany

Bahl D, Athar F, Soares PBM, Sá SM, Moreira MRD, Srivastava MR, Leite ACL, Azam A (2010) Structure-activity relationship of mononuclear metal-thiosemicabazone complexes endowed with potent antiplasmodial and antiamoebic activities. Bioorg Med Chem 18:6857–6864

Barends M, Jaidee A, Khaohirum N, Singhasivanon P, Nosten F (2007) In vitro activity of ferroquine (SSR97193) agaisnt *Plasmodim falciparum* isolates from the Thai-Burmese border. Malaria J 6:1–5

Beagley P, Blackie MAL, Chibale K, Clarkson C, Moss JR, Smith PJ (2002) Synthesis and antimalarial activity in vitro of new ruthenocene-chloroquine analogues. Dalton Trans 23:4426–4433

Biot C, Glorian G, Maciejewski LA, Brocard JS, Domarle O, Blampain G et al (1997) Synthesis and antimalarial activity in vitro and in vivo of a new ferrocene-chloroquine analogue. J Med Chem 40:3715–3718

Biot C, Delhaes L, Abessolo H, Domarle O, Maciejewski LA, Mortuaire M, Delcourt P, Deloron P, Camus D, Dive D, Brocard JS (1999) Novel metallocenic compounds as antimalarial agents. Study of the position of ferrocene in chloroquine. J Organomet Chem 589:59–65

Biot C, Taramelli D, Forfar-Bares I, Maciejewski L, Boyce M, Nowogrocki G, Brocard JS, Basilico N, Olliaro P, Egan TJ (2005) Insights into the mechanism of action of ferroquine. Relationship between physicochemical properties and antiplasmodial activity. Mol Pharm 2:185–196

Biot C, Pradines B, Sergeant MH, Gut J, Rosenthal PJ, Chibale K (2007) Design, synthesis, and antimalarial activity of structural chimeras of thiosemicarbazone and ferroquine analogues. Bioorg Med Chem Lett 17:6434–6438

Biot C, Delhaes L, Maclejewski AL (2000) Synthetic ferrocene mefloquine and quinine analogues as potential antimalarial agents. Eur J Med Chem 35: 7–8

Biot C, Nosten F, Fraisse L, Ter-minassian D, Khalife J, Dive D (2011) The antimalarial ferroquine: from bench to clinic. Parasite 18:207–214

Biot C, Castro W, Botté YC, Navarro M (2012) The therapeutic potential of metal-based antimalarial agents: implications for the mechanism of action. Dalton Trans 21:6321–6580

Biot C, Delhaes L, Maclejewski AL, Mortuaire M, Camus D, Dive D, Brocard S J (2000) Synthetic ferrocenic mefloquine and quinine analogues as potential antimalarial agentes. Eur J Med Chem 35:707–714

Biot C, Daher W, Ndiaye C M, Melnyk P, Pradines B, Chavain N, Pellet A, Fraisse L, Pelinski L, Jarry C, Brocard J, Khalife J, Forfar-Bares I, Dive D (2006) Probing the role of the covalent linkage of ferrocene into a chloroquine template. J Med Chem 49:4707–4714

Blackie ALM, Chibale K (2008) Metallocene antimalarials: the continuing quest. Metals Based Drug 1:1–10

Blackie ALM, Beagley CK, Clarkson C, Hutton TA, Moss RJ, Smith JP (2003) Synthesis and antimalarial activity in vitro of new heterobimetallic complexes: Rh and Au derivatives of chloroquine and a series of ferrocenyl-4-amino-7-chloroquines and a series of ferroceny-4-amino-7-chloroquines. J Organomet Chem 688:144–152

Boss C, Richard-Bildstein S, Weller T, Fischli W, Meyer S, Binkert C (2003) Inhibitors of the *Plasmodium falciparum* parasite aspartic protease plasmepsin II as potential antimalarial agents. Curr Med Chem 10:883–907

Brittenham GM (1988) Iron chelating agentes. Curr Ther Hematol Oncol 3:149–153

Bruce-Chwatt LJ (1988) History of malaria from prehistory to eradication. In: Wernsdorfer WH, McGregor I (eds) Malaria: principles and practice of malariology. Churchill Livingstone, Edinburgh, pp 1–59

Cabantchik ZI, Glickstein H, Golenser J, Loyevsky M, Tsafack A (1996) Iron chelators: mode of action as antimalarials. Acta Haematol 95:70–77

Celli A (1925) *Storia della malaria nell'agro romano*. Roma, Academia dei Lincei

Centers for Disease Control and Prevention (2006) Malaria: topic home. In: http://www.cdc.gov/malaria/

Chavain N, Biot C (2010) Organometallic complexes: new tools for chemotherapy. Curr Med Chem 17:2729–2745

Chevion M, Chuang L, Golenser J (1995) Effects of zinc-desferrioxamine on *Plasmodium falciparum* in culture. Antimicrob Agents Chemother 39:1902–1905

Correa SR, Silva MM, Graminha EA, Meira SC, Santos FAJ, Moreira MRD, Soares PBM, Poelhsitz VG, Castellano EE, Bloch C Jr, Batista RM, Cominetti AA (2016) Ruthenium (II) complexes of 1,3-thiazolidine-2-thione: cytotoxicity against tumor cells and anti-*Trypanosoma cruzi* activity enhanced upon combination with benzidazole. J Inorg Biochem 156:153–163

Crumbliss AL (1990) Iron bioavailability and the coordination chemistry of hydroxamic acids. Coord Chem Rev 105:155

Cunico W, Carvalho AS, Gomes CRB, Marques GH (2008) Fármacos antimalariais—história e perspectives. Revista Brasileira de Farmácia 89:49–55

Daher W, Pelinski L, Klieber S, Sadoun F, Meunier V, Bourri M, Biot C, Guilou F, Fabre G, Brocard J, Fraisse L, Maffrand J, Khalife J, Dive D (2006) *In vitro* metabolism of ferroquine (SSR97193) in animal and human hepatic models and antimalarial activity of major metabolites on *Plasmodium falciparum*. Drug Metab Dispos 34:667–682

Despomnier DD, Gwadz RW and Hotez PJ (2006) Parasitic diseases 5th In: http://www.medicalecology.org/pdf/pd_malaria.pdf

Donnici LC, Araujo HM, Oliveira SH, Moreira MRD, Pereira ARV, Souza AM, Castro BACM, Leite LCA (2009) Ruthenium complexes endowed with potent anti-*Trypanosoma cruzi* activity: synthesis, biological characterization and structure-activity relationships. Bioorg Med Chem 17:5038–5043

Duffy J (1953) Epidemics in Colonial América. Lousiana State University Press, Baton Rouge

FioCruz—Malaria (2017) In: http://www.cpqrr.fiocruz.br/informacao_em_saude/CICT/malaria/malaria.htm

Foley M, Tilley L (1998) Quinoline antimalarials: mechanisms of action and resistance and prospects for new agents. Pharmacol Ther 79:55–87

Fouda MFR, Abd-Elzaher MM, Abdelsamaia RA, Labib AA (2007) On the medicinal chemistry of ferrocene. Appl Organomet Chem 21:613–625

França TCC, Santos MG, Figueroa-Villar JD (2008) Malária: aspectos históricos e quimioterapia. Quim Nova 5:1271–1278

Fricker PS, Mosi MR, Cameron RB, Baird I, Zhu Y, Anastassov V, Cox J, Doyle SP, Hansell E, Lau G, Langille J, Olsen M, Qin L, Skerlj R, Wong RSY, Santucci Z, Mckerrow HJ (2008) Metal compounds for the treatment of parasitic diseases. J Inorg Biochem 102:1839–1845

Furrer J, Süss-Fink G (2016) Thiolato-bridged dinuclear arene rutheium complexes and their potential as anticaner drug. Coordination Chem 309:36–50

Gambino D, Otero L (2012) Perspectives on what ruthenium-based compounds could offer in the development of potential antiparasitic drugs. Inorg Chim Acta 393:103–114

Glickstein H, Breuer B, Loyevsky M, Konijn A, Libman J, Shanzer A, Cabantchik ZI (1996) Differential cytotoxicity of iron chelators on malaria-infected cells versus mammalian cells. Blood 87:4871–4878

Gokhale HN, Padhye BS, Croft LS, Kendrick DH, Davies W, Anson EC, Powell KA (2003) Transition metal complexes of buparvaquone as potent new antimalarial agents Synthesis, X-ray crystal-structures, electrochemistry and antimalarial activity against *Plasmodium falciparum*. J Inorg Biochem 95:249–258

Gokhale HN, Shirisha K, Padhye BS, Croft LS, Kendrick DH, Mckee V (2006) Metalloantimalarials: Synthesis, x-ray Crystal structure of potent antimalarial copper(II) complex of arylazo-4-hydroxy-1,2-naphthoquinone. Bioorg Med Chem Lett 16:430–432

Goodwin JF, Whitten CF (1965) Chelation of ferrous sulfate solutions by desferrioxamine B. Nature 205:281–283

Hawass Z, Gad YZ, Ismail S, Khairat R, Fathalla D, Hasan N, Ahmed A, Elleithy H, Ball M, Gaballah F, Wasef S, Fateen M, Amer H, Gostner P, Selim A, Zink A, Pusch CM (2010) Ancestry and pathology in King Tutankhamun's family. JAMA 7:638–647

Haynes R (2001) Artemisia and derivatives: the future of malaria treatment. Curr Opin Inf Dis 14:719–726. http://rollbackmalaria.org. Accessed on 25 Nov 2017

Keeble TW (1997) A cure for the ague: the contribuition of Robert Talbor (1642–81). J R Soc Med 90:285–290

Khanye DS, Smith SG, Lategan C, Smith JP, Gut J, Rosenthal JP, Chibale K (2010) Synthesis and *in vitro* evaluation of gold(I) thiosemicarbazone complexes for antimalarial activity. J Inorg Biochem 104:1079–1083

Korolkovas A, Burckhalter JH (1982) Química Farmacêutica. São Paulo, Guanabara Dois

Lee MR (2002) Plants against malaria Part 1: Chinchona or Peruvian Bark. J Roy Coll Phys Edinburg 32:189–196

Leovac MV, Jovanovic SL, Jevtovic SV, Pelosi G, Bisceglie F (2007) Transition metal complexes with thiiosemicarbazide-based ligand—Part LV: Synthesis and X-ray structural study of novel Ni(II) complexes with pyridoxal semicarbazone and pyridoxal thiosemicabazone. Polyhedron 26:2971–2978

Lessa AJ, Parrilha LG, Beraldo H (2012) Gallium complexes as new promising metallodrugs candidates. Inorg Chim Acta 393:53–63

Levina A, Mitra A, Lay AP (2009) Recent developments in ruthenium anticancer drugs. Metallomics 1:458–470

Li Y, Wu YL (1998) How Chinese scientists discovered qinghaosu (artemisinin) and developed its derivatives? What are the future perspectives? Med Tropicale (Mars) 58(3 Suppl):9–12

Lima GR, Rodrigues SRB, Silva SR, Bendhack ML (2014) Ruthenium complexes as no donors for vascular relaxation induction. Molecules 19:9628–9654

Loyevsky M, Lytton SD, Mester B, Libman J, Shanzer A, Cabantchik ZIJ (1993) The Antimalarial action of deferral involves a direct access route to erythrocytic (*Plasmodium falciparum*) parasites. Clin Inv 91:218–224

Lytton SD, Mester B, Dayan I, Glickstein H, Libman J, Shanzer A, Cabantchik ZI (1993) Mode of action of iron (III) chelators as antimalarials: I. Membrane permeation properties and cytotoxic activity. Blood 81:214–221

Mabeza FG, Loyevsky M, Victor R, Gordeuk RV, Weiss G (1999) Iron chelation therapy for malaria: a review. Pharmacol Ther 81:53–75

Martínez A, Rajapakse CSK, Naoulou B, Kopkalli Y, Davenport L, Sánchez-Delgado RA (2008) The mechanism of antimalarial action of the ruthenium(II)-chloroquine complex $[RuCl_2(CQ)]_2$. J Biol Inorg Chem 13:703

Martínez A, Suárez J, Shand T, Magliozzo SR, Sánchez-Delgado AR (2011) Interactions of arene-Ru(II)-chloroquine complexes of know antimalarial and antitumor activity with human sérum albumin (HSA) and transferrin. J Inorg Biochem 105:39–45

Mazuryk O, Lomzik M, Martineau D, Beley M, Brendell M, Stochel G, Gros CP (2016) Anticancer activity of ruthenium(II) polypyridine complexes bearing pyrrolidine substituents. Inorg Chimica Acta 443:86–90

Meunier B (2008) Hybrid molecules with a dual mode of action: dream or reality. Acc Chem Res 41:69–77

Miessler LG, Tarr AD (2004) Inorganic chemistry, 3rd edn. Minnesota, Pearson

Modell B, Berdoukas V (1984) The clinical approach to Thalassemia. Grune and Stratton, London

Navarro M (2009) Gold complexes as potential anti-parasitic agentes. Coord Chem Rev 253:1619–1626

Navarro M, Pérez H, Sanchez-Delgado RA (1997) Toward a novel metal-based chemotherapy against tropical diseases. 3. Synthesis and antimalarial activity in vitro and in vivo of the new gold-chloroquine complex $[Au(PPh_3)(CQ)]PF_6$. J Med Chem 40:1937–1939

Navarro M, Vásquez F, Sánchez-Delgado RA, Pérez H, Sinou V, Schrével J (2004) Toward a novel metal-based chemotherapy against tropical diseases. 7. Synthesis and in vitro antimalarial activity of new gold-chloroquine complexes. J Med Chem 21:5204–5209

Navarro M, Gabbiani C, Messori L, Gambino D (2010) Metal-based drugs for malaria, trypanosomiasis and leishmaniasis: recent achievements and perspectives. Drug Discovery Today 15:1070–1078

Navarro M, Castro W, Martínez A, Sánchez Delgado RA (2011) The mechanism of antimalarial action of $[Au(CQ)(PPh)_3]PF_6$: structural effects and increased drug lipophilicity enhance heme aggregation inhibition at lipid/water interfaces. J Inorg Biochem 105:276–282

Nzila A (2006) The past, present and future of antifolates in the treatment of *Plasmodium falciparum* infection. J Antimicrob Chemother 57:1043–1054

Ockenhouse CF, Magill A, Smith D, Milhous W (2005) History of U.S. Military contributions to study of malaria. Mil Med 170:6–12

Pangjit K, Banjerdpongchai R, Phisalaphong C, Fucharoen S, Xie YY, Lu ZD, Hider RC, Srichairatanakool S (2015) Characterisation of a novel oral iron chelator: 1-(N-Acetyl-6-Aminohexyl)-3-Hydroxy-2-Methylpyridin-4-one. J Pharm Pharmacol 67:703–713

Ponka P, Richardson DR, Edward JT, Chubb FL (1994) Iron chelators of the pyridoxal isonycotinoyl hydrazone class. Relationship of the lipophilicity of the apo chelator to its ability to mobilize iron from reticulocyte in vitro. Can J Physiol Pharmacol 72:659–666

Prince R (2000) Artemisinin drugs: novel antimalarial agents. Expert Opin Investig Drugs 9:1815–1827

Quirante J, Ruiz D, Gonzalez A, López C, Cascante M, Cortés R, Messeguer R, Calvis C, Baldoma L, Pascual A, Guérardel Y, Pradines B, Font-Bardía M, Calvet T, Biot C (2011) Platinum(II) and palladium(II) complexes with (N, N′) and (C, N, N′) ligands derived from pyrazole as anti-cancer and antimalarial agents: Synthesis, characterization and in vitro activities. J Inorg Biochem 105:1720–1728

Rabinovitch L, Silva CMB, Alves RSA (1999) Controle biológico de vetores de doenças tropicais utilizando Bacillus entomopatogênicos. In: Melo IS, Azevedo JL (eds) Controle biológico. Jaguariúna, EMBRAPA Meio Ambiente

Rai MK, Ingle AP, Paralikar P, Gupta I, Medici S, Santo CA (2017) Recent Advances in use of silver nanoparticles as antimalarial agents. Int J Pharm 526:254–270

Ridley RG (2002) Medical need, specific opportunity and the drive for antimalarial drugs. Nature 415:686–693

Robert A, Benoii-Vical F, Dechy-Cabaret O et al (2001) From classical antimalarial drugs to new compounds based on the mechanism of action of artemisinin. Pure Appl Chem 73:1173–1188

Rocha MNA, Ferreira EAP, Souza JM (2006) Aspecto histórico da malária. Rev Para Med 20:81–82

Russel PF (1968) The United States and malaria: debits and credits. Bulletin of the New York Academy of Medicine. 44:623

Salas FP, Herrmann C, Orvig C (2013) Metalloantimalarials. Chem Rev 113:3450–3492

Sanchez-Delgado R, Navarro M, Perez H, Urbina JA (1996) Toward a novel metal-based chemotherapy against tropical diseases. 2. Synthesis and antimalarial activity in vitro and in vivo of new ruthenium and rhodium-chloroquine complexes. J Med Chem 39:1095–1099

Scheibel LW, Rodriguez S (1989) Anti-malarial activity of selected aromatic chelators. V. Localization of 59Fe in *Plasmodium falciparum* in the presence of oxines. Prog Clin Biol Res 313:119–149

Seuanes GC, Moreira MB, Petta T, Moraes DMPF, Moraes LAB, Oliveira ARM, Naal GZMR, Nikolaou S (2015) Novel binuclear μ-oxo diruthenium complexes combined with ibuprofen and ketoprofen: interaction with relevant target biomolecules and anti-allergic potential. J Inorg Biochem 153:178–185

Sharma V (2005) Therapeutic drugs for targeting chloroquine resistance in malaria. Mini-Rev Med Chem 5:337–351

Sibley CH, Ringwald PA (2007) Database of antimalarial drug resistance. In http:www.malariajournal.com/ content/5/1/48

Silva THA, Oliveira MT, dos Santos HF, de Oliveira AB, de Almeida WB (2005) Estudo de modelagem molecular de complexos ferriprotoporfirina IX e quinolinocarbinolaminas antimaláricos: Proposta de um farmacóforo. Quim Nova 28:244–249

Souza BN, Carmo LMA, Lagatta CD, Alves MJM, Fontes SPA, Coimbra SE, Silva DA, Abramo C (2011) 4-aminoquinoline analogues and its platinum (II) complexes as antimalarials agents. Biomed Pharmacother 65:313–316

Tapanelli S, Habluetzel A, Pellei M, Marchió L, Tombesi A, Capparé A, Santini A (2017) Novel metalloantimalarials: Transmission blocking effects of water soluble Cu (I), Ag(I) and Au(I) phosphane complexes on the murine malaria parasite *Plasmodium berghei*. J Inorg Biochem 166:1–4

Van Schalkuyk DA, Walder JC, Smith PJ (2001) Reversal of chloroquine resistance in *Plasmodium falciparum* using combinations of chemosensitizers. Antimicrob Agents Chemotherapy 45:593–597

Van-Staveren DR, Metzler-Nolte N (2004) Bioorganometallic chemistry of ferrocene. Chem Rev 104:5931–5986

Vieites M, Smircich P, Guggeri L, Marchán E, Gónrez-Barrio A, Navarro M, Garat B, Gambino D (2009) Synthesis and characteization of a pyridine-2-thiol N-oxide gold(I) complex with potent antiproferative effect against *Trypanosoma cruzi* and *Leishmania* sp insight into its mechanism of action. J Inorg Biochem 103:1300–1306

Wallace DJ (1989) The use of quinacrine (atrabine) in rheumatic diseases: a reexamination. Semin Arthritis Rheu 18:282–297

Wani AW, Jameel E, Baig U, Mumtazuddin S, Hun TL (2015) Ferroquine and its derivatives: new generation of antimalarial agents. Eur J Med Chem 01:534–551

Wasi N, Singh HB, Gajanana A, Raichowdhary AN (1987) Synthesis of metal complexes of antimalarial drugs and in vitro evaluation of their activity against *Plasmodium falciparum*. Original Inorg Chimica Acta 135:133–137

WHO (2017) http://www.who.int/malaria/en/

WHO Facts on ACTs (Artemisinin-based Combination Therapies) (2007) In:http://rbm.who.int/cmc_upload/ 0/000/015/364/RBMInfosheet_9.htm

Yalcindag E, Elguero E, Arnathau C, Durand P, Akiana J, Anderson TJ, Aubouy A, Balloux F, Besnard P, Bogreau H, Carnevale P, D'Alessandro U, Fontenille Gamboa D, Jombart T, Le Mire J, Leroy E, Maestre A, Mayxay M, Ménard D, Musset L, Newton PN, Nkoghé D, Noya O, Ollomo B, Rogier C, Veron V, Wide A, Zakeri S, Carme B, Legrand E, Chevillon C, Ayala FJ, Renaud F, Prugnolle F (2012) Multiple independent introductions of *Plasmodium falciparum* in South America. Proc Nat Acad Sci 109:511–516

Zhang C, Han B, Zeng C, Lai S, Li W, Tang B, Wan D, Jiang G, Liu Y (2016) Synthesis characterization in vitro cytotoxicity and anticancer affects of ruthenium(II) complexes on BEL-7402 cells. J Inorg Biochem 157:62–72

Chapter 9
Metal-Based Therapy in Traditional and Modern Medicine Systems

Reetika Singh and Bechan Sharma

Abstract Traditional medicine system is an integral part of therapy due to high extent of reliability, efficiency and cost-effectiveness. Ayurveda is the oldest traditional medicine system in India having a long history of use of metals in the form of Bhasma for the cure of various diseases. In addition to different other factors, the human metabolism needs various gases, elements and metals for the proper functioning. These metals are required in the adequate quantity for a specific physiological function of the body in order to ensure healthy and long life. Any imbalance in the levels of these metals results into alterations in the normal biochemical, physiological and behavioural functions leading to the onset of several diseases. The metals such as cobalt, copper, iron, selenium, zinc, etc. are the essential part of some enzymes and proteins called metalloenzymes and metalloproteins, and actively involved in the body metabolisms. These metals like selenium, copper and gold have also been successfully used in cancer therapy. There is a need of conducting extensive research in this area to establish appropriate formulation and application of different metals and metal-based nanomaterials to get the desired results with least side effects.

Keywords Herbal medicines · Metals · Modern medicines · Therapeutic value

9.1 Introduction

Medicine can be defined as any substance, compound or a mixture of substances or compounds that has the ability to cure a particular disease. On the basis of different nature of substance or compounds or the source of it, medicine system has been divided into different branches such as Traditional, Herbal, Ayurvedic, Homoeopathic, Unani, Siddha, Allopathic medicine system, etc. All the medicine

R. Singh · B. Sharma (✉)
Department of Biochemistry, University of Allahabad,
Allahabad 211002, Uttar Pradesh, India
e-mail: sharmabi@yahoo.com

M. Rai et al. (eds.), *Biomedical Applications of Metals*,
https://doi.org/10.1007/978-3-319-74814-6_9

systems are mutually correlated to each other for the resources and basic knowledge for development of a new drug (Afzal and Afzal 2016).

Use of metals for the therapeutic purpose is a very old concept. The concept of Bhasma is a very established and reliable mode of medicine in Ayurveda. Bhasma is prepared through a specific process known as shodhan, by burning of metals such as gold, silver, iron, etc. Based on current research report, it is clear that the scientific community showing their interest in the use of metal hyper-accumulating plants in phytoremediation has increased. Metal-accumulating plants have a broader potential as a way to improve nutrient content and, even to create foods that fight against cancer (Salt 2001).

In recent years, researchers are paying attention on the toxicity of trace metals on human health and the environment. Plants are the main link in the transfer of heavy metals from the contaminated soil to humans. Heavy metals may accumulate in the food chain and have low excretion rates through the kidney which could result in damaging effects on humans even at very low concentrations. However, an increase in their intake above certain permissible limits can become toxic (Korfali et al. 2013a, b). Generally, excessive uptake of dietary heavy metals causes a number of health risks such as cardiac dysfunction, foetal malformation, decrease in immunological defences, impaired psychosocial and neurological behaviour, gastrointestinal cancer, etc. (Singh et al. 2011; Mahan et al. 2012).

The composition of a human body can be analysed in terms of either tissue type (such as bones, muscles, organs, etc.) or molecular type (water, fat, carbohydrate, lipid, protein, DNA etc.) or percentage of different elements. The major part of a human body (96%) is made up of oxygen (65%), carbon (18%), hydrogen (10%) and nitrogen (3%) (Wikipedia 2017a, b). Biological functioning and metabolism of human body is a tough task to understand due to participation of several enzymes and molecules. Remaining 4% of human body comprises of the several elements. Calcium and phosphorus comprise 1.5 and 1%, respectively, and sodium, potassium, magnesium, sulphur and chlorine comprise only about 0.85% (Fig. 9.1). Inorganic elements act as cofactors in enzymes called metalloproteins and also essential for organic life. When metals are scarce or are in high quantities, equilibrium is set out of balance. Equilibrium (natural state) of these metals must be maintained via interventional and natural method (Wikipedia 2017a, b).

Metals such as zinc, copper, iron, manganese and chromium are essential nutrients and are important for the physiological and biological functions of the human body. Copper is an essential component of many enzymes and plays a significant role in various physiological processes including free radicals elimination, melanin production, iron utilization, bone and connective tissues development and many others (Johnson 1998; Martin and Griswold 2009; Maobe et al. 2012). Sodium and potassium are important elements for the normal metabolism of the human body and they are the important components of Na^+/K^+ ATPase. Sodium maintains the electrolyte balance in the body and regulates the transportation of water across the membrane. Sodium ions are present inside the nerve cells. Potassium ions are present inside the cells and act as cofactor for the certain enzymes. Potassium ions (K^+) maintain the osmolarity of the cell.

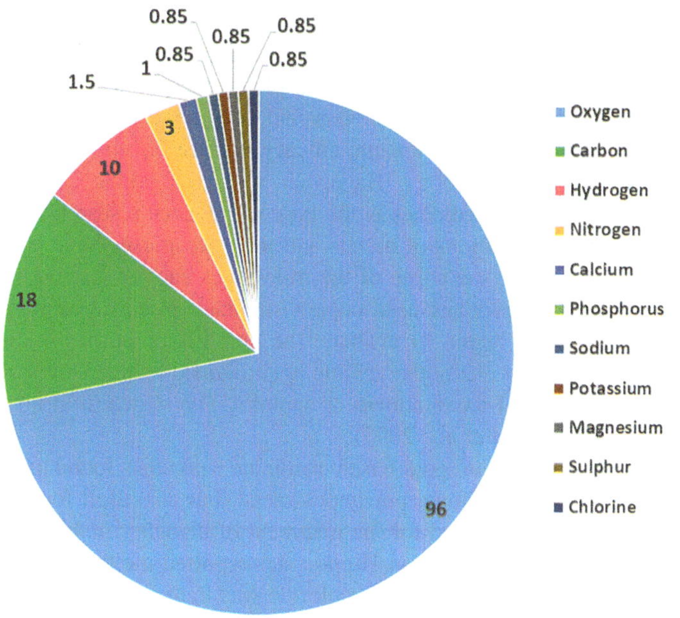

Fig. 9.1 Percentage of various elements and metals in human body

The trace elements play significant role in the normal physiological functions. Some important examples are: (1) Selenium acts as an antioxidant and anticancer, (2) Zinc mediates in the process of wound healing and sustained release of Insulin, (3) Copper participates in the formation of skin pigment (melanin), (4) Iron is an important component of haemoglobin (present in blood) and essential for carrying oxygen. Iron deficiency in blood causes anaemia and it is one of the major causes of maternal mortality. Gold in colloidal form is used for the cure of rheumatoid arthritis (www.healingbase.com; Sarkar et al. 2010). Copper (Cu) is an essential part of several proteins and vital enzymes such as copper cytochrome c oxidase, superoxidase, lysyl oxidase, and participated in the process of ATP synthesis and reduction of oxygen to water, etc. Dietary copper and the health-related issue are summarized by Bost et al. (2016). Selenium (Se) and selenoprotein play a crucial role for the proper functioning of brain (Solovyev 2015). In the diabetic patients, Se actively involved in the defence mechanism and antioxidant enzymes (Othman et al. 2017). The aim of this review is to summarize the comprehensive data about the role of metals in medicine and their toxicity.

9.2 Role of Metals in Traditional Medicine System

Ayurveda is most ancient medicine system and played an important role for the cure of various diseases since ancient time. It is believed that Chinese, Tibetan and Greek traditional medicine systems have been evolved from the Indian traditional medicine system. The increasing realization of the health hazards and toxicity associated with the indiscriminate use of synthetic drugs and antibiotics have renewed the interest in the use of plants and plant-based drugs.

Many elements and minerals have been included in the form of *Rasaushadhis*. *Rasashastra* highlighted the therapeutic efficacy of these *Rasaushadhis* to cure the ailments and rejuvenate the body (Bagewadi and Kumbhojkar 2015). Presently, knowledge of traditional medicines is the base of advance research in the field of medicine. Medical applications of metals and their complexes have been reported since ancient time. There are some of the milestones such as in 3000 BC for the sterilization of water Egyptians used copper sulphate. In early twentieth century, scientific approach has begun to evaluate the curative properties of metal complexes. In 1909, the first chemotherapeutic agent named arsphenamine (salvarsan) was discovered and used for treatment of syphilis. The structure of arsphenamine was determined by Lloyd et al. (2005).

Around 2500 BC use of gold-based medicine was also found in China and Arabia. Arsenic is a well-known poisonous metal, but also used for curative purposes. Arsenic is recommended for the treatment of diabetes, malaria, rheumatism and tuberculosis. Ancient physician Hippocrates reported the therapeutic nature of arsenic sulphides. In Europe, mercuric chloride was traditionally used as a diuretic and laxative and also used for the cure of syphilis since sixteenth century. By the nineteenth century, mercuric chloride was incorporated in a tonic known as 'blue mass' and used to treat many ailments including such diverse conditions as constipation, toothache and depression. Due to poisonous properties, the use of mercury is limited, but they are still found in traditional therapies Chinese, Tibetan and Ayurvedic medicine system. Romans used zinc for healing wound throughout the history.

Bhasmas are metal-based Ayurvedic drugs prepared by the different methods of bhasmikaran. Different processes are involved in bhasma preparation which include shodhana (purification), Bhavana, Jarana, Putapak, Marana (calcination) (Rasheed and Shivashankar 2015). These processes are applied on the basis of nature of materials. Ayurvedic healers suggested the specific type of bhasma to cure a particular ailment. Gold, silver, iron, copper, etc., are the metals that are commonly used for the bhasma preparation. In modern medicine also, several metals such as calcium, copper, gold, silver, zinc and so many others are used as bhasma with no side effects (Subrahmanian et al. 2002).

9.3 Therapeutic Uses of Metals in Modern Medicine System

In modern medicine system, metals are used as therapeutic agent in various ways. Radioactive metals are mostly used for diagnostic purpose. Other type of metals are also used for the cure of various ailments depending on their particular properties.

9.3.1 *Metals Used for Diagnostic*

In modern medicine system, metal ions are often used for diagnostic medical imaging (Wikipedia 2017a, b). In diagnostic, metals and their complexes are used either for radioisotope imaging (from their emitted radiation) or as contrast agents, for example, in magnetic resonance imaging (MRI). These imaging may be enhanced by altering the ligands in a metal complex to produce specificity. Therefore, the complex is taken up by a certain cell or organ type and a clear and specific image is produced (Lippard 1994; Dabrowiak 2012). So, important metals used for diagnosis include the following.

9.3.1.1 Cobalt(III)

Bleomycin is an antibiotic, when it is used with the ^{57}Cobalt(III) to selectively be taken up by tumour or cancer cells. The use of cobalt results in the best blood-to-tumour distribution ratio, but its half-life is too long to be conducive for imaging purposes. EDTA moiety is attached to the terminal thiazole ring of bleomycin, radiolabeled so that the entire complex can be easily traceable. This method can locate the tumour resulting into the early detection. It may be more useful in the diagnostic purpose in the future (Lippard 1994).

9.3.1.2 Gadolinium (III), Iron (III) and Manganese (II)

These three paramagnetic metals have the ability to alter the tissue relaxation times and produce a contrast image. In MRI imaging, these metals are useful to produce a contrast image.

9.3.1.3 Technetium

Technetium (^{99m}Tc) is the most commonly used radioisotope agent for imaging purposes. Due to short half-life, it emits only gamma ray photons (do not emit beta or alpha particles, which are more damaging to surrounding cells), so that it is particularly suitable as an imaging radioisotope.

9.3.2 *Metals Used for Treatment of Various Diseases*

Metals have been used in treatments since ancient times. In 1500 BC, The Ebers Papyrus is the first written document of the use of metals for the cure of various diseases and describes the use of copper to reduce inflammation and the use of iron to treat anaemia. Since, early twentieth century, sodium vanadate has been used for the treatment rheumatoid arthritis. Recently, metals have been used to treat cancer, by specifically attacking cancer cells and interacting directly with DNA (Table 9.1).

Table 9.1 Therapeutic use of metals and their complex for the treatment of various diseases

S. No.	Metal	Name/form (common/trade name)	Use/treatment
1	Aluminium (Al)	Hydroxide (Gaviscon)	Heartburn
		Silicate (Kaolin)	Diarrhoea
2	Antimony (Sb)	Sodium stibogluconate	Leishmaniasis
3	Arsenic (As)	Organic arsenic compound (Melarsoprol)	Sleeping sickness
4	Bismuth (Bi)	Bismuth complex	Heartburn, diarrhoea, peptic ulcer
5	Calcium (Ca)	Carbonate	Heartburn, peptic ulcer, diarrhoea
6	Copper (Cu)	Histidine complex	Menkes disease
7	Galadium (Ga)	Galadium (III) complex	Cancer
8	Gold (Au)	Gold (III) complex	cancer
		Gold (I) complex	Arthritis
9	Iron (Fe)	Iron complex	Hypertension
10	Lithium (Li)	Lithium carbonate	Manic depressive illness
11	Magnesium (Mg)	Magnesium sulphate (Epsom salts)	Constipation
		Magnesium hydroxide (milk of magnesia)	Heartburn
12	Platinum	Platinum (II) complex—Ag/Hg amalgam	Cancer dental amalgams
		Platinum (IV) complex	Cancer
13	Rhenium (Re)	Rhenium complex	Bone cancer
14	Ruthenium (Ru)	Ruthenium complex	Cancer, parasitic diseases
15	Samarium (Sm)	Samarium complex	Bone cancer
16	Silver (Ag)	Silver sulfadiazine	Burns
		Silver complex	Cancer, antimicrobial
17	Sodium (Na)	Sodium bicarbonate (Alka-seltzer)	Heartburn
18	Stronium (Sr)	Strontium complex	Bone cancer
19	Titanium (Ti)	Titanium alloy	Hip and knee replacement
		Oxide	Sunblock
20	Vanadium (V)	Vanadium complex	Diabetes
21	Yttrium (Y)	Yttrium complex	Bone and liver cancer
22	Zinc (Zn)	Oxide	Sunblock
		Oxide with Fe_2O_3 (Calamine lotion)	Antimicrobial agent
		Zn complex	Wound healing
23	Zerconium (Zr)	Zr (IV) glycinate	Antiperspirant

9.3.3 Therapeutic Uses of Metals Against Cancer

Cancer is a most common, dangerous and life-threatening disease. Cancer is a condition in which cells multiplied rapidly without any regulation and invades to adjacent healthy tissue and caused damage. Several factors may be responsible for the cause of cancer such as, genetic changes in DNA, age of candidate, epigenetic changes, exposure to any chemical or biological carcinogen, infection with virus, abnormality in DNA repair system, changes in cell cycle regulation protein, etc. Finally, all the factors cause genetic changes and at the gene level, two types of genes, i.e. oncogenes are responsible for the growth of cancer cells and tumour suppressor genes prevent the cancer development (Knudson 2001). Cancer treatment through chemotherapy, radiotherapy, hyperthermia and surgery is often painful and caused significant side effects which may be long term or short term (Irvine et al. 1994). Use of metals in cancer therapy has a long history. Initially, the platinum and gold were used for cancer therapy. Recently, a number of metals and their complexes are used for the treatment of cancer: chemotherapy or radiotherapy (Fig. 9.2).

9.3.3.1 Arsenic and Antimony

Arsenic compounds are the natural substances, having the long history of medical use in China. The patient suffering from acute promyelocytic leukaemia (APL) is treated with arsenic trioxide (As_2O_3) for more than 20 years (Desoize 2004).

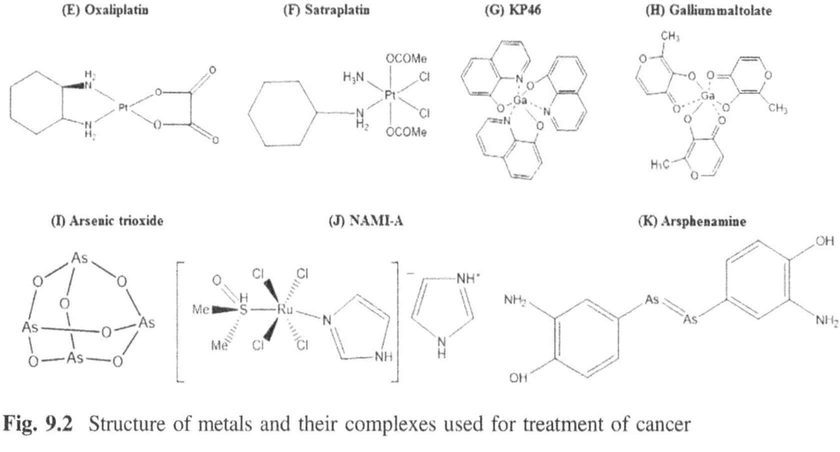

Fig. 9.2 Structure of metals and their complexes used for treatment of cancer

Arsenic trioxide is a safe and effective compound not for only the leukaemia but also for other types of cancers (Feng et al. 2002). The expected mechanism of action of arsenic is the activation of caspase 8 or caspase 9 which further induces the p53 gene dependent G1 or G2/M cell cycle arrest (Liu et al. 2003). The anti-cancer activity of arsenic compounds may be involved in the induction of apoptosis. Shen et al. (2003) also reported the higher concentration of As (5 μM/l) was responsible for the initiation of apoptosis. Zhao et al. (2002) reported the simultaneous up-regulation of BAX gene and down-regulation of bcl-2 gene, these regulations also may be the reason for the apoptosis.

Structurally arsenic trioxide and antimony trioxide are similar but antimony trioxide (Sb_2O_3) is less toxic in comparison to the arsenic trioxide (Desoize 2004). When a mice with S180 solid tumours treated with Antimony (III) complexes with polydentate carboxylic acids showed the antitumour activity (Hu et al. 1997). Anticancer activity of potassium antimony tartrate is very significant in lymphoid carcinoma (Lecureur et al. 2002; Sampayo-Reyes et al. 2000). Triphenylantimony (V) polyamines showed a significant toxicity against several cancer cell lines (Tiekink 2002a, b).

9.3.3.2 Cobalt and Copper

Characteristically, Cobalt-60 emits gamma rays, and therefore is used as radio-therapeutic agent in cancer. Since 1950, it is used for radiotherapy. Because of the emission of gamma rays, it is more effective than X-rays. Half-life of Co-60 is 5.3 years so it needs to be replaced occasionally (Wikipedia 2017a, b).

Copper is an essential element so it may be less toxic than non-essential elements such as ruthenium, vanadium, platinum, etc. (Marzano et al. 2009). The antitumor activity of copper complexes was reported and many new complexes of copper have great antitumor potential. Copper complexes may have relatively lower side effects than platinum-based drugs, and are suggested to be able to overcome inherited or acquired resistance of cisplatin (Marzano et al. 2009). In this overview, the most recent advances in copper homeostasis, copper-related chelation therapy and design of copper-based antitumor complexes were summarized by Wang and Guo (2006).

9.3.3.3 Gold

Chinese and Arabic physicians used gold for treatment of several diseases. Few years back, the anti-tumour activity of gold was recognized (Desoize 2004). Gold nanoparticles have been reported for the detection and treatment for cancer (Brigger et al. 2002). The main application of gold complex is for the cure of rheumatoid arthritis and as antitumor agents (McKeage et al. 2002). Many compounds of gold such as phosphine-gold (I) thiolates showed noteworthy celltoxicity (Tiekink 2002a, b) and tetrahedral gold (I) compounds showed similar result against several cancer cell line (Berners-Price et al. 1986).

9.3.3.4 Platinum

Platinum is the most frequent used metals in popular anticancer drugs and anticancer metal-containing complex to be found in the twentieth century. Cisplatin is one of the most frequently used platinum-containing anticancer drugs. Its anticancer activity was discovered serendipitously by Barnett Rosenberg in the 1960s and it is also used for the treatment of testicular cancer and some other cancers (Marzano et al. 2006). Cisplatin, cis-diamminedichloro-platinum (II), is one of most widely used anticancer drugs for which it has a greater than 90% cure rate. Cisplatin enters into cells by passive diffusion (Jamieson and Lippard 1999).

9.3.3.5 Ruthenium

Recently, Ruthenium is identified as a potent anticancer agent. Similar to the other metal drugs, the activity of the ruthenium compounds depends on both the oxidation state and the ligands. By modification in oxidation states and ligands, ruthenium-based drugs are formed against malaria, bacterial infections and immunosuppression. The presence of some unique properties like many oxidation states, rate of ligand exchange and the ability to mimic the iron to bind with certain biological molecules, makes it more suitable for medical use. Many complexes of Ru(I), Ru(II), Ru(III), Ru(IV), with amine, dimethylsulfoxide, imine, polyaminopolycarboxy-late and N-heterocyclic ligands have been reported to bind with DNA (Claire and Paul 2001). However, many of these compounds are less soluble in H_2O, which is necessary for the efficient transportation within the human body. Claire and Paul (2001) have reported that the solubility of these compounds can be increased by using dialkylsulfoxide derivatives, such as [*trans*-$RuCl_4$(DMSO)Im][ImH], NAMI-A, which is known to act as the most successful ruthenium-based anticancer compound.

9.3.3.6 Selenium

Selenium (Se) appears to function as an antimutagenic agent, it is preventing the transformation of normal cells into malignant cells. These protective effects of Se seem to be primarily associated with its presence in the glutathione peroxidases (GSH-Pxs) and thioredoxin reductase. GSH-Pxs is an antioxidant enzyme known to protect DNA and other cellular components from oxidative stress (Trueba et al. 2004; Schrauzer 2000). It induced the apoptosis and in another way, it inactivates the oncogenes. Low level of Se and GSH-Px was found in the patients suffering with cervical cancer (Valko et al. 2006).

Researchers reported that in in vitro studies, selenium compounds inhibit oxidative stress-induced DNA damage and carcinogen-induced covalent DNA adduct formation. Further, in vitro studies showed that selenium also induced cell apoptosis and inhibited transformed cells growth (Sinha et al. 1996). Cell apoptosis is induced by the activation of *p53* gene so, it is clear that selenium compounds have ability to induce the *p53* gene. Makropoulos et al. (1996) have reported the involvement of in signal transduction. Selenium activates MAPKs and transcription factors such as AP-1, NF-B. The activation of these two factors influenced gene expression and cell growth. Growth inhibition and induction of apoptosis were observed in the premalignant human breast cancer cells, when it was treated and incubated with methylselenic acid. Selenium directly affects the molecular processes involving cell signalling and apoptosis occurs mainly via a redox-dependent mechanism (Valko et al. 2006).

9.4 Mechanism of Actions of Metals Against Various Diseases

Most of the metals possess positive charges and can interact with the phosphate backbone of DNA (negative charge). Some drugs are developed that include metals that interact directly with other metals already present in protein active sites, while other drugs can use metals to interact with amino acids with the highest reduction potential. Most of the metals and their complexes follow a common pathway in cancer cells (Fig. 9.3). Metals used in treatment of different diseases and their mechanism of actions are summarized in Table 9.2 (Wikipedia 2017a, b; Wang and Guo 2006).

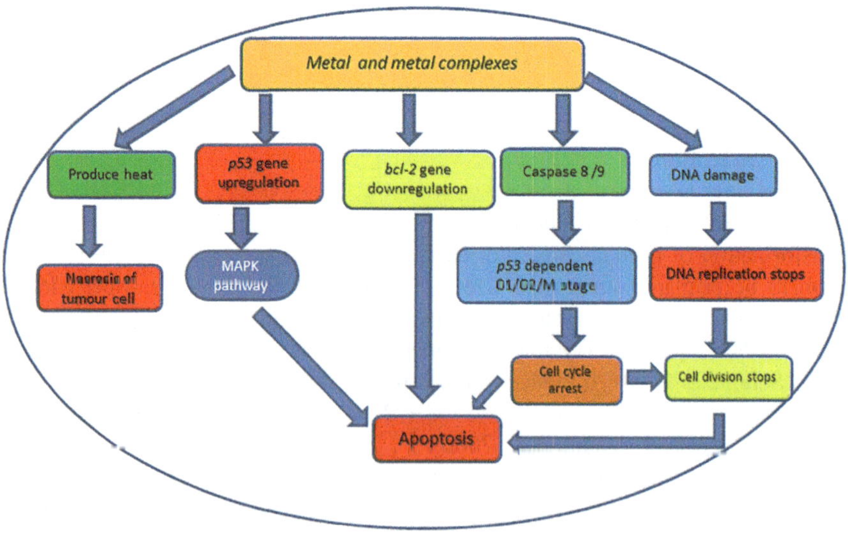

Fig. 9.3 Common mechanism of actions of metals and their complexes used in cancer therapy

Table 9.2 Use of metals for the treatment of various diseases and their mechanisms of actions

Metals	Used in diseases	Mechanism of action
Gold	Rheumatoid arthritis, immune response, cancer	Interact with albumin and eventually be taken up by immune cells, triggering anti-mitochondrial effects and cell apoptosis
Lanthanum	Chronic Kidney disease	Lanthanum used as a phosphate binder in patients suffering from Chronic Kidney disease
Lithium (Li_2CO_3)	Prophylaxis of manic depression behaviour, mental health	Not known
Platinum	Head and neck tumour	Act to cross-link DNA in tumour cells
Silver	Burning, cancer	Prevent infection at the burn site for burn wound patients
Titanium and Vanadium, iron	Cancer	React with DNA specifically in tumour cells
Zinc	Wound healing, Herpes virus infection	Not known

Copper can be considered as most important essential transition metals because of involvement of copper in various biological processes such as connective tissue formation, nerve cell function, temperatures control and embryo development. Therapeutic role of copper and its complexes have been shown in Wilson's and Menkes diseases and some neurological disorders. Copper chaperones, Menkes and Wilson proteins and Copper-transporting P-type ATPases have been identified and characterized at the molecular level and it is considered as novel components of copper homeostasis (Wang and Guo 2006). The role of copper deficiency or copper toxicity in physiological and pathological conditions can be better understood by these research findings.

9.5 Limitations of Metals Used in Medicine System

Although the metals are essential for healthy and wealthy human life, but excessive intake of metals may cause serious adverse effect on metabolisms of human, finally causing several diseases. Every metal causes toxicity beyond the permitting limit (PL) (Table 9.3). Ayurveda and Siddha used metals and minerals in their medicines. According to the Indian medicine system, after proper purification and processing, use of metals and minerals was permitted and helps in the recovery of patients but it should be up to permissible limits. However, dangerously high level of heavy metals was found in the final product due to improper manufacturing

Table 9.3 Heavy metals poisoning and their permitting limits by WHO in herbal medicine

Metals	Permissible value ($mg\text{-}kg^{-1}$)	Symptoms/ adverse effects	Organs affected	Reference
Cadmium	0.3	Liver damage, vascular abnormality	Kidney, liver and vascular system	Martin and Griswold (2009), Li et al. (2012), Maobe et al. (2012)
Lead	10	Hearing and vision impairments, poor muscle coordination	Nervous system, kidney, immune system, skeletal, reproductive system	Johnson (1998), Anonymous (2007)
Zinc	50	Not available	Immune system	Fosmire (1990)
Copper	20 and 150[a]	Dermatitis, abdominal pain, irritation in the respiratory tract	Skin, respiratory system	Johnson (1998), Martin and Griswold (2009), Maobe et al. (2012)
Iron	Not available	Nausea, vomiting, diarrhoea, joint pain and liver damage	Cardiovascular system and metabolic functions	Martin and Griswold (2009)

[a]Limit was set by China and Singapore, respectively

processes. Heavy metals may accumulate in vital organs and cause various health problems (WHO 2005). Children and pregnant women are more susceptible to the heavy metals toxicity. Arsenic, lead and mercury toxicity is more dangerous in comparison to the other heavy metals. The toxicity of these heavy metals may cause dizziness, insomnia, nausea, abdominal pain, vomiting, weight loss, anaemia, muscle cramps, tremors, swelling of the brain and paralysis, heart abnormalities, liver damage, memory loss, reduced motor nerve function and reduced mental function (Anonymous 2005; Sharma et al. 2014; Gupta et al. 2015). In some Ayurvedic medicines, presence of lead, arsenic and mercury was found beyond permitting limit (Saper et al. 2004). In recent years, several reports are available of heavy metal poisoning after the use of Ayurvedic medicines (Lynch and Braithwaite 2005).

In 2005, Canadian government analysed few Ayurvedic drugs present in the market which contained high levels of lead, mercury and/or arsenic and banned these drugs for public use (Table 9.4). The toxicity of different metals is discussed below:

Table 9.4 List of drugs having the heavy metals beyond permitting limit

S. No.	Product name	Manufacturer company	Manufacturer Country
1	Karela tablets	Shriji Herbal Products	India
2	Karela capsules	Himalaya Drug Co., Charantia, UK (specifically batch #12011)	UK
3	Maha Sudarshan Churna powder	Zandu Pharmaceuticals, D & K Pharmacy, Dabur India Ltd., Chhatrisha, Lalpur	India
4	SAFI liquid	Hamdard-WAKF	India, Pakistan
5	Yograj Guggul tablets	Zandu Pharmaceuticals	India
6	Sudarshan tablets	Zandu Pharmaceuticals	India
7	Shilajit capsules	Dabur India Ltd.	India

9.5.1 *Cadmium*

For cadmium, FAO/WHO decided the 0.3 mg-kg^{-1} as the permissible limit (PL) set for medicinal herbs and plants in different countries (WHO reports 2005, 2006). The high concentrations of cadmium in the blood result in a serious toxicological effect on human health. At high levels, cadmium produces serious effects on vascular and immune system, and the liver (Maobe et al. 2012). Kidney is the primary and critical target organ in the exposed population. Excretion of cadmium from human body is very slow. Cadmium accumulates relatively for a longer time in kidney which produces adverse effect on the impairment of the renal tract (Martin and Griswold 2009; Li et al. 2012; Maobe et al. 2012).

9.5.2 *Lead*

Lead is considered as one of the highly toxic environmental pollutants and a major health hazard. Lead can form complex with various biomolecules and unfavourably may affect their functions (Dghaim et al. 2015). Exposure of lead can produce adverse effect on the various organs and organ system of the human body such as blood, nervous, immune, renal, skeletal, muscular, reproductive and cardiovascular systems causing poor muscle coordination, gastrointestinal symptoms, brain and kidneys damage, hearing and vision impairments and reproductive defects (Johnson 1998; Anonymous 2007). In early childhood and prenatally period, exposures of lead are associated with slowed cognitive development, learning deficits and many other effects (Johnson 1998; Anonymous 2007).

9.5.3 Iron

The FAO/WHO has not been set the PL for iron yet. Different herb samples showed the variations in iron content. These results are comparable to values of iron found in Egyptian spices and medicinal plants that ranged between 26.96 and 1046.25 mg-kg^{-1} (Abou-Arab and Abou-Donia 2000). Iron has several key functions in the human body including oxygen supply, energy production and immunity. Excessive intake of iron may produce the symptoms of nausea and vomiting, diarrhoea, joints pain, shock and liver damage. Toxicity of iron may produce an adverse effect on cardiovascular system and various metabolic functions and (Martin and Griswold 2009).

9.5.4 Copper and Zinc

Excessive intake of copper can cause dermatitis, irritation of the upper respiratory tract, abdominal pain, nausea, diarrhoea, vomiting and liver damage (Johnson 1998; Martin and Griswold 2009; Maobe et al. 2012). Zinc is an essential trace element required for proper growth, blood clotting and thyroid function. It also plays an important role in DNA and protein synthesis. However, high intake of zinc produces toxic effects on the blood lipoprotein levels, copper level and immune system (Fosmire 1990).

9.6 Conclusions

Metals and non-metals both are essential for the human life but these are needed in the proper quantity. Metals are playing an important role in cancer chemotherapy. After crossing the permitting limit, these metals cause toxicity and start acting as major factors for the initiation of several diseases. Before the clinical use, toxicity of every drug (either of plant origin or synthetic origin) should be evaluated after several stage of clinical trials. For the use of metals in the advance modern drugs, more organized, intense comprehensive research should be done. In future, metals may be used as a more powerful medical tool for the development of new drugs.

Acknowledgements RS wishes to acknowledge the Department of Science & Technology—Science and Engineering Research Board (DST-SERB), Government of India, New Delhi for providing financial support as National Post-Doctoral Fellowship (N-PDF, File No. PDF/2016/000061). Authors wish to acknowledge Mr. Abhishek Kumar for drawing the chemical structure of the compounds.

References

Abou-Arab AA, Abou Donia MA (2000) Heavy metals in Egyptian spices and medicinal plants and the effect of processing on their levels. J Agric Food Chem 48(6):2300–2304

Afzal A, Afzal M (2016) Herbal medicine: past, present and future with emphasis on the use of some common species. In: Armstrong D, Stratton RD (eds) Oxidative stress and antioxidant protection: the science of free radical biology and disease, 1st edn, pp 471–482

Anonymous (2005) Press release. Health Canada warns consumers no to use certain Ayurvedic medicinal products. 2005–2080

Anonymous (2007) Agency for toxic substances and disease registry (ATSDR), toxicological profile for lead (Update). Public Health Service, U.S. Department of Health and Human Services, Atlanta, GA, USA

Bagewadi SS, Kumbhojkar VF (2015) Role of metals and minerals in ayurvedic therapeutics. Int Ayurvedic Med J 3:1–4

Berners-Price SJ, Mirabelli CK, Johnson RK, Mattern MR, McCabe FL, Faucette LF, Sung CM, Mong SM, Sadler PJ, Crooke ST (1986) *In vivo* antitumor activity and *in vitro* cytotoxic properties of bis[1,2-bis(diphenylphosphino)ethane]gold(I) chloride. Cancer Res 46: 5486–5493

Bost M, Houdart S, Oberli M, Kalonji E, Huneau JF, Margaritis I (2016) Dietary copper and human health: current evidence and unresolved issues. J Trace Elem Med Biol 35:107–115

Brigger I, Dubernet C, Couvreur P (2002) Nanoparticles in cancer therapy and diagnosis. Adv Drug Delivery Rev 54:631–651

Claire SA, Paul JD (2001) Ruthenium in medicine: current clinical uses and future prospects. Platin Metals Rev 45(2):62–69

Dabrowiak JC (2012) Metals in medicine. Inorganic Chemica Acta. Preface

Desoize B (2004) Metals and metal compounds in cancer treatment. Anticancer Res 24:1529–1544

Dghaim R, Khatib SA, Rasool H and Khan MA (2015) Determination of heavy metals concentration in traditional herbs commonly consumed in the United Arab Emirates. J Environ Public Health. Article ID 973878, 6 pages http://dx.doi.org/10.1155/2015/973878

Feng CQ, Ma WL, Zheng WL (2002) Research advances on effect of arsenic trioxide on tumor. Ai Zheng 21:1386–1389

Fosmire GJ (1990) Zinc toxicity. Am J Clin Nutr 51(2):225–257

Gupta VK, Singh S, Agrawal A, Siddiqi NJm Sharma B (2015) Phytochemicals mediated remediation of neurotoxicity induced by heavy metals. Biochem Res Int, Article ID 534769. http://dx.doi.org/10.1155/2015/534769

Hu SZ, Fu YM, Yu WJ (1997) Studies of the antitumor antimony(III) triaminocarboxylic complexonates. Crystal structures of $NH_4[Sb(Hdtpa)].H_2O$ and $Na[Sb(Hdtpa)].4.5H_2O$ (dtpa = diethylenetriamine-pentaacetic acid). Main Group Metal Chem 20:169–180

Irvine D, Vincent L, Graydon JE, Bubela N, Thompson L (1994) Prevalence and correaltes of fatigue in patients receiving treatment with chemotherapy and radiotherapy: a comparison with fatigue experienced by healthy individuals. Cancer Nurs 17(5):367–378

Jamieson ER, Lippard SJ (1999) Structure, recognition, and processing of cisplatin-DNA adducts. Chem Rev 99:2467–2498

Johnson FM (1998) The genetic effects of environmental lead. Mutat Res 410(2):123–140

Knudson AG (2001) Two genetic hits (more or less) to cancer. Nat Rev Cancer 1:157–162

Korfali SI, Hawi T, Mroueh M (2013a) Evaluation of heavy metals content in dietary supplements in Lebanon. Chem Central J 7:10. https://doi.org/10.1186/1752-153X-7-10

Korfali SI, Mroueh M, Al-Zein M, Salem R (2013b) Metal concentration in commonly used medicinal herbs and infusion by Lebanese population: health impact. J Food Res 2(2):70–80

Lecureur V, Le Thiec A, Le Meur A, Amiot L, Drenou B, Bernard M, Lamy T, Fauchet R, Fardel O (2002) Potassium antimonyl tartrate induces caspase- and reactive oxygen species-dependent apoptosis in lymphoid tumoral cells. Br J Haematol 119:608–615

Li SM, Fang Y, Ning HM, Wu YX (2012) Heavy metals in Chinese therapeutic foods and herbs. J Chem Soc Pak 34(5):1091–1095

Lippard SJ (1994) Metals in medicine. Bioinorganic chemistry. University Science Books, Mill City, pp 505–583

Liu Q, Hilsenbeck S, Gazitt Y (2003) Arsenic trioxide-induced apoptosis in myeloma cells: p53-dependent G1 or G2/M cell cycle arrest, activation of caspase 8 or caspase 9 and synergy with APO2/TRAIL. Blood 101:4078–4087

Lloyd NC, Morgan HW, Nicholson BK, Ronimus RS (2005) The composition of Ehrlich's salvarsan: resolution of a century-old debate. Angew Chem Int Ed 44(6):941–944

Lynch E, Braithwaite R (2005) A review of the clinical and toxicological aspects of 'traditional' (herbal) medicines adulterated with heavy metals. Expert Opin Drug Safety 4(4):769–778

Mahan L, Escott-Stump S, Raymond L (2012) Krause's food and nutrition care process. In: Alexopoulos Y (ed), 13th edn. Saunders, St. Louis, Mo, USA

Martin S, Griswold W (2009) Human health effects of heavy metals. Center for Hazardous Substance Research, Manhattan, Kan, USA. Environ Sci Technol Briefs Citizens 15:1–6

Maobe MAG, Gatebe E, Gitu L, Rotich H (2012) Profile of heavy metals in selected medicinal plants used for the treatment of diabetes, malaria and pneumonia in Kisii Region southwest Kenya. Glob J Pharmacol 6(3):245–251

Makropoulos V, Bruning T, Schulze-Osthoff K (1996) Selenium mediated inhibition of transcription factor NF-kappa B and HIV-1 LTR promoter activity. Arch Toxicol 70:277–283

Marzano C, Pellei M, Colavito D, Alidori S, Lobbia GG, Gandin V, Tisato F, Santini C (2006) Synthesis, characterization, and in vitro antitumor properties of tris (hydroxymethyl) phosphine copper(I) complexes containing the new bis (1,2,4-triazol-1-yl) acetate ligand. J Med Chem 49(25):7317–7324

Marzano C, Pellei M, Tisato F, Santini C (2009) Copper complexes as anticancer agents. Anti-Cancer Agents Med Chem 9:185–211

McKeage MJ, Maharaj L, Berners-Price SJ (2002) Mechanisms of cytotoxicity and antitumor activity of gold(I) phosphine complexes: the possible role of mitochondria. Coord Chem Rev 232:127–135

Othmana FB, Mohamed HJBJ, Sirajudeen KNS, Noh MFM, Rajabe NF (2017) The influence of selenium status on body composition, oxidative DNA damage and total antioxidant capacity in newly diagnosed type 2 diabetes mellitus: a case-control study. J Trace Elem Med Biol 43:106–112

Rasheed SP, Shivashankar M (2015) Evaluation of herbo mineral formulations (bhasma): an overview. Int J Res Ayurveda Pharm 6:382–386

Salt DE (2001) Disease-fighting foods may be derived from plants. Science Daily www.sciencedaily.com/releases/2001/08/0108150815082019.htm

Sampayo-Reyes A, Zakharyan RA, Healy SM, Aposhian HV (2000) Monomethylarsonic acid reductase and monomethylarsonous acid in hamster tissue. Chem Res Toxicol 13:1181–1186

Saper RB, Kales SN, Paquin J, Burns MJ, Eisenberg DM, Davis RB, Phillips RS (2004) Heavy metal content of Ayurvedic Herbal medicine product. J Am Med Assoc 292(23):2868–2873

Sarkar PK, Das S, Prajapati PK (2010) Ancient concept of metal pharmacology based on Ayurvedic Literature. Ancient Sci Life 29(4):1–6

Schrauzer GN (2000) Anti-carcinogenic effects of selenium. Cell Mol Life Sci 57:1864–1873

Sharma B, Singh S, Siddiqi NJ (2014) Biomedical implications of heavy metals induced imbalances in redox systems. Biomed Res Int 2014: Article ID 640754. https://doi.org/10.1155/2014/640754

Shen ZY, Shen WY, Chen MH, Shen J, Zeng Y (2003) Reactive oxygen species and antioxidants in apoptosis of esophageal cancer cells induced by As_2O_3. Int J Mol Med 11:479–484

Sinha R, Said TK, Medina D (1996) Organic and inorganic selenium compounds inhibit mouse mammary cell growth in vitro by different cellular pathways. Cancer Lett 107:277–284

Singh R, Gautam N, Mishra A, Gupta R (2011) "Heavy metals and living systems: an overview. Indian J Pharmacol 3(3):246–253

Solovyev ND (2015) Importance of selenium and selenoprotein for brain function: from antioxidant protection to neuronal signalling. J Inorg Biochem 153:1–12
Subrahmanian CVS, Setty JT, Suresh S, Devi VK (2002) Size reduction, 2nd edn. Vallabh Prakashan, Delhi, p 148
Tiekink ER (2002a) Antimony and bismuth compounds in oncology. Crit Rev Oncol Hematol 42:217–224
Tiekink ER (2002b) Gold derivatives for the treatment of cancer. Crit Rev Oncol Hematol 42: 225–248
Trueba GP, Sanchez GM, Giuliani A (2004) Oxygen free radical and antioxidant defense mechanism in cancer. Front Biosci 9:2029–2044
Valko M, Rhodes CJ, Moncol J, Izakovic M, Mazur M (2006) Free radicals, metals and antioxidants in oxidative stress-induced cancer. Chemico-Biol Inter 160:1–40
Wang T, Guo Z (2006) Copper in medicine: homeostasis, chelation therapy and antitumor drug design. Curr Med Chem 13(5):525–537
Wikipedia (2017a) Composition of the human body. Accessed 25 May 2017
Wikipedia (2017b) Cobalt therapy. Wikipedia. Accessed 20 June 2017
World Health Organization (2005) WHO drug information 19(3):215–216
www.healingbase.com, The use of metals and minerals in Ayurvedic and Siddha Medicine. Accessed 25 May 2017
Zhao Z, Huang C, Wang J, Jiang H, Li J, Wang X (2002) Effect of arsenic trioxide on inhibition of restenosis after rabbit vascular injury and its mechanism. Chin Med J 115:1608–1614 (English)

Chapter 10
Mechanism of Action of Anticancer Metallodrugs

Carmen Mejía, Said Ortega-Rosales and Lena Ruiz-Azuara

Abstract Herein the anticancer mechanisms of action from platinum and essential metals compounds are discussed. In the second half of last century, the cytotoxic activity of the cisplatin [cis-dichloro, diamin platinum (II)] was discovered and the use as anticancer drugs of this compound was proposed. For several decades, the inorganic anticancer drug seemed excellent. Nevertheless, undesired side effects such as toxicity and resistance to the drug shadowed its success. To accomplish an increased anticancer activity and a lower toxicity, several analogues such as carboplatin and oxaliplatin were developed as antineoplastic drugs. Research in the platinum metal group was developed rapidly; palladium, ruthenium, osmium, and rhodium. However, an innovative approach was developed by the use of essential metals compounds as an alternative to reduce the toxicity and resistance induced by the platinum compounds. Iron and copper were the first essential metal compounds studied. The term "metals" in medicine was emerging at that moment and later on, the term *Metallodrug* was acquired. Some other essential metals have been studied and proposed as metallodrugs. Regarding the mechanism of action, at first, interaction with DNA was thoroughly studied and research leads to the proposal of adducts formation by direct bond between platinum and DNA bases mainly. Later on, cell death by means of apoptosis was mentioned, and therefore, the formation of reactive species of oxygen was proposed.

C. Mejía (✉)
Facultad de Ciencias Naturales, Universidad Autónoma de Querétaro, Avenida de las Ciencias S/N Juriquilla, Delegación Santa Rosa Jáuregui, 76230 Querétaro, México
e-mail: maria.c.mejia@uv.es

S. Ortega-Rosales · L. Ruiz-Azuara
Departamento de Química Inorgánica y Nuclear, Laboratorio de Química Inorgánica Medicinal. Facultad de Química, Universidad Nacional Autónoma de México, Av. Universidad 3000, 04510 Mexico City, Mexico
e-mail: said.orosales@gmail.com

L. Ruiz-Azuara
e-mail: lenar701@gmail.com

M. Rai et al. (eds.), *Biomedical Applications of Metals*,
https://doi.org/10.1007/978-3-319-74814-6_10

Keywords Metals · Metallodrugs · Anticancer · Mechanism of action
Essential metals

10.1 Introduction

Since the discovery of cisplatinum (CDDPt) as a cytotoxic and antineoplastic compound, the interest on the research of coordination compounds as metallodrugs has been increased over the years. The medicinal inorganic chemistry discipline has been a growing field with direct impact on therapy of several diseases, mainly cancer, and also in diagnostic tools (Palermo et al. 2016). Nowadays, several Pt-based drugs are widely used in the treatment of cancer such as cisplatin, carboplatin, oxaliplatin, and nedaplatin (Dilruba et al. 2016). However, the clinical success of these compounds is limited by significant side effects and intrinsic or acquired resistance (Johnstone et al. 2016). Therefore, a rapid expansion in the development of novel metal-based anticancer drugs (metallodrugs) has been achieved (Barry et al. 2014) since 25 years ago, principally those involving essential metals, in order to improve clinical effectiveness, reduce general toxicity and broaden the activity spectrum (Nardon et al. 2014; Mari and Gasser 2015).

An innovative approach was to consider the possibility of introducing complexes containing essential metals under the hypothesis of decreased toxicity. Titanocene (dichloro, biscyclopentadienyl titanium (IV)) was developed and reached clinical trials (Buettner and Valentine 2012). One of the essential metal ions which has been profoundly explored is copper (Ruiz-Azuara and Bravo 2010; Santini et al. 2014). Copper's toxicity comes from its ability to produce reactive oxygen species (ROS), and direct cleavages of DNA and RNA (Linder 2002; García-Ramos et al. 2017). Direct cleavage of DNA comes as the product of interactions of metallodrugs with DNA followed by ROS formation (García-Ramos et al. 2017).

Among the essential metals, iron, cobalt, nickel, and zinc compounds had been investigated, also vanadium compounds have been tested for anticancer activity although early studies supported their antidiabetic activity. In this chapter, we concentrated mainly on the mechanism of action of the metallodrugs as anticancer compounds.

10.2 Nonessential Metal Compounds

10.2.1 Platinum Complexes

The discovery of cisplatin [*cis*-di-amminedichloridoplatinum(II)] as an antiproliferative compound (Rosenberg et al. 1965), positioned it as a successful anticancer drug. Since then, it has been used in tumors such as ovarian, testicular, head and neck, and lung (Wheate et al. 2010; Spreckelmeyer et al. 2014). Although more than 4000 platinum compounds have been tested as anticancer drugs, only carboplatin [*cis*-diammine (1,1-cyclobutanedicarboxylato)platinum(II)] and oxaliplatin [*R,R*-cyclohexane-1,2-diammineoxalatoplatinum(II)] have been approved by the FDA (1989 and 2002, respectively). Other three platinum compounds, nedaplatin, lobaplatin, and heptaplatin were approved only in some countries (Wheate et al. 2010) (Fig. 10.1).

The mechanisms of action of metal-based drugs by which they produce cytotoxicity are not fully elucidated and, in most cases, include a variety of biological targets. Once the drug has entered into the cell, it reacts with cellular components such as nucleic acids, proteins, membrane phospholipids, and thiol-containing molecules (glutathione or metallothioneins). Proteins that can bind to metal-based drugs include repair enzymes, transcription factors, histones, and HMG (high motility group) domain proteins, which can function as antioxidants, exchange electrons, repair DNA, or transporters of Cu (Ctrs), organic cation (OCT), solute carriers (SLC), or ATP binding cassette (ABC) (Burger et al. 2011; Casini and Reedijk 2012; Giacomini et al. 2013).

A biological target of cisplatin is DNA, and its mechanism of action includes changes in the structure of nucleic acids due to the increased formation of adducts, which represent a steric blockade so that RNA polymerase II is translocated on the adduct to synthesize new chains of RNA. The DNA adducts most frequently induced by cisplatin are the intrastrand cross-links where platinum is coordinated to the N7 positions of the imidazole ring of two adjacent guanines (60–65%), adenine and guanine ($\sim$20%), or the adducts of the same strand ($\sim$2%) (Lemaire et al. 1991; Brabec 2000). Another consequence of the formation of the DNA adducts is a distortion of the double helix conformation that gives rise to a structural motif recognized by several damaged DNA binding proteins and transcription factors, which may affect replication and transcription, ultimately resulting in cell death by apoptosis (Fig. 10.2) (Cohen 2001; Todd and Lippard 2009; Johnstone et al. 2016).

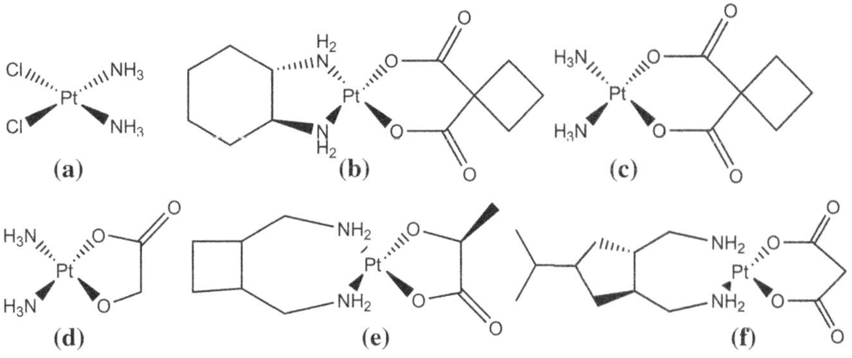

Fig. 10.1 **a** Cisplatin, **b** Oxaliplatin, **c** Carboplatin, **d** Nedaplatin, **e** Lobaplatin and **f** Heptaplatin

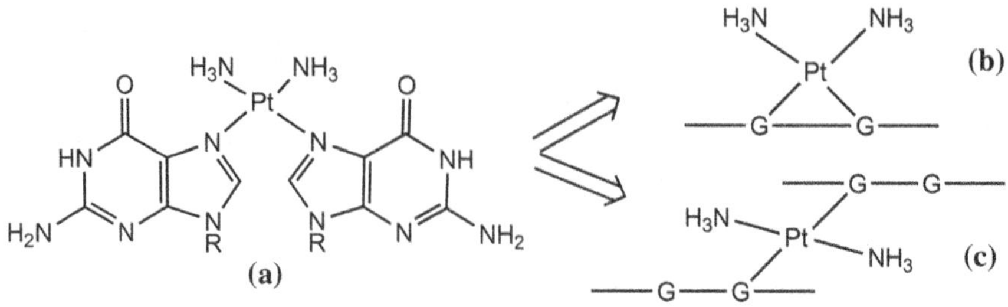

Fig. 10.2 **a** Guanine N(7)—cisplatin adduct which cause **b** Intrastrand cross-links and **c** Interstrand cross-links

Despite the success of cisplatin-based drugs, various mechanisms of resistance of cancer cells have been identified, including reduction of uptake or increase of drug outflow, complexation to sulfur ligands such as metallothionein or glutathione, low apoptosis due to hypermethylation of gene promoters, or cleavage of the Pt from DNA and damage repair, or increased DNA adduct bypass activity (Martin et al. 2008; Nijwening et al. 2011; Espina et al. 2017). Therefore, there is a need to design alternative metal-based anticancer drugs that can overcome the problems of cancer cell selectivity, resistance and side effects of platinum complexes including nephrotoxicity, ototoxicity, and peripheral neurotoxicity (Wheate et al. 2010).

Recently, it has been shown that the photoactivation of the platinum compounds may be the solution to these drawbacks. The rationale is that the application of irradiation may be restricted to tumor tissues only in such a way that the resulting effects could be much more selective for tumor cells, thereby minimizing the side effects (Farrer et al. 2009). Moreover, it has been observed that the biological mechanism of cisplatin is not significantly affected by irradiation with UVA, visible light (Heringova et al. 2006; Kasparkova et al. 2015), or even more with red light (Zhang and Dong 2009, Zhang et al. 2015).

On the other hand, the effect of a new bifunctional and mononuclear Pt(II) compound, trans-[$PtCl_2(NH_3)(L)$] (L = 1-methyl-7-azaindole) was investigated (Pracharova et al. 2016). To establish the photocytotoxic effect of UVA radiation, the human cell lines of ovarian carcinoma A2780 (parent cisplatin-sensitive) and prostate adenocarcinoma LNCaP were treated with this compound. It was found that after UVA radiation, both cell lines suffered dose-dependent apoptosis. This type of cell death can generate singlet oxygen responsible for DNA cleavage (Pracharova et al. 2016)

In the search for more active and less toxic compounds against cancer, several platinum (IV) compounds have been explored. It is known that octahedral compounds $5d^6$ of low spin Pt^{IV}, unlike the square planar complexes Pt^{II}, are largely inert due to the substitution of ligands, so it is probable that the drugs will experience fewer reactions to penetrate the cancerous cell. However, Pt^{IV} complexes can be activated chemically by reduction (Bramwell et al. 1985; van der Veer et al. 1986; Anderson et al. 1988), although their effect will depend on the abundance and local concentration of reductants such as glutathione and ascorbate. Another factor that may explain the selective activation of Pt^{IV} as prodrugs is hypoxia, which may favor a reducing microenvironment. Advantages of Pt^{IV} over platinum(II) complexes include a higher aqueous solubility (Braddock et al. 1975), as well as a reduced probability of deactivation of the compounds as anticancer prodrugs (Barry and Sadler 2013; Butler and Sadler 2013; Johnstone et al. 2013; Smith and Sadler 2013), due to their inertness before undergoing reduction.

Following these arguments, the group of (Mackay et al. 2007) developed a general method for the photoactivation of Pt^{IV}-diazido complexes containing different monodentate and chelated diamine ligands which allow a specific site supply, greatly reducing the possibility of undesired effects including mechanisms of cell resistance.

Some examples of these Pt^{IV}-diazido complexes include the *trans, trans, trans*-$[Pt(N_3)_2(OH)_2(NH_3)(pyridine)]$ complex that contains an octahedral Pt^{IV} center with linear azido ligands, which is very stable in darkness when accompanied by millimolar concentrations of glutathione. This combination can undergo photoinduction of ligand substitution and photoreduction, promoting an increase in toxicity by cellular photoactivation, as was observed in cisplatin-resistant human ovarian cancer cells (Mackay et al. 2007). Other compounds were *trans-dihydroxide* $[Pt(N_3)_2(OH)_2(NH_3)(X)]$ (X = alkyl or aryl amine) platinum(IV) diazido complexes. These complexes were investigated to determine the influence of *cis–trans* isomerism, showing that *trans* isomers of aliphatic or aromatic amine-containing complexes are more photocytotoxic than their *cis* isomers (Farrer et al. 2009). The novel platinum(IV) diazido *trans, trans, trans*-$[Pt(N_3)_2(OH)_2(pyridine)_2]$ is another complex synthesized by this group. The novelty of this bis-pyridine complex includes photoactivation at low doses of UVA, visible blue, and green light. The last two radiation energies showed cytotoxicity in keratinocytes and ovarian cancer cell lines at micromolar doses, showing an increased antiproliferative activity (Farrer et al. 2010). The resulting cell death is not an apoptotic process (Westendorf et al. 2012) because its stability in aqueous solution can protect the cells of reactive oxygen species (ROS), mainly through detoxification by GSH that leads to the deactivation of platinum (Petzold and Sadler 2008).

Another photoactivatable Pt(IV) prodrug is *trans, trans, trans*-$[Pt(N_3)_2(OH)(OCOCH_2CH_2CONH\text{-}TEMPO)(Py)_2]$ (Pt-TEMPO, where TEMPO = 2,2,6,6-tetramethylpiperidine 1-oxyl). Photoactivation of this complex with visible blue light produced Pt(II) and azidyl radicals as well as nitroxyl. It also showed cytotoxicity toward A2780 human ovarian cancer cells in a manner similar to chlorpromazine (a clinical photosensitizer) (Venkatesh et al. 2016). On the other hand, nitroxyl radicals are permeable to the membrane and also possess antioxidant activity mimicking superoxide dismutase (SOD) (Offer et al. 2000), which has been shown active in a variety of cancer cell lines (Suy et al. 1998; Arion et al. 2012) (Fig. 10.3).

Considering that tumor cells overexpress different factors due to the cell growth process, transmembrane heterodimeric glycoproteins have become another relevant subject of study (Auzzas et al. 2010). Currently, peptides containing metal-based drug-bound RGD (-Arg-Gly-Asp-) sequences (Mukhopadhyay et al. 2008;

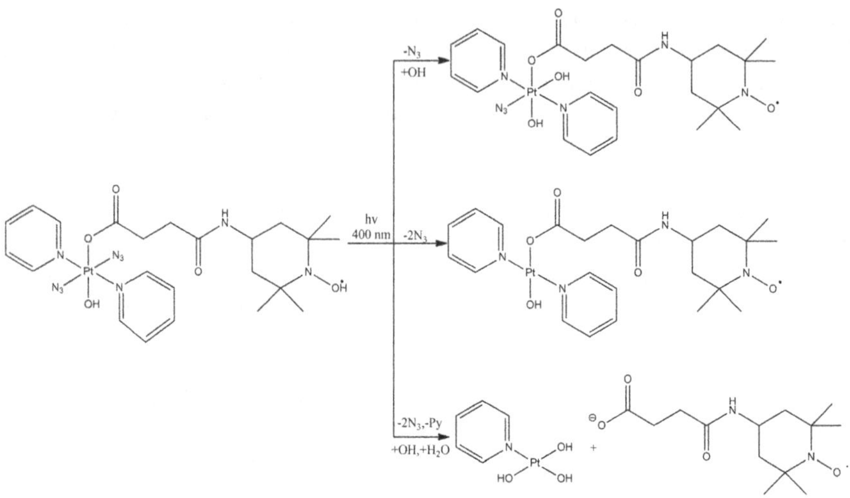

Fig. 10.3 Photoreaction pathways for Pt-TEMPO, (0.1 mm in H_2O) on irradiation with blue visible light, 400 nm, showing the products of the reaction

Barragán et al. 2011; Yuan et al. 2013; Massaguer et al. 2015) have been explored for their toxicity in cancer cells (Temming et al. 2005; Liu 2006; Danhier et al. 2012). Thus, the anticancer agent was synthesized based on the conjugation of a photoactivable *trans, trans, trans*- $[Pt(N_3)_2(OH)_2(py)_2]$ prodrug to a cyclic RGD sequence (-Arg-Gly-Asp-), which is selectively recognized by integrins $\alpha_v\beta3$ and $\alpha_v\beta5$. As was demonstrated in SK-MEL-28 melanoma cancer cells overexpressing $\alpha_v\beta_3$ integrin compared to DU-145 human prostate carcinoma cells as a consequence of the phototoxicity of the complex induced by visible light irradiation (Gandioso et al. 2015).

Despite the success of platinum compounds on various tumors, the extensive knowledge of its mechanism of action, and even more so as its suitability to reduce the multiple undesirable effects, research on different metal drugs such as ruthenium is more active never.

10.2.2 Ruthenium Complexes

In the fight against cancer, metal-based compounds are still under investigation. Thus, ruthenium-based compounds have been developed (Süss-Fink et al. 2010). These metal-based drugs may be useful in the treatment of platinum-drug-resistant tumors (Bergamo and Sava 2011; Heffeter et al. 2014).

Ruthenium complexes can readily be obtained in two oxidation states (II and III) and are susceptible to ligand exchange. Currently, two rhutenium (III) complexes have completed Phase I clinical trials (Heffeter et al. 2014), [ImH]

[trans-$RuCl_4$(DMSO)Im)](DMSO)(Im)(Im=imidazole) also called (NAMI-A) (Fig. 10.4a) and *trans*-[tetrachlorobis(iH-indazole)ruthenate (III)] or (KP1019) (Fig. 10.4b). Both compounds have shown low dose toxicity and high selectivity for metastasis of solid tumors (Bergamo and Sava 2007). For its part, NKP-1339, a sodium salt analogue of KP1019 is a strong candidate for clinical trials because of the cytotoxicity shown in various tumors and specifically in cisplatin-resistant human colon carcinoma cell lines. A third group of Ru complexes included RAPTA-C, RM175, and RAPTA-T (Fig. 10.4c, d, e respectively) are in preclinical phase due to their activity against primary tumors and metastasis (Bergamo et al. 2012) by G2/M cell cycle arrest (Babak et al. 2015).

Other four ruthenium(II)-based complexes with N-(acyl)-N′,N′-(disubstituted), thiourea derivatives (Th) were synthesized. The compounds with a general trans [$Ru(PPh_3)_2$(Th)(bipy)] PF_6 formula can bind to bovine serum albumin (BSA) and DNA. Additionally, they were shown to be more cytotoxic on DU-145 (prostate) and A549 (lung) cancer cells compared to normal cells (L929) (Correa et al. 2015).

Some compounds that have shown to be a promising alternative against cancer are the organometallic arene Ru(II) complexes [(η6-biphenyl)Ru(en) $Cl]^+$ (en = ethylenediamine) (Wang et al. 2003), and [(η6-p-cymene)Ru(PTA)Cl_2] (p-cymene = para-cymene and PTA = 1,3,5-triaza-7-phosphaadamantane) (Pernot et al. 2012; Romero-Canelón et al. 2013). The activity of arene osmium half-sandwich analogous has been extensively studied in vitro and in vivo to explain anticancer activity (Fu et al. 2011; Barry and Sadler 2012). These metal-based drugs show interactions between the Ru-Cl reactive linker complexes

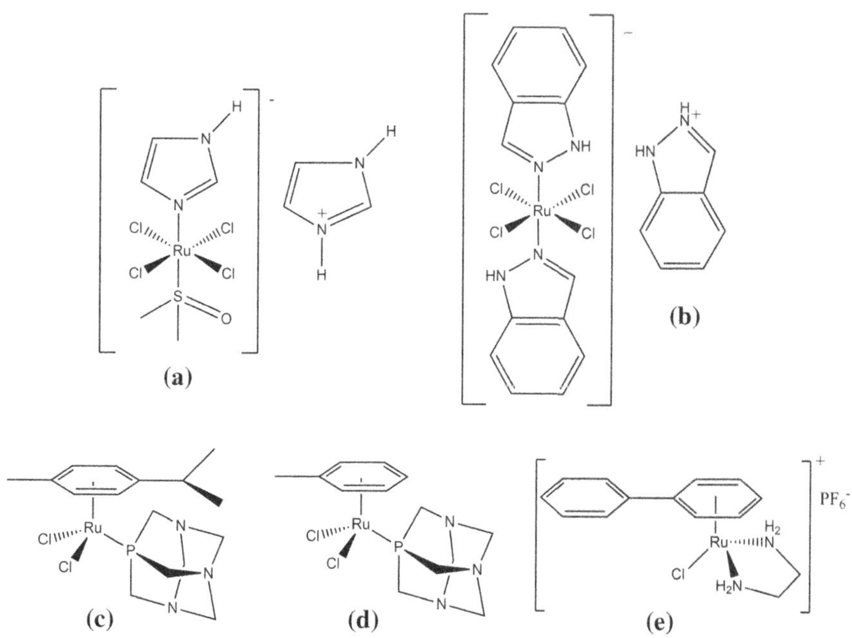

Fig. 10.4 **a** NAMI-A, **b** KP1019, **c** RAPTA-C, **d** RAPTA-T, **e** RM175

bonds and the nuclear DNA by hydrolysis, by developing intermediary aqua complexes able to ruthenate DNA at guanine residues (Chen et al. 2002). Other RuII arene complexes of mono- and bidentate N-donor ligands with carboxyl or ester groups and chlorido ancillary ligands were synthesized by the group of Richter et al. (2016). Its antitumor activity was measured in different cell lines, but only in human breast cancer (MCF-7) it was more effective, as demonstrated through inhibition of cell division and caspase-dependent apoptosis.

New ruthenium(II) and iron(II) organometallic compounds of general formula [(η5-C5H5)M(PP)Lc][PF_6], bearing carbohydrate derivative ligands (Lc), were synthesized and their biological activity was investigated in colon cancer HCT116. Their effects include significantly more cytotoxic than oxaliplatin, elevated levels of caspase-3 and -7, and finally dose-dependent apoptosis (Florindo et al. 2015).

The ruthenium(II) [Ru(h_2- $O_2CCH_2CH_3$)$(dppe)_2$]PF_6 complex containing dppe and the propionate anion was synthesized and characterized recently. When their biological activity was measured, a higher cytotoxicity was in murine sarcoma (S-180) than in human cells (HepG2 hepatocellular carcinoma, MCF-7 breast adenocarcinoma, MO59J glioblastoma, and GM07492A normal lung fibroblasts). Recently, new cycloruthenated [Ru(bpy)(phpy)(dppz)]+(bpy = bipyridine, dppz = dipyridophenazine) complex was synthesized by replacing the bpy ligand with the cycloruthenated ligand, phpy (2-phenylpyridine), from the molecule [Ru (bpy)2(dppz)]2+. The compound showed a higher cytotoxity than cisplatin and easily penetrated the nucleus (Huang et al. 2014). Mari and Gasser et al. (2015) observed that $[Ru(dppz)_2(CppH)]^{2+}$ (1a, CppH = 2-(20-pyridyl)-pyrimidine-4-carboxylic acid) accumulates in mitochondria as well as shows important tumor selectivity. As compared to cisplatin on A2780 cancer cells, their activity is similar (IC50 2.8 and 2.9 mM, respectively), but it is less toxic in healthy MRC-5 cells (Dickerson et al. 2014; Zeng et al. 2017).

A group of diruthenium (II, III) metallodrugs containing the nonsteroidal anti-inflammatory drug (NSAID), Ru_2(NSAID) have shown important anticancer activity. These metallodrugs containing ibuprofen (HIbp), [$Ru_2(Ibp)_4Cl$] or RuIbp, and also the new analogue of naproxen (HNpx), [$Ru_2(Npx)_4Cl$] or RuNpx, were encapsulated in novel injectable solid polymer–lipid nanoparticles (SPLNs). The Ru_2(NSAID)-SPLNs showed increased cytotoxicity (IC50 at 60–100) with respect to their corresponding Ru_2(NSAID) metallodrugs in EMT6 and MDA-MB-231 (both breast) and DU145 (prostate) cancer cells. The cell viability of both metallodrug nanoformulations was also compared with those of the parent NSAIDs, HIbp and HNpx, and their corresponding NSAID-SPLNs. In vivo and ex vivo experiments revealed good biodistribution and high tumor accumulation of fluorescence-labeled SPLNs following injection in an orthotopic breast tumor model. On the other hand, when RuIbp metallodrug was tested in a C6 rat orthotopic glioma model, it showed great efficiency by decreasing the tumor area in addition to affecting the cell cycle proteins p21, p27, p53, Bax, and COX-1. Likewise, inhibition of cellular proliferation in the U138MG glioma cell line (p53 mutant type) was higher compared to U87MG and A172 (p53 wild type) cell lines, suggesting that p53 and COX-1 may play a key role in the mechanism of action of

RuIbp. Whereas RuIbp and aqua-RuNpx only weakly affected the proliferation of human colon carcinoma cells (HT-29 and Caco-2) and had no significant effect on Hep2 human larynx or T24/83 human bladder tumor (Alves et al. 2017).

As with other metal-based anticancer drugs, tumor selectivity is an important factor to consider among the Ru complexes. To solve this, photocaged Ru complexes have been proposed (Siewert et al. 2016; Sun et al. 2017). The ability of Ru complexes to absorb visible or near-infrared (NIR) light penetrates the tissue causing less damage to biological systems than UV light. Photocaged Ru complexes can be activated by NIR light through a process of one photon or a photon upconversion. This gives the photocaged Ru complexes a higher activity in vitro over in vivo because of their rapid urine excretion in mice. On the other hand, Sun et al. (2017) synthesized a novel Ru containing block copolymer (PolyRu) as a photoactivated polymetallodrug. Experiments in mice showed that PolyRu allowed inhibition of tumor growth after light irradiation, further showing minimal systemic toxicity. The red light irradiation of the nanoparticles in cancer cells HeLa, PC3, and HepG2 increased the antitumour activity of the Ru compounds. For the photoactivation (with red light) the cancer cells with the nanoparticles where incubated for 24 h (Sun et al. 2017). Another work describes two novel photopharmacological ruthenium prodrugs based on the tetrapyridyl biqbpy ligand (6,60-bis[N-(isoquinolyl)-1-amino]-2,20-bipyridine), which can be activated by green light. Its biological activity was investigated in the A431 and A549 cancer cell lines, which showed an increase up to 22-fold in cytotoxicity as well as cell death by apoptosis after green light irradiation (520 nm, 75 J cm^{-2}) (Siewert et al. 2016).

A novel study was focused on looking for apoptosis-independent drugs for which they were given the task of synthesizing 195 organoruthenium complexes. These compounds were screening in sensitive HCT116 colorectal carcinoma, and apoptosis-resistant TC7 cells (Violette et al. 2002). It was thus found that two Re (V) oxo complexes exhibited necroptosis, a form of cell death where necrosis is mediated by the RIP1/RIP3 kinase complex (Suntharalingam et al. 2015), while other Ru(II) complexes underwent another non-apoptotic cell death (Soldevila-Barreda et al. 2015; Yuan et al. 2015; Siewert et al. 2016). It is important to establish the type of cellular death because the multidrug-resistant phenotype (MDR) becomes highly refractory to treatments and thus to die by apoptosis (Fulda et al. 2009; Hervouet et al. 2013)

Finally, to study the possible pathways for accumulation of metal-based Ru (Romero-Canelón et al. 2013) two iminopyridine ruthenium(II) arene complexes were investigated, which differ in their halide ligands, Ru(η6-*p*-cymene)(*N*,*N*-dimethyl-*N*′-[(*E*)-pyridine-2-ylmethylidene]benzene-1,4-diamine)X]PF6 (X = Cl, I) (Romero-Canelon et al. 2012). To test this, human ovarian cancer A2780 cells were co-incubated with the compounds and different concentrations of verapamil (competitor for efflux via P-gp), oubain (inhibition of Na+/K+pump), $CuCl_2$ (competitor for transport via hCtr1), antimycin A (ATP depletion), amphotericin B (membrane disruption and model for protein-mediated transport), and methyl ß-cyclodextrin (caveolae endocytosis). It was noted that by changing from a chloro to an iodo ligand, the mechanism of uptake varied from being active to mainly passive diffusion (Ca 40% and Cl 26%, respectively) through the cell membrane. In addition, it seems that the endocytosis pathway is not involved in the uptake of Ru complexes as shown by co-incubation experiments with methyl β-cyclodextrin (Romero-Canelon et al. 2012). These results showed that the accumulation pathways for Ru compounds include the cell type, the type of ligand set stabilizing the metal center, the oxidation state of the metal, the possible effects of the compounds on the transporters distribution and expression, as well as the metal complex speciation pathways (Spreckelmeyer et al. 2014). Characteristics that must be taken into account for this metal-based Ru can be used effectively against different tumors.

10.3 Essential Metal Compounds

The use of metals has not only spread to the treatment of various diseases but also to antitumorals, it has also been diversified to consider essential metals such as titanium (IV), the compounds of titanium are titanocene [$cp_2Ti\ Cl_2$] and [(bzac)2Ti $(OEt)_2$], which were the first molecules without platinum to reach Clinical Phase I (Buettner and Valentine 2012).

10.3.1 *Iron Complexes*

The coordination compounds of iron, another relevant essential metal, present different biological targets. Among these, enzymes and their inhibition results particularly important. In addition, nuclease activity has been observed (Araujo et al. 2016). One example of this type of behavior is the bimetallic Fe(III) complex with the ligand 2,6-bis(1,4,7-triazacyclonon-1-ylmethyl)-4-methylphenol (bcmp) has been synthesized and studied. The geometry of the coordination environment of the two iron atoms is octahedral in the complex, [Fe_2-{bcmp(-H)}(μ-OH)Cl_2]Cl_2, and the metal atoms are bounded to the two triaza-cyclononane rings of bcmp and the sixth coordination position contains one chlorine, one bridging phenolate oxygen, and one bridging hydroxide group. The di-iron complex has been obtained unfortunately; attempts to obtain a crystal were unsuccessful. Mössbauer spectroscopic investigations confirmed the presence of only Fe(III) centers; no signals of Fe(II) species were detected. In aqueous solution, the two chloride ligands are replaced by water ligands as confirmed by the ESI mass spectrum (Araujo et al. 2016).

The family of the metallo-nucleases, which are able to hydrolyze the phosphodiester bonds of DNA and RNA, is of particular interest, since the phosphate diester linkages in DNA are extremely resistant to spontaneous hydrolysis; at neutral pH and 25 °C, the half-life for the hydrolysis of the bond is more than hundreds of thousands of years. The interaction of [Fe_2{bcmp(-H)}(μ-OH)Cl_2]Cl_2 compound with CT DNA was studied by electronic absorption spectroscopy and gel electrophoresis. Notably, the complex relaxes supercoiled pUC19 DNA into the nicked form at low micromolar concentration (10 μM) in the presence of an external reducing agent (ascorbic acid). Finally, the in vitro antiproliferative activity of $[Fe_2\text{-}\{bcmp(\text{-}H)\}(\mu\text{-}OH)_{C12}]Cl_2$ was assessed on a panel of human cancer cell lines and results revealed that the complex exhibited a significant cytotoxic effects in particular versus colon LoVo cancer cells, with IC50 value 2.5 times lower than that shown by the reference metallodrug cisplatin (3.54 vs. 8.53 lM). DNA binding activity of the Fe(III) compound supports the hypothesis that its molecular mechanism and cytotoxic potential is related to its DNA cleavage ability. (Araujo et al. 2016).

Artificial metallonucleases are metal complexes that catalyze phosphate diester hydrolysis, mimic the function of the nucleases, and can be employed as biomimetic systems to elucidate the mechanisms of natural enzymes. Dinuclear complexes of Cu(II) and Zn(II) have shown interesting biological properties such as DNA cleavage activity and in vitro cytotoxicity against different cancer cell lines. These results triggered interest in using Fe(III) instead of Cu(II) and Zn(II), where the higher oxidation state of iron could lead to stronger binding interaction with negatively charged phosphate diester backbone of DNA and thus higher biological activity. It has been found as well that a bimetallic complex based on two Fe(III) ions is able to cleave DNA and catalyze oxidation of catechol.

10.3.2 Nickel and Zinc Complexes

Chemokine receptors are signaling proteins located on the cellular surface, which have specific physiological roles like recruitment of leukocytes to sites of infection and the trafficking of stem cells for organ formation at the embryonic stage. There are currently 19 known chemokine receptors with a confirmed role. There are only two clinically approved drugs targeting the-mokine receptors: maraviroc, which targets the CCR5 receptor and is used to treat HIV infection and plerixafor, which targets the CXCR4 chemokine receptor, which is used for haemato-poietic stem cell mobilization to allow harvesting in patients with B-cell non-Hodgkin's lymphoma and multiple myeloma prior to immuno-compromising treatment. The CXCR4 receptor is also linked with many diseases, such as arthritis, asthma, HIV infection, and various types of cancer.

It is possible to take advantage of the properties of transitions metals, such as nickel(II), which is particularly interesting due to its varying coordination preferences. It can form diamagnetic square planar complexes or expand its coordination sphere to incorporate additional donors. Plerixafor is a cyclam-based compound that contains two macrocyclic rings with an ideal ring size cavity for binding to first row transition metals. The only nickel(II) complex investigated as a CXCR4 antagonist is the plerixafor/AMD3100 complex (Smith et al. 2012)

The anti-HIV data on $[Ni_2AMD3100]^{4+}$ shows that the compound has a very similar potency to the free ligand and is lower than the equivalent zinc(II) complexes. Nevertheless, previous studies on configurationally restricted macrocyclic zinc(II) complexes showed increased potency, relative to both plerixafor and its complexes, and for this reason, the study has been extended to nickel(II) with the cyclam ligands.

The most striking structure in the database for comparison is one where two C-alkylated cyclam nickel(II) complexes are bridged by a bis-carboxylate. This contains one metal center which is six coordinate with a coordinated water molecule and a monodentate acetate ligand and a second metal centre which is six coordinate with a bidentate acetate.

The biological assays were based on calcium signaling and anti-HIV activity. An initial screen of the compounds was carried out using a calcium signaling assay in response to stimulation by the chemokine protein binding partner of the CXCR4 receptor, CXCL12. The concentration of intracellular calcium released was measured and the abrogation of this flux by the antagonists was recorded at a series of concentrations to give a value whereby a 50% reduction was observed. The bis ring nickel(II) complexes show a higher potency than the mono ring compound $[Ni_2]^{2+}$, only active at a micromolar level. The para side bridged compound $[Ni_2]^{4+}$ was significantly more active than the meta one, cross-bridged compound and 2-fold more active than plerixafor. The cytotoxicity of the three nickel(II) complexes was measured in MT-4 cells as IC50 and in all cases was greater than 125 μM, the maximum value tested. Nickel(II) complexes can have low cytotoxicity and high potency against HIV, which makes them highly selective. The flexible coordination sphere of nickel(II) is a good match for introducing strong binding interactions with the protein amino acid residues and offers significant scope for the future development of metallodrugs (Smith et al. 2012)

Low selectivity, toxicity, and drug resistance are associated with the use of zinc(II) thiosemicarbazone complexes $[Zn(atc\text{-}Et)_2]$ and $[Zn(atc\text{-}Ph)_2]$ (atc-R: monovalent anion of 2-acetylpyridine N4-R-thiosemicarbazone) were synthesized and fully characterized in the solid state and in solution via elemental analysis, Fourier transform infrared (FTIR), ultraviolet–visible (UV–Vis) and proton nuclear magnetic resonance (1H NMR) spectroscopy, conductometric and single-crystal X-ray diffraction. The cytotoxicity of these complexes was evaluated in the HepG2, HeLa, MDA-MB-231, K-562, DU 145, and MRC-5 cancer cell lines. The strongest antiproliferative results were observed in MDA-MB-231 and HepG2 cells, in which these complexes displayed significant selective toxicity (3.1 and 3.6, respectively) compared with their effects on normal MRC-5 cells. In vivo studies were performed using an alternative model (*Artemia salina* L.) to assure the safety of these complexes, and the results were confirmed using a conventional model (BALB/c mice). Tests of oral bioavailability showed maximum plasma concentrations of 3029.50 and 1191.95 g/L for complexes $[Zn(atc\text{-}Et)_2]$ and $[Zn(atc\text{-}Ph)_2]$, respectively. According to all obtained results, both compounds could be considered as prospective antiproliferative agents that warrant further research (Lopes et al. 2016).

10.3.3 Copper Complexes

The first copper mixed chelate complexes that have synthesized, characterized, and patented as antineoplastic agents is a series of based on copper (II) mixed chelates registered under the trademark Casiopeínas® (Fig. 10.5a) (Ruiz-Azuara 1992, 1996, 1997), with general formulas [Cu (NN) (aminoacidato)] NO_3 and [Cu (N-N) (OO)] NO_3, where the donor NN is a substituted aromatic diimine (1,10-phenanthroline or 2,2′-bipyridine) and the oxygen donor (OO) is acetylacetonate (acac) or salicylaldehyde (salal) (Fig. 10.5b).

By monocrystal X-ray diffraction, the crystal structures were obtained and it is observed that this type of compound has square-shaped pyramid geometry slightly distorted with a water molecule in the apical position, as seen in Fig. 10.6 (García-Ramos et al. 2017).

Currently, more than 100 Casiopeínas have been synthesized, which are divided into different groups according to the binders they present in their structure by first and secondary ligands combination. The design of Casiopeínas® takes into consideration molecules that provide to copper the possibility of producing cytotoxicity by means of different mechanisms of action. In the case of copper, it is known that this metal is involved in various biological processes (Da Silva and Williams 1991; Arredondo and Nuñez 2005). However, this does not prevent it from presenting toxic effects, among which the generation of ROS (reactive species of oxygen) (Gaetke and Chow 2003; Klaunig and Kamendulis 2004), which can cause damage through the oxidation of cellular components, alters the oxidation–reduction balance in the cell or interferes with the mechanisms of cellular signaling related to the redox state (Huang et al. 2005). On the other hand, the binders modify the transport properties of the cationic copper, the electronic properties of the central metal, and the molecular recognition.

Several studies such as antiproliferative activity in cell cultures, antineoplastic activity over murine tumors, and xenograft human tumors into nu/nu mice have

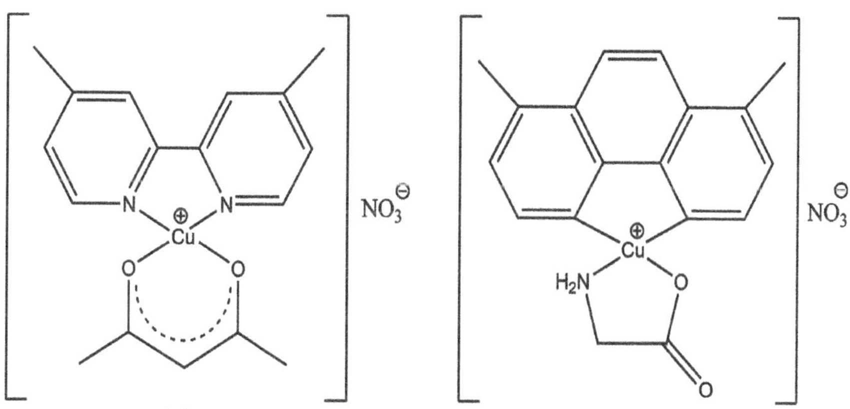

(a) (b)

Fig. 10.5 **a** Casiopeína [Cu(4,4′dm-bpy)(acac)]NO_3 and, **b** [Cu(4,7-dmphen)(gly)]

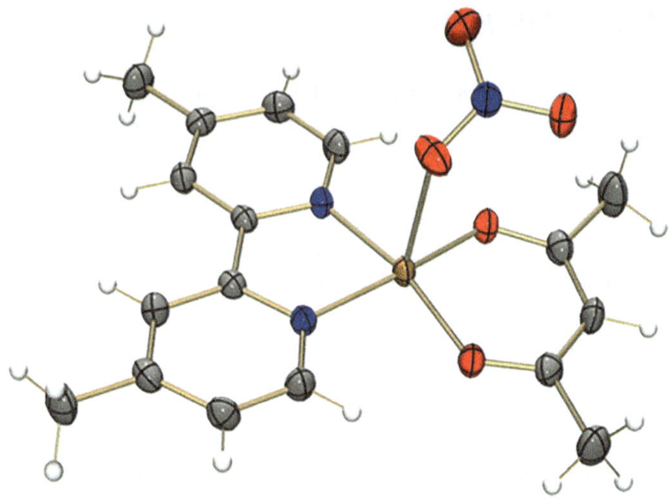

Fig. 10.6 [Cu (4,4′-dimethyl-2,2′-bipyridine)(acetylacetonate)(NO_3)] $(H_2O)_3$ (Cas III-ia)

been performed. On the other hand, survival was evaluated in murine models: L1210 (leukemia), S180 (sarcoma), B16 (melanoma) (Ruiz-Azuara and Bravo 2010). QSAR studies has shown that the half-wave potential and aromatic ring in the molecule are relevant for activity of the compounds, (Bravo-Gómez et al. 2009). Also secondary ligand effect has being studied with the observation that the secondary ligand does not impact the degree of activity but the selectivity (Bravo-Gómez et al. 2012). When several cell lines were tested with mixed chelate complexes, the depletion of glutathione was observed, suggesting the importance of Cu(II) being reduced to Cu(I) inducing mitochondrial damage and therefore DNA damage (Fig. 10.7).

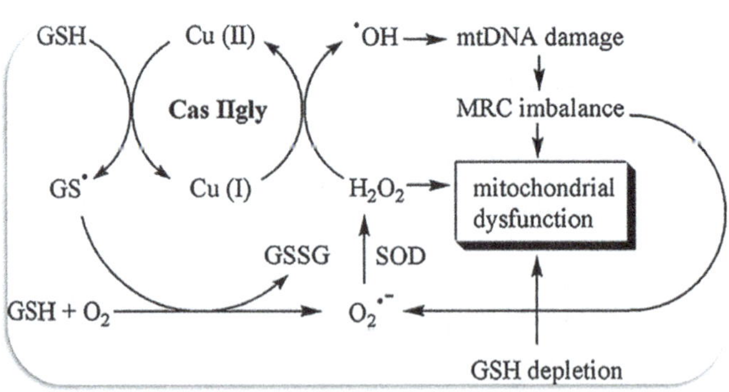

Fig. 10.7 Glutathione depletion and mechanism of action proposed for Casiopeina IIgly (Kachadourian et al. 2010)

Therefore, it was observed that Casiopein III-ia decreased cell viability and induced apoptosis on HCT-15 in vitro and in vivo, in a dose-dependent manner and independent cell cycle, through the activation of Bax and caspases, apparently via the pathway intrinsic. In the xenotransplanted (nu/nu) mouse model with HCT-15 and administered at a dose of 6 mg/kg, there was an increase in the relative tumor volume delay, as well as in the time of tumor duplication; the mitotic index decreased, while the apoptotic index increased with respect to the results observed for the negative control and the positive control administered with cisplatin (Carvallo-Chaigneau et al. 2008; Bravo-Gómez et al. 2013).

On the other hand, in the case of non-tumor cells, the mean inhibitory concentration of this compound was determined in lymphocytes, with a concentration of 4.7 mM, approximately 250 times higher than that observed in tumor lines (García-Ramos et al. 2017). These results, together, suggest an increase in the in vivo activity of the compound CasIII-ia, with respect to the activity observed in vitro, and having the cisplatin as a positive control evaluated in the same system.

With respect to in vivo toxicity, in general for this family of compounds, it was found that they present lethal doses higher than that of cisplatin, where Casiopein III-ia was one of the least toxic, in congruence with the observed effect of the activity in vitro. In a study of the hematotoxicity of the compound in Wistar rats, it was found that the administration of DL10 (3 mg/kg or 6.74 μmol/kg) produces acute hemolytic damage of low severity 24 h after the administration of the same, manifested as the significant decrease in hemoglobin, hematocrit, mean corpuscular volume (MCV), increase in morphological alterations of erythrocytes, and the presence of hematuria and hemoglobinuria, said damage being reversible at 21 days post administration of the compound, so it was concluded that the 6.74 μmol/kg dose of Casiopein III-ia is hematologically safe in the protocol proposed for the start of Clinical Phase I. The type of damage is a consequence of the generation of reactive oxygen species and is similar to the damage caused by the toxicity associated with copper (Serment-Guerrero et al. 2017).

The interactions of DNA with several casiopeinas has been studied using both experimental and theoretical models. It has been found that the mixed chelate complexes interact initially with the oxygen of phosphate group in minor groove of DNA, and depending on the substituents in the diamine ligand and nature of secondary ligand it can stay, or intercalate between the bases in DNA opening the H bonds between bases, mainly due to steric effects (Becco et al. 2012; Galindo-Murillo et al. 2012, 2015). A study of chemical correlation between structure, EPR and electrochemical behavior, supported by DFT calculation can predict the degree of activity of mixed chelate copper complexes (García-Ramos et al. 2014).

Other transition metal ions such as manganese, iron, copper, zinc, and molybdenum are well known catalytic centers in several metalloenzymes, and small molecular mass complexes of transition metals display similar catalytic activities. These compounds are referred to as catalytic metallodrugs; taking these into account, several metallodrugs have been prepared with such essential metals. The amino terminal Cu(II) and Ni(II) (ATCUN) binding motif has emerged as a suitable template to design catalytic metallodrugs with nuclease and protease activities.

The ATCUN motif is a small tripeptide metal-binding site found in the N-terminus of many naturally occurring proteins, such as albumin, histatins-5, and the neuropeptide neuromedin-C. The high affinities for Cu(II), for instance, make it possible to administer them in a metal-free state for subsequent recruitment from the labile pool of intracellular metal ions in bacteria or cancer cells, avoiding the toxicity and regulatory problems that might stem from the delivery of exogenous metal cofactors. The stereochemistry of the a-carbon of the amino acids that make up the motif as well as their hydrophobicity or bulkiness and the choice of metal ion provide a means to fine-tune the catalytic activity of the ATCUN–metal complex (Agbale et al. 2016).

As a consequence, these metallodrugs exhibit low toxicity and employ novel mechanisms to irreversibly inactivate disease-associated genes or proteins, which could be a channel to circumvent the rapid emergence of chemoresistance. The ATCUN motif presents novel strategies for the treatment of many diseases including cancers, HIV, and infections caused by drug-resistant bacteria at the genetic level. Details of the ROS generating mechanism, following binding of the ATCUN motif to Cu(II) and Ni(II) ions, have been deciphered. Earlier studies using various approaches confirmed Fe and not Cu as the main driver of oxidative damage within cells. Binding of the ATCUN motif to Cu(II) forms a redox-active complex that promotes the formation of ROS in the presence of H_2O_2, a by-product of cellular aerobic respiration (Agbale et al. 2016).

Compared to other chelates, the peptide backbone of ATCUN motifs permits easy conjugation to a bioactive peptide to provide target specificity. Conjugation to target domains promises to be an improved means of drug delivery, with reduced toxicity and minimum adverse effects. Targeting exploits the high affinity of cell-surface-targeted and DNA-targeted ligands.

Many studies have aimed at understanding the factors that modulate the reactivity and specificity of DNA strand scission chemistry by changing the stereochemistry and positioning of amino acids in the motif as well as the Cu(II) and Ni(II) metal centers. Miyamoto et al., recently reported that the reactivity of the catalytic metal center is determined by the hydrophobicity and bulkiness of individual amino acids in the motif indicating that, for example, the Cu(II)–Val–Iso–His motif should be more reactive than Cu(II)–Gly–Gly–His due to greater stabilization of the Cu(II)/Cu(III) transition state by the former. The motif has undergone a series of chemical modifications to improve its metal binding, selectivity and DNA/RNA cleavage compared to the linear analogues (Agbale et al. 2016).

10.4 Conclusions

Coordination complexes of transition metals were designed specifically to inactivate therapeutically important targets through various mechanisms. These mechanisms include generation of reactive oxygen species (ROS), enzyme inhibition, and intercalation of DNA or the formation of DNA adducts. The above interactions lead finally to cell death, depending on the oxidation state of the metal and the steric effect of the ligands.

The main pathway to act as anticancer agents for coordination compounds is to induce cell death by apoptosis. Other important point to consider is the difference between nonessential and essential metals in terms of toxicity to normal cells. The essential metals have natural chaperone proteins and elimination rates that make them to be less toxic.

References

Agbale CM, Cardoso MH, Galyuon IK, Franco OL (2016) Designing metallodrugs with nuclease and protease activity. Metallomics 8(11):1159–1169

Alves SRR, Abbasi AZ, Ribeiro G, Ahmed T, Wu XY, de Oliveira Silva D (2017) Diruthenium (II, III) metallodrugs of ibuprofen and naproxen encapsulated in intravenously injectable polymer-lipid nanoparticles exhibit enhanced activity against breast and prostate cancer cells. Nanoscale 9(30):10701–10714

Anderson H, Wagstaff J, Crowther D, Swindell R, Lind MJ, McGrego RJ, Timms MS, Brown D, Palmer P (1988) Comparative toxicity of cisplatin, carboplatin (CBDCA) and iproplatin (CHIP) in combination with cyclophosphamide in patients with advanced epithelial ovarian cancer. Eur J Cancer Clinical Oncology 24(9):1471–1479

Araujo TP, Gandin V, Kavanagh P, Braude JP, Nodari L, Montagner D, Erxleben A (2016) DNA binding, cleavage and cytotoxicity of a novel dimetallic Fe(III) triaza-cyclononane complex. Inorg Chim Acta 452:170–175

Arion VB, Dobrov A, Göschl S, Jakupec MA, Keppler BK, Rapta P (2012) Ruthenium- and osmium-arene-based paullones bearing a TEMPO free-radical unit as potential anticancer drugs. Chem Commun 48(68):8559–8561

Arredondo A, Nuñez M (2005) Iron and copper metabolism. Mol Aspects Med 26:313–325

Auzzas L, Zanardi F, Battistini L, Burreddu P, Carta P, Rassu G, Curti C, Casiraghi G (2010) Targeting αvβ3 integrin: design and applications of mono-and multifunctional RGD-based peptides and semipeptides. Curr Med Chem 17(13):1255–1299

Babak MV, Plażuk D, Meier SM, Arabshahi HJ, Reynisson J, Rychlik B, Błauż A, Szulc K, Hanif M, Strobl S, Roller A, Keppler BK, Hartinger CG (2015) Half-sandwich ruthenium(II) biotin conjugates as biological vectors to cancer cells. Chemistry 21(13):5110–5117

Barragán F, López-Senín P, Salassa L, Betanzos-Lara S, Habtemariam A, Moreno V, Sadler PJ, Marchán V (2011) Photocontrolled DNA binding of a receptor-targeted organometallic ruthenium (II) complex. J Am Chem Soc 133(35):14098–14108

Barry NP, Sadler PJ (2012) Dicarba-closo-dodecarborane-containing half-sandwich complexes of ruthenium, osmium, rhodium and iridium: biological relevance and synthetic strategies. Chem Soc Rev 41(8):3264–3279

Barry NP, Sadler PJ (2013) Challenges for metals in medicine: how nanotechnology may help to shape the future. ACS Nano 7(7):5654–5659

Barry NP, Sadler PJ (2014) 100 years of metal coordination chemistry: from Alfred Werner to anticancer metallodrugs. Pure Appl Chem 86(12):1897–1910

Becco L, García-Ramos JC, Ruiz-Azuara L, Gambino D, Garat B (2012) New achievements on biological aspects of copper complexes Casiopeínas®: interaction with DNA and proteins and anti-*Trypanosoma cruzi* activity. J Inorg Biochem 109:45–49

Bergamo A, Sava G (2007) Ruthenium complexes can target determinants of tumour malignancy. Dalton Trans 13:1267–1272

Bergamo A, Sava G (2011) Ruthenium anticancer compounds: myths and realities of the emerging metal-based drugs. Dalton Trans 40(31):7817–7823

Bergamo A, Gaiddon C, Schellens JH, Beijnen JH, Sava G (2012) Approaching tumour therapy beyond platinum drugs: status of the art and perspectives of ruthenium drug candidates. J Inorg Biochem 106(1):90–99

Brabec V (2000) Chemistry and structural biology of 1,2-interstrand adducts of cisplatin. In: Kelland LR, Farrell NP (eds) 2000 Platinum-based drugs in cancer therapy. Humana Press Inc, Totowa/NJ, pp 37–61

Braddock PD, Connors TA, Jones M, Khokhar AR, Melzack DH, Tobe ML (1975) Structure and activity relationships of platinum complexes with anti-tumour activity. Chem Biol Interact 11 (3):145–161

Bramwell VH, Crowther D, O'Malley S, Swindell R, Johnson R, Cooper EH, Thatcher N, Howell A (1985) Activity of JM9 in advanced ovarian cancer: a phase I-II trial. Cancer Treat Rep 69(4):409–416

Bravo-Gómez ME, Dávila-Manzanilla S, Flood-Garibay J, Muciño-Hernández MA, Mendoza A, García-Ramos JC, Moreno-Esparza R, Ruiz-Azuara L (2012) Secondary ligand effects on the cytotoxicity of several Casiopeína's group II compounds. J Mex Chem Soc 56:85–92

Bravo-Gómez ME, García-Ramos JC, Gracia-Mora I, Ruiz-Azuara L (2009) Antiproliferative activity and QSAR study of copper(II) mixed chelate [Cu(N-N) (acetylacetonate)] NO_3 and [Cu(N-N)(glycinate)] NO_3 complexes, (Casiopeínas®). J Inorg Biochem 103:299–309

Bravo-Gómez ME, Hernández de la Paz AL, Gracia-Mora I (2013) Antineoplastic evaluation of two mixed chelate copper complexes (Casiopeínas®) in HCT-15 xenograft model. J Mexican Chem Soc 57(3):205–211

Buettner KM, Valentine AM (2012) Bioinorganic chemistry of titanium. Chem Rev 112(3):1863–1881

Burger H, Loos WJ, Eechoute K, Verweij J, Mathijssen RHJ, Wiemer EAC (2011) Drug transporters of platinum-based anticancer agents and their clinical significance. Drug Resist Updates 14:22–34

Butler JS, Sadler PJ (2013) Targeted delivery of platinum-based anticancer complexes. Curr Opin Chem Biol 17(2):175–188

Carvallo-Chaigneau F, Trejo-Solís C, Gómez-Ruiz C, Rodríguez-Aguilera E, Macías-Rosales L, Cortés-Barberena E, Cedillo-Peláez C, Gracia-Mora I, Ruiz-Azuara L, Madrid-Marina V, Constantino-Casas F (2008) Casiopeina III-ia induces apoptosis in HCT-15 cells in vitro through caspase-dependent mechanisms and has antitumor effect in vivo. Biometals 21:17–28

Casini A, Reedijk J (2012) Interactions of anticancer Pt compounds with proteins: an overlooked topic in medicinal inorganic chemistry. Chem Sci 3:3135–3144

Chen H, Parkinson JA, Parsons S, Coxall RA, Gould RO, Sadler PJ (2002) Organometallic ruthenium(II) diamine anticancer complexes: arene-nucleobase stacking and stereospecific hydrogen-bonding in guanine adducts. J Am Chem Soc 124(12):3064–3082

Cohen SM (2001) Alternative models for carcinogenicity testing: weight of evidence evaluations across models. Toxicological Pathology 29(Suppl):183–190

Correa RS, de Oliveira KM, Delolo FG, Alvarez A, Mocelo R, Plutin AM, Cominetti MR, Castellano EE, Batista AA (2015) Ru(II)-based complexes with N-(acyl)-N', N'-(disubstituted) thiourea ligands: synthesis, characterization, BSA- and DNA-binding studies of new cytotoxic agents against lung and prostate tumour cells. J Inorg Biochem 150:63–71

Da Silva JJRF, Williams JRP (1991) The biological chemistry of the elements. Oxford University Press, Canada

Danhier F, Le Breton A, Préat V (2012) RGD-based strategies to target alpha(v) beta(3) integrin in cancer therapy and diagnosis. Mol Pharm 9(11):2961–2973

Dickerson M, Sun Y, Howerton B, Glazer EC (2014) Modifying charge and hydrophilicity of simple Ru(II) polypyridyl complexes radically alters biological activities: old complexes, surprising new tricks. Inorg Chem 53(19):10370–10377

Dilruba SG, Kalayda V (2016) Platinum-based drugs: Past, present and future. Cancer Chemother Pharmacol 77:1103–1124

Espina M, Corte-Rodríguez M, Aguado L, Montes-Bayón M, Sierra MI, Martínez-Camblor P, Blanco-González E, Sierra LM (2017) Cisplatin resistance in cell models: evaluation of metallomic and biological predictive biomarkers to address early therapy failure. Metallomics 9:564

Farrer NJ, Salassa L, Sadler PJ (2009) Photoactivated chemotherapy (PACT): the potential of excited-state d-block metals in medicine. Dalton Trans 48:10690–10701

Farrer NJ, Woods JA, Salassa L, Zhao Y, Robinson KS, Clarkson G, Mackay FS, Sadler PJ (2010) A potent trans-diimine platinum anticancer complex photoactivated by visible light. Angewandte Chemie Int Ed (English) 49(47):8905–8908

Florindo PR, Pereira DM, Borralho PM, Rodrigues CM, Piedade MF, Fernandes AC (2015) Cyclopentadienyl-ruthenium(II) and iron(II) organometallic compounds with carbohydrate derivative ligands as good colorectal anticancer agents. J Med Chem 58(10):4339–4347

Fu Y, Habtemariam A, Basri AM, Braddick D, Clarkson GJ, Sadler PJ (2011) Structure-activity relationships for organometallic osmium arene phenylazopyridine complexes with potent anticancer activity. Dalton Trans 40(40):10553–10562

Fulda S (2009) Tumor resistance to apoptosis. Int J Cancer 124(3):511–515

Gaetke LM, Chow CK (2003) Copper toxicity, oxidative stress, and antioxidant nutrients. Toxicology 189:147–163

Galindo-Murillo R, Garcia-Ramos JC, Ruiz-Azuara L, Cheatham TE, Cortes-Guzman F (2015) Intercalation processes of copper complexes in DNA. Nucleic Acids Res 43:5364–5367

Galindo-Murillo R, Ruiz-Azuara L, Moreno-Esparza R, Cortés-Guzmán F (2012) Molecular recognition between DNA and a copper-based anticancer complex. Phys Chem Chem Phys 14:15539

Gandioso A, Shaili E, Massaguer A, Artigas G, Gonzalez-Canto A, Woods JA, Sadler PJ, Marchán V (2015) An integrin-targeted photoactivatable Pt(IV) complex as a selective anticancer pro-drug: synthesis and photoactivation studies. Chem Commun 51:9169

García-Ramos JC, Galindo-Murillo R, Tovar-Tovar A, Alonso-Saenz AL, Gómez-Vidales V, Flores-Alamo M, Ortiz-Frade L, Cortes-Guzmán F, Moreno-Esparza R, Campero A, Ruiz-Azuara L (2014) The p-back-bonding modulation and its impact in the electronic properties of CuII antineoplastic compounds: an experimental and theoretical study. Chem Euro J 20(42):13730–13741

García-Ramos JC, Gutiérrez A, Vázquez-Aguirre A, Toledano-Magaña Y, Alonso-Sáenz AL, Gómez-Vidales V, Flores-Alamo M, Mejía C, Ruiz-Azuara L (2017) The mitochondrial apoptotic pathway is induced by Cu(II) antineoplastic compounds (Casiopeínas®) in SK-N-SH neuroblastoma cells after short exposure times. Biometals 30:43–58

Giacomini KM, Balimane PV, Cho SK, Eadon M, Edeki T, Hillgren KM, Huang SM, Sugiyama Y, Weitz D, Wen Y, Xia CQ, Yee SW, Zimdahl H, Niemi M (2013) International Transporter Consortium commentary on clinically important transporter polymorphisms. Clin Pharmacol Ther 94(1):23–26

Heffeter P, Riabtseva A, Senkiv Y, Kowol CR, Körner W, Jungwith U, Mitina N, Keppler BK, Konstantinova T, Yanchuk I, Stoika R, Zaichenko A, Berger W (2014) Nanoformulation improves activity of the (pre)clinical anticancer ruthenium complex KP1019. J Biomed Nanotechnol 10(5):877–884

Heringova P, Woods J, Mackay FS, Kasparkova J, Sadler PJ, Brabec V (2006) Transplatin is cytotoxic when photoactivated: enhanced formation of DNA cross-links. J Med Chem 49 (26):7792–7798

Hervouet E, Cheray M, Vallette FM, Cartron PF (2013) DNA methylation and apoptosis resistance in cancer cells. Cells 2(3):545–573

Huang H, Zhang P, Yu B, Chen Y, Wang J, Ji L, Chao H (2014) Targeting nucleus DNA with a cyclometalated dipyridophenazineruthenium(II) complex. J Med Chem 57(21):8971–8983

Huang R, Wallqvist A, Covell DG (2005) Anticancer metal compounds in NCI's tumor screening database: putative mode of action. Biochem Pharmacol 69:1009–1039

Johnstone TC, Kulak N, Pridgen EM, Farokhzad OC, Langer R, Lippard SJ (2013) Nanoparticle encapsulation of mitaplatin and the effect thereof on in vivo properties. ACS Nano 7(7):5675–5683

Johnstone TC, Suntharalingam K, Lippard SJ (2016) The next generation of platinum drugs: targeted Pt(II) agents, nanoparticle delivery, and Pt(IV) prodrugs. Chem Rev 116(5):3436–3486

Kachadourian R, Brechbuhl HM, Ruiz-Azuara L, Gracia-Mora I, Day BJ (2010) Casiopeína IIgly-induced oxidative stress and mitochondrial dysfunction in human lung cancer A549 and H157 cells. Toxicology 268:176–183

Kasparkova J, Kostrhunova H, Novakova O, Křikavová R, Vančo J, Trávníček Z, Brabec V (2015) A photoactivatable platinum(IV) complex targeting genomic DNA and histone deacetylases. Angew Chem Int Ed Engl 54(48):14478–14482

Klaunig JE, Kamendulis LM (2004) The role of oxidative stress in carcinogénesis. Annu Rev Pharmacol Toxicol 44:239–267

Lemaire MA, Schwartz A, Rahmouni AR, Leng M (1991) Interstrand cross-links are preferentially formed at the d(GC) sites in the reaction between cis-diamminedichloroplatinum (II) and DNA. Proc National Acad Sci USA 88(5):1982–1985

Linder MC (2002) Biochemistry and molecular biology of cooper in mammals. In: Massaro EJ (ed) Handbook of copper pharmacology and toxicology. Humana Press New Jersey, USA, pp 3–32

Liu S (2006) Radiolabeled multimeric cyclic RGD peptides as integrin alphavbeta3 targeted radiotracers for tumor imaging. Mol Pharm 3(5):472–487

Lopes EDO, Oliveira CGD, Silva PBD, Eismann CE, Suárez CA, Menegário AA, Pavan FR (2016) Novel zinc(II) complexes [Zn(atc-Et)2] and [Zn(atc-Ph)2]: in vitro and in vivo antiproliferative studies. Int J Mol sciences 17(5):781

Mackay FS, Woods JA, Heringová P, Kaspárková Pizarro AM, Moggach SA, Parsons S, Brabec V, Sadler PJ (2007) A potent cytotoxic photoactivated platinum complex. Proc National Acad Sci USA 104(52):20743–20748

Mari C, Gasser G (2015) Lightening up ruthenium complexes to fight cancer? Chimia (Aarau) 69 (4):176–181

Martin LP, Hamilton TC, Schilder RJ (2008) Platinum resistance: the role of DNA repair pathways. Clin Cancer Res 14(5):1291–1295

Massaguer A, González-Cantó A, Escribano E, Barrabés S, Artigas G, Moreno V, Marchán V (2015) Integrin-targeted delivery into cancer cells of a Pt(IV) pro-drug through conjugation to RGD-containing peptides. Dalton Trans 44(1):202–212

Mukhopadhyay S, Barnés CM, Haskel A, Short SM, Barnes KR, Lippard SJ (2008) Conjugated platinum(IV)-peptide complexes for targeting angiogenic tumor vasculature. Bioconjug Chem 19(1):39–49

Nardon C, Boscutti G, Fregona D (2014) Beyond platinums: gold complexes as anticancer agents. Anticancer Res 34(1):487–492

Nijwening JH, Kuiken HJ, Beijersbergen RL (2011) Screening for modulators of cisplatin sensitivity: unbiased screens reveal common themes. Cell Cycle 10(3):380–386

Offer T, Russo A, Samuni A (2000) The pro oxidative activity of SOD and nitroxide SOD mimics. FASEB J 14(9):1215–1223

Palermo G, Magistrato A, Riedel T, von Erlach T, Davey CA, Dyson PJ, Rothlisberger U (2016) Fighting cancer with transition metal complexes: from naked DNA to protein and chromatin targeting strategies. ChemMedChem 11(12):1199–1210

Pernot M, Bastogne T, Barry NP, Therrien B, Koellensperger G, Hann S, Reshetov V, Barberi-Heyob M (2012) Systems biology approach for in vivo photodynamic therapy optimization of ruthenium-porphyrin compounds. J Photochemistry Photobiology B 117:80–89

Petzold H, Sadler PJ (2008) Oxidation induced by the antioxidant glutathione (GSH). Chem Commun (Cambridge) 37:4413–4415

Pracharova J, Radošová-Muchová T, Tomastikova ED, Intini FP, Pacifico C, Natile G, Kasparkovab J, Brabec V (2016) Anticancer potential of a photoactivated transplatin derivative containing the methylazaindole ligand mediated by ROS generation and DNA cleavage. Dalton Trans 45:13179–13186

Richter S, Singh S, Draca D, Kate A, Kumbhar A, Kumbhar AS, Maksimovic-Ivanic D, Mijatovic S, Lönneckea P, Hey-Hawkins E (2016) Antiproliferative activity of ruthenium(II) arene complexes with mono- and bidentate pyridine-based ligands. Dalton Trans 45:13114–13125

Romero-Canelón I, Pizarro AM, Habtemariam A, Sadler PJ (2012) Contrasting cellular uptake pathways for chlorido and iodido iminopyridine ruthenium arene anticancer complexes. Metallomics 4(12):1271–1279

Romero-Canelón I, Salassa L, Sadler PJ (2013) The contrasting activity of iodido versus chlorido ruthenium and osmium arene azo- and imino-pyridine anticancer complexes: control of cell selectivity, cross-resistance, p53 dependence, and apoptosis pathway. J Med Chem 56(3):300–1291

Rosenberg B, Vancamp L, Krigas T (1965) Inhibition of cell division in *Escherichia coli* by electrolysis products from a platinum electrode. Nature 13(205):698–699

Ruiz-Azuara L (1996) Process to obtain new mixed copper aminoacidate from methylate phenanthroline complexes to be used as anticancerigenic agents. USA, Patent No. 5,576,326 (07/628,628). 1992

Ruiz-Azuara L (1997) Process to obtain new mixed copper amino acidatecomplexes from phenylatephenanthroline to be used as anticancerigenic agents. Patent No. 07/628843, US5107005 A, 1992, RE 35458, US RE35, 458E

Ruiz-Azuara L, Bravo ME (2010) Copper compounds in cancer chemotherapy. Curr Med Chem 17(31):3606–3615

Santini C, Pellei M, Gandin V, Porchia M, Tisato F, Marzano C (2014) Advances in copper complexes as anticancer agents. Chem Rev 114:815–862

Serment-Guerrero J, Bravo-Gomez ME, Lara-Rivera E, Ruiz-Azuara L (2017) Genotoxic assessment of the copper chelated compounds casiopeinas: clues about their mechanisms of action. J Inorg Biochem 166:68–75

Siewert B, van Rixel VH, van Rooden EJ, Hopkins SL, Moester MJ, Ariese F, Siegler MA, Bonnet S (2016) Chemical swarming: Depending on concentration, an amphiphilic ruthenium polypyridyl complex induces cell death via two different mechanisms. Chem Euro J 22 (31):10960–10968

Smith NA, Sadler PJ (2013) Photoactivatable metal complexes: from theory to applications in biotechnology and medicine. Philos Trans Mathe Phys Eng Sci 371. https://doi.org/10.1098/rsta.2012.0519

Smith R, Huskens D, Daelemans D, Mewis RE, Garcia CD, Cain AN, Freeman TN, Pannecouque C, De Clercq E, Schols D, Hubin TJ, Archibald SJ (2012) CXCR4 chemokine receptor antagonists: nickel(II) complexes of configurationally restricted macrocycles. Dalton Trans 41(37):11369–11377

Soldevila-Barreda JJ, Romero-Canelón I, Habtemariam A, Sadler PJ (2015) Transfer hydrogenation catalysis in cells as a new approach to anticancer drug design. Nat Commun 6:6582. https://doi.org/10.1038/ncomms7582

Spreckelmeyer S, Orvig Ch, Casini A (2014) Cellular transport mechanisms of cytotoxic metallodrugs: an overview beyond cisplatin. Molecules 19:15584–15610

Sun W, Li S, Häupler B, Liu J, Jin S, Steffen W, Schubert US, Butt HJ, Liang XJ, Wu S (2017) An amphiphilic ruthenium polymetallodrug for combined photodynamic therapy and photochemotherapy in vivo. Adv Mater 29(6). https://doi.org/10.1002/adma.201603702

Suntharalingam K, Awuah SG, Bruno PM, Johnstone TC, Wang F, Lin W, Zheng YR, Page JE, Hemann MT, Lippard SJ (2015) Necroptosis-inducing rhenium(V) oxo complexes. J Am Chem Soc 137(8):2967–2974

Süss-Fink G (2010) Arene ruthenium complexes as anticancer agents. Dalton Trans 39(7): 1673–1688

Suy S, Mitchell JB, Ehleiter D, Haimovitz-Friedman A, Kasid U (1998) Nitroxides tempol and tempo induce divergent signal transduction pathways in MDA-MB 231 breast cancer cells. J Biol Chem 273(28):17871–17878

Temming K, Schiffelers RM, Molema G, Kok RJ (2005) RGD-based strategies for selective delivery of therapeutics and imaging agents to the tumour vasculature. Drug Resistance Update 8(6):381–402

Todd RC, Lippard SJ (2009) Inhibition of transcription by platinum antitumor compounds. Metallomics 1(4):280–291

van der Veer JL, Peters AR, Reedijk J (1986) Reaction products from platinum(IV) amine compounds and 5′-GMP are mainly bis(5′-GMP)platinum (II) amine adducts. J Inorg Biochem 26(2):137–142

Venkatesh V, Wedge CJ, Romero-Canelón I, Habtemariama A, Sadler PJ (2016) Spin-labelled photo-cytotoxic diazido platinum(IV) anticancer complex. Dalton Trans 45:13034–13037

Violette S, Poulain L, Dussaulx E, Pepin D, Faussat AM, Chambaz J, Lacorte JM, Staedel C, Lesuffleur T (2002) Resistance of colon cancer cells to long-term 5-fluorouracil exposure is correlated to the relative level of Bcl-2 and Bcl-X(L) in addition to Bax and p53 status. Int J Cancer 98(4):498–504

Wang F, Chen H, Parsons S, Oswald ID, Davidson JE, Sadler PJ (2003) Kinetics of aquation and anation of ruthenium(II) arene anticancer complexes, acidity and X-ray structures of aqua adducts. Chemistry 9(23):5810–5820

Westendorf AF, Woods JA, Korpis K, Farrer NJ, Salassa L, Robinson K, Appleyard V, Murray K, Grünert R, Thompson AM, Sadler PJ, Bednarski PJ (2012) Trans, trans, trans-[PtIV(N3)2(OH) 2(py)(NH3)]: a light-activated antitumor platinum complex that kills human cancer cells by an apoptosis-independent mechanism. Mol Cancer Ther 11(9):1894–1904

Wheate NJ, Walker S, Craig GE, Oun R (2010) The status of platinum anticancer drugs in the clinic and in clinical trials. Dalton Trans 39:8113–8127

Yuan J, Lei Z, Wang X, Zhu F, Chen D (2015) Ruthenium complex Λ-WH0402 induces hepatocellular carcinoma LM6 (HCCLM6) cell death by triggering the beclin-1-dependent autophagy pathway. Metallomics 7(5):896–907

Yuan Y, Chen S, Paunesku T, Gleber SC, Liu WC, Doty CB, Mak R, Deng J, Jin Q, Lai B, Brister K, Flachenecker C, Jacobsen C, Vogt S, Woloschak GE (2013) Epidermal growth factor receptor targeted nuclear delivery and high-resolution whole cell X-ray imaging of Fe_3O_4@TiO_2 nanoparticles in cancer cells. ACS Nano 7(12):10502–10517

Zeng L, Gupta P, Chen Y, Wang E, Ji L, Chao H, Chen ZS (2017) The development of anticancer ruthenium (ii) complexes: from single molecule compounds to nanomaterials. Chem Soc Rev 46(19):5771–5804

Zhang Z, Dong X (2009) Interaction of DNA with a novel photoactive platinum diimine complex. Biometals 22(2):283–288

Zhang Z, Dai R, Ma J, Wang S, Wei X, Wang H (2015) Photoinduced DNA damage and cytotoxicity by a triphenylamine-modified platinum-diimine complex. J Inorg Biochem 143:64–68

Part II
Toxicity of Metals

Chapter 11
Toxicity of *Bhasmas* and Chelating Agents Used in *Ayurveda*

Shruti Pandey and Anand Chaudhary

Abstract The use of metals in medicine is not new to this world. It has been used by both modern and traditional systems of medicines. Perhaps, the *Ayurveda* stood first for using metals in medicine. The *Ayurvedic* pharmaceutical processes are used to convert metallic properties of metals into medicinal properties defined as *Bhasma* in *Ayurveda*. If these metals in their ionic/metallic forms accumulate in body tissues, then severe damage and toxicity may occur. But *Ayurveda acharyas* proposed some therapy and agents like cilantro, boron, and garlic which were used to remove toxins, produced from intake of improperly prepared *Bhasma*. These so-called agents may be termed as chelating agents of *Ayurveda* because certain researches showed that these agents help to chelate metal ions from the body. These herbs have antioxidant property which helps to chelate these metallic ions as well as helps to restore the normal functioning of tissues.

Keywords *Ayurveda* · *Bhasmas* · Toxicity · Chelating agents
Antioxidants

11.1 Introduction

The Indian traditional system of medicine, i.e., *Ayurveda* dating back to about 5000 years B.C., has literature which states that drugs originated from plant, animal, metal, and mineral sources were used in healthcare system (Galib et al. 2011). The use of different forms of metals to restore the normal, healthy physiology of the body either by direct administration of essential metals or by chelating out excess metals, or using them as carriers for targeted drug delivery or for targeting biomolecule for diagnostic, are all techniques that may be classified under the general headings of metallo-pharmacology. Metallo-pharmacology is an area of thrust

---

S. Pandey (✉) · A. Chaudhary
Department of Rasa Shastra and Bhaishjya Kalpana, Faculty of Ayurveda,
Institute of Medical Sciences, Banaras Hindu University, Varanasi 221005, India
e-mail: shruayu@gmail.com

M. Rai et al. (eds.), *Biomedical Applications of Metals*,
https://doi.org/10.1007/978-3-319-74814-6_11

where clinical trials are being conducted worldwide for the use of metals in therapeutics. For example, clinical trials for silver and zinc biotics have been carried out to assess its efficacy for a wide variety of human problems like malaria, burn wounds respiratory tract infections, etc. (Pathad and Lokhande 2014). On the requirement of metals for the body physiological functions, these can be classified into two categories—essential and nonessential. Lemire et al. (2013) classified metals into essential and nonessential on the basis of their utilization for body. Essential metals that are required for the normal physiology and function of organisms these include sodium, magnesium, calcium, iron, copper, zinc, etc. while non-essential metals have no known biological function for an organism these include mercury, arsenic, lead etc. Any reason, either environmental or medicinal which disturbs the homeostatic balance of essential metal ion in the body, can result in a shift from that equilibrium state to a condition of either shortage or excess and it is a latter state that causes the toxicity of essential metals. Toxicity is a measurement to which any substance or mixture of substance can harm or damage an organism. Metal toxicity is the harmful effect of certain metals in certain dose on an organism. Metal toxicity occurs when metals form poisonous soluble compounds in living body (Flora and Pachuari 2010). However, if these metals accumulate in the body, in concentrations sufficient to cause poisoning, then serious damage may occur. Some metals are toxic when they form poisons soluble compounds. Often heavy metals are thought as synonymous of toxins, but lighter metals may also be toxic in certain circumstances (Lemire et al. 2013).

Ayurveda is the science made up of *Veda* (knowledge) and *Ayush* (life), i.e., knowledge of life. An *Ayurvedic* system adopts a holistic approach toward health care by balancing the physical, mental, and spiritual functions of the human. The use of metallic preparations to cure diseases is a precise characteristic of this system. The metallic preparations play a vital role in the treatment of different diseases. Processed metals like mercury, gold, silver, lead, zinc, copper, etc. were used very frequently by *Ayurvedic acharyas* in different disease conditions with great authority. It is mentioned in the *Ayurvedic* texts that these elements either essential metals or non essential metals (Table 11.1) are detoxified during the highly complex manufacturing processes (*Sodhana*—purification process, *Marana*—incinerated ash) before the use of therapeutic purpose. *Charaka Samhita*, one of the pioneer texts of *Ayurveda*, has indicated ample of references regarding the use of metals in different forms for different clinical purposes. These metallic preparations are termed as *Bhasma*. *Rasashastra* (*vedic-chemistry*) is one of the parts of *Ayurveda*, which deals with herbomineral/metals/nonmetals preparations called *Bhasma*. *Rasayana* (immunomodulation and antiaging

Table 11.1 List of essential and nonessential metals

S. No.	Name of metals	
	Essential metals	Nonessential metals
1	Calcium	Mercury
2	Zinc	Lead
3	Copper	Gold
4	Iron	Silver

quality) and *yogavahi* (ability to target drugs to the site) are characteristics of a properly made herbomineral/metals/nonmetals preparation, which is also nontoxic, gently absorbable, adaptable, and digestible in the body. *Bhasma* is an *Ayurvedic* metallic/mineral preparation, treated with herbal juices or decoction and exposed for certain quantum of heat as per *puta* system of *Ayurveda*, which itself is well known in Indian medicine system since eighth century A.D. and widely recommended for the treatment of many disease conditions. *Bhasma* is claimed to be biologically produced mixtures of nanoparticles and macroparticles, which are prescribed with several other medicines of *Ayurveda* (Chaudhary and Singh 2010). These *Bhasma*s prescribed to patients either in single form or in combination with herbal preparations (Herbomineral formulations). They are given to patients in the very low dose form (Galib et al. 2011). These *Bhasmas* do contain metals as an integral component; if not used by following proper *Ayurvedic* pharmaceutics processes, then it may show symptoms of toxicity. The *Ayurvedic* Seers were well versed about this fact and documented the toxic effects in their respective classics.

In contemporary science, there is an alternative for treatment of metal poisoning namely chelation therapy, which is a technique that involves the administration of chelating agents to remove metals from the body. In this therapy, there is the use of chelating agents to detoxify poisonous metal agents such as mercury, arsenic, iron, etc. by converting them to a chemically inert form that can be excreted without further interaction with the body. Chelation therapy is a medical procedure that involves the administration of chelating agents to remove metals or heavy metals from the body. The few chelating agents which are used in contemporary sciences are EDTA, 2,3-Dimercaprol, and meso-2,3-dimercaptosuccinic acid. Chelating agents must be administered with care as it has a number of possible side effects including death. Some of the risks while using chelating agents in contemporary science (Angle 1996) are as follows:

1. Chelators bind to heavy metal or metal particles, but they can also bind to important minerals in the body, such as calcium and iron, which are essentials for human body.
2. Although chelating agents can be beneficial in cases of heavy metal poisoning, sometimes these may be critical if acts otherwise. The use of disodium EDTA instead of calcium EDTA has resulted in fatalities due to hypocalcemia.
3. Side effects of chelation therapy include dehydration, low blood calcium, harm to kidneys, increased enzymes as would be detected in liver function tests, allergic reactions, and lowered levels of dietary elements.
4. When administered inappropriately, chelation therapy brings the risk of cancer, neurodevelopment disorder, and even death.

Ayurveda viewed health as a state of many-sided equilibrium. It is achieved through dietary regimen and medications. The ancient scholars of *Ayurveda* while practicing these *Bhasmas* came to know about the ill effects of these medicines on human body, which may be caused due to the use of *Bhasmas*, made from improper processed metals and minerals. Sometimes, these *Bhasma*s show toxic signs in the body if not used by following proper *Ayurvedic* pharmaceutics processes. The ancient seers of *Ayurveda* at the same time advised to administer various natural substances in the form of antidotes such as honey, ghee, cow's milk, garlic, coriander, turmeric, and coconut water to remove ill effects or toxicity occurred from these medicines, i.e., *Bhasmas* (Choube 2000). These natural antidotes may be considered as chelating agents of *Ayurveda*, which are not only helpful to remove the toxic effects of metal and minerals without causing any side effects but also protect the loss of essential elements from the body.

This chapter mainly emphasized on procedures of *Ayurveda* used for removal of metal and mineral toxicity caused by improperly prepared medicines of *Ayurveda*, i.e., *Bhasmas*. This chapter deals with all the process of *Ayurvedic* clinical practices and pharmaceutical process, and diet regimen given to the patients while treatment. These are aimed to maintain the balance of human body to keep it free from disease and related adverse effects of medicines. All these processes of *Ayurveda* are closer or equivalent to chelation therapy of contemporary sciences.

11.2 Assertions of Contemporary Science, *Ayurvedic* Pharmaceutics and Therapeutics for Chelation

11.2.1 Remedies for Removal of Toxic Element/Metal Poisoning

There are certain methods through which toxicity of metals can be removed from body (Pandey and Chaudhary 2016).

11.2.1.1 Chelation

Certain foods, herbal drinks, and herbs actively bind to a range of minerals or metals. They are then excreted or washed away from the body.

11.2.1.2 Saturation

Sufficient and wide range of minerals in the diet and cells becomes saturated with the variety of minerals they need. Toxic minerals are then likely to be excreted rather than taking up. Some minerals are also antagonistic to each other, and a high level of one prevents the uptake of another.

11.2.1.3 Antioxidants

A diet high in antioxidant nutrients and enzymes protect from toxic minerals.

11.3 General Antidotes or Chelating Agent of Ayurveda

Tankan (borax), *Gandhak* (sulfur), *Saindhava Lavana* (rock salt), *Churnodaka* (limewater), *Triphala Kwath*, *Arjuna* (*Terminalia arjuna*), *Maricha* (black pepper), *Kumari Swarasa* (aloe vera juice), coriander, ginger juice honey, turmeric, lemon juice, cow's milk, goat's milk, cow's ghee, cow's urine, etc. are some common antidotes, which are used to subside the toxic symptoms and to remove the toxic effects of administration of improper processed metals and minerals (Choube 2000).

11.4 Purification Materials (*Shodhana* Drugs) Versus Chelating Agents

The use of metals as medicine is a multistep process. Metals need to be treated with various natural agents, including heat in various complex and multistep processes, and then only a metal is converted into a medicine (Chaudhary and Singh 2010). First, these metals are detoxified during the highly complex manufacturing processes (*Sodhana*- purification/potentiation processes) by different natural agents from herbal, animal, and mineral origin which are described in *Ayurvedic* texts (Choube 2000) (Table 11.2). The respective branch of *Ayurveda* where these processes take place called *Rasa Shastra* (Metallic *Ayurvedic* pharmaceutics). General rule for removing toxic elements from the human body is quite logical in *Ayurveda;* any substance used for the purification of metals automatically has potent antidote properties attached to it. So, for removing toxicity of metals from body, same purification agents are used. For example,

Table 11.2 Drugs used in purification process of metals (*Shodhana process*) versus chelating agents

S. No.	Metals	Drugs used for purification process of metals
1.	*Swarna* (Gold)	*Saindhava lavan* (Rock salt), *Swarna gairik* (Ochre), *and Nimbu swaras* (Lemon juice)
2.	*Raupya* (Silver)	*Agastya swaras* (Juice of *Sesbania grandiflora* Pers.), *Nimbu swarasa*, Lead, and Borax
3.	*Tamra* (Copper)	*Nimbu swarasa*, *Saindhava lavan*, *Nirgundi* (*Vitex negundo* Linn.) *swarasa*, *Ark milk* (milky latex of *Calotropis gigantea* R.Br.ex Ait.), Cow's urine
	Swarnamakshika (Copper pyrite)	*Nimbu swarasa*, *Triphala*[*]
	Tuttah (Copper sulfate)	*Nimbu Swarasa*, *Cow's urine*

(continued)

Table 11.2 (continued)

S. No.	Metals	Drugs used for purification process of metals
4.	*Lauha* (Iron)	*Triphala decoction, Sea salt, Cow's urine*
	Mandur (Iron oxide)	*Cow's urine, Triphala decoction*
	Vimal (Iron pyrite)	*Meshashringi, nimbu swarasa*
	Gairik (Haematite)	Cow's milk and Cow ghrita (Clarified butter)
	Kasisa (Ferrous sulfate)	*Nimbu swarasa, Bhringaraj swarasa* (Juice of *Eclipta alba* Hassk)
5.	*Yasad* (Zinc)	*Limewater, Nirgundi root swarasa, Ark milk, Cow's milk*
6.	*Parad* (Mercury)	*Garlic* (*Allium sativum*), *Limewater*
	Hingul (Cinnabar)	*Nimbu swarasa, Adraka swarasa* (Juice of *Zingiber officinale*)
7.	*Naag* (Lead)	*Nirgundi swarasa, churnodaka (limewater) Haridra powder* (*Curcuma longa*), Cow's urine, *Cow's ghee,* Honey
8.	Arsenic	
	Hartala (orpiment)	*Kushmand swarasa* (Juice of *Benincasa hispida* Cogn.), Limewater, Borax, *Nimbu swarasa, Triphala decoction,* Sesame oil
	Manhashila (Realger)	*Adraka swarasa, Bhringraj swarasa, Goat urine. Limewater, Nimbu swarasa*
	Gauripasan (Arsenious oxides)	*Karvellaka* (*Momordica charantia* Linn.), *Cow's milk,* Borax water

*Triphala (Three fruits)—Fruit of *Terminalia chebula* Retz., *Terminalia belerica* Roxb., *Emblica officinalis* Gaertn—all taken in equal quantities.

1. Raw *Vimal* (Iron pyrite) gets purified in *Meshshringi* (*Gymnema sylvestre*) juice while performing the pharmaceutical process of *Shodhana*. If its toxicity occurs in the body, then *Meshshringi* is recommended with sugar for 3 days to remove its toxicity from the body (Choube 2000).
2. Raw *Hartala* (Arsenic trioxide; As_2S_3) gets purified with *Kushmand Swarasa* (*Benincasa hispida Juice*) and to remove its toxicity *Kushmand Swarasa* is recommended with *Jeerak* (*Carum carvi*) and honey (Sharma 1998).
3. Raw *Gauripasan* (Arsenious oxide; As_2O_3) gets purified with *Tankan* (borax) and cow's milk and to remove its toxicity from body, the same is recommended (Sharma 1998; Jha 2000).

11.5 Ayurvedic Concepts Concerning Metal Pharmacology

The pharmacology of metals, which are used as medicine, has been described in *Ayurvedic* treasures. Some of them are mentioned here in terms of their pharmacological actions, related adverse effect, and its management (Upadhyay 1994; Sharma 1998; Choube 2000).

11.5.1 Rasa Aushadhi (Mercurial/Metallic/Mineralic Medicinal Compounds)

11.5.1.1 Pharmacological Actions

Aphrodisiac, Antiaging, Immunomodulator, Increases Intellect, Memory, Tissue Element, and eradicate disease caused by vitiated *doshas* (Humoral Principles, Viz., *Vata, Pitta, Kapha*).

11.5.1.2 Adverse Effects

Fainting, Vomiting, Diarrhea, Dyspnoea, etc. even Death.

11.5.1.3 Management of Adverse Reactions

Coriander sativum with sugar candy and *Piper nigrum* with clarified butter should be repeated for 7 days.

11.5.2 Swarna Bhasma (Medicinal Gold Preparations)

11.5.2.1 Pharmacological Actions

Aphrodisiac, Cardiac Stimulant, Immunomodulator, it increases Longevity, Memory, Attentiveness, and eradicate the diseases caused by all three vitiated *Doshas*.

11.5.2.2 Adverse Reactions

Illness, Weakness, Impotency, and leads to imbalance of homeostasis and even Death.

11.5.2.3 Management of Adverse Reactions

Powder of *Terminalia chebula* with sugar candy for 3 days.

11.5.3 *Raupya Bhasma (Medicinal Silver Preparations)*

11.5.3.1 Pharmacological Actions

Aphrodisiac, Antiaging, and Immunomodulator. It increases Potentiality, Intellect complexion.

11.5.3.2 Adverse Reactions

Anemia, Fever, Weakness, Itching, Constipation, Headache, Cervical Lymphadenopathy, Oligospermia, and reduce Potency.

11.5.3.3 Management of Adverse Reactions

Honey and sugar for 3 days.

11.5.4 *Tamra Bhasmas (Medicinal Copper Preparations)*

11.5.4.1 Pharmacological Actions

Rejuvenator, Wound healer, Emaciator, Purgative, Immunomodulator. Alleviates disorder caused by *Kapha* and *Pitta*.

11.5.4.2 Adverse Reactions

Vomiting, Fainting, Hallucination, Skin Disorders, Spasmodic Pain, Hyperlipidimia, Delirium, Anorexia, Impotency, and even Death.

11.5.4.3 Management of Adverse Reactions

Coriandrum sativum with *Sesbania grandiflora* given with sugar candies.

11.5.5 *Lauha Bhasmas (Medicinal Iron Preparations)*

11.5.5.1 Pharmacological Reactions

Aphrodisiac, Antiaging, Emaciating, Immunomodulator. Increase Complexion, Appetite, Potentiality, and eradicate diseases caused by vitiated *Kapha* and *Pitta*.

11.5.5.2 Adverse Reactions

Angina, Skin Disorders, Urolethiasis, Spasmodic Pain, Burning Sensation, Weakness, and even Death.

11.5.5.3 Management of Adverse Reactions

Powder of *Embelia ribes* with juices of *Sesbania grandiflora* and patients should be exposed to sunlight. Fruit pulp of *Cassia fistula* and powder of *Elettaria cardamomum* seeds should be given repeatedly.

11.5.6 Naag Bhasmas (Medicinal Lead Preparations)

11.5.6.1 Pharmacological Actions

Appetizer, Aphrodisiac, Immunomodulator, Urinary tract disease, and in disease caused by vitiated *Vata* and *Kapha.*

11.5.6.2 Adverse Reactions

Emaciation, Jaundice, Oedema, Peri-Anal Fistula, and Dyspepsia.

11.5.6.3 Management of Adverse Reactions

Swaran Bhasma and *Terminalia chebula* with sugar candy for 3 days.

11.5.7 Yasad Bhasmas (Medicinal Zinc Preparations)

11.5.7.1 Pharmacological Actions

Ophthalmic Nourisher, Immunomodulator, Increase Strength, Potentiality, Intellectual Power and disease caused by vitiated *Kapha* and *Pitta.*

11.5.7.2 Adverse Reactions

Diabetes, Indigestion, Vomiting, and Hallucination.

11.5.7.3 Management of Adverse Reactions

Terminalia chebula with sugar candies for 3 days.

11.5.8 Haratala Bhasmas (Medicinal Orpiment Preparations) (Arsenic Compounds)

11.5.8.1 Pharmacological Actions

Immunomodulator, Increase Strength and Digestive Power, Rejuvenative, and Increase Complexion.

11.5.8.2 Adverse Reactions

Diabetes, Pyrexia, Blisters on skin, and even Death.

11.5.8.3 Management of Adverse Reactions

Cumin seeds and sugar candies for 3 days.

11.5.9 Manhashila Bhasmas (Medicinal Realgar Preparations)

11.5.9.1 Pharmacological Actions

Immunomodulator, Increase Strength and Digestive Power, Rejuvenative, and Increase Complexion.

11.5.9.2 Adverse Reactions

Calculi, Dysuria, Burning Micturition, and Constipation.

11.5.9.3 Management of Adverse Reactions

Cow's milk with honey for 3 days.

11.5.10 Gauripasan Bhasmas (Medicinal Arsenious Oxides Preparations)

11.5.10.1 Pharmacological Actions

Respiratory disorders, Aphrodisiac, Digestive disorders, and Fevers.

11.5.10.2 Adverse Reactions

High dose can cause death.

11.5.10.3 Management of Adverse Reactions

Tankan (Borax), *Godudha* (Cow's milk) with *Goghrita* (Cow's *Ghee*), and *Karvelaka* (*Momordica charantia*).

11.6 *Pathya and Apathya* (Wholesome Diet and Unwholesome Diet) and Chelating Concepts

The ancient seers of *Ayurveda* found that drugs of different origins (herbal, metal, or animal) in addition to codes of conduct and dietary regulations are suitable tools to maintain health and eradicating disease (Galib et al. 2011). There is a concept of wholesome diet and unwholesome diet, which go along with the treatment (Choube 2000). These diets somehow reduce the chances of toxicity of metals or heavy metals. It is a method for reducing heavy metal or metal exposure via the inhibition of absorption from the gastrointestinal tract. They have a key role in reducing the gastrointestinal tract absorption of these elements. These herbal diets may actively encourage mobilization and excretion of metals which further give a hand in reducing an individual's overall exposure. Hence, the underlying principle behind using herbal diet is as follows.

1. Lessen gastrointestinal uptake of free metal ions (when taken with wholesome diet).
2. Passively assist excretion of toxic intermediates/elements from the body.
3. Diets which are contraindicated may boost the uptake by making more soluble intermediate products or may cause any adverse reaction with the metal ions in the body.

11.6.1 Description of Definitive Diets in Ayurveda *While Treatment with* Bhasmas-*Specific Metallic Preparations*

11.6.1.1 *Rasa Aushadhis* (Medicinal Mercurial/Metals/ Minerals Preparations)

Wholesome diet: Milk, Rock salt, Clarified butter, Curd, Butter, *Phaseolus aureus* seeds, *Crocus sativus* stigma, *Zingiber officinale* rhizome, and *Cyperus rotundus* root.
Unwholesome diet: These herbs are strictly avoided during mercurial therapy. *Benincasa cerifera* fruit, *Dolichus biflorus* seeds, *Cucumis utilissimus* fruit, *Solanum nigrum* fruit, *Momordica charantia* fruit, *Carthamus tinctorius* seeds, *Citullus vulgaris* fruit, and *Musa sapientum* fruit.

11.6.1.2 *Swarna Bhasmas* (Medicinal Gold Preparations)

Wholesome diet: Milk, Sugar unctuous foodstuffs.
Unwholesome diet: *Aegel marmelous* fruit and all herbs included in mercury unwholesome diet.

11.6.1.3 *Tamra Bhasmas* (Medicinal Copper Preparations)

Wholesome diet: Milk with sugar candies, sweet food with clarified butter.
Unwholesome diet: Sour foodstuffs are strictly avoided.

11.6.1.4 *Lauha Bhasmas* (Medicinal Iron Preparations)

Wholesome diet: Honey, Milk, Sweet food, Clarified butter, Triphala (Three fruits —Fruit of *Terminalia chebula* Retz., *Terminalia bellerica* Roxb., and *Emblica officinalis* Gaertn—all taken in equal quantities.).
Unwholesome diet: Sesame oil, Wine, Sour food, Fish, Brinjal, Bitter gourd.

11.6.1.5 Medicinal Arsenic Preparations

Wholesome diet: Sweet food and rock salt (in place of other salts).
Unwholesome diet: Salt, sour, pungent, and exposure to sunlight.

11.7 Researches on References of Ayurvedic Chelating Agents

Each and every medicine system has its own line of the treatment for removing toxin or poison caused by their respective medicines or by any other mean, present in the body. In *Ayurveda*, poisoning/toxicity can be treated by some of the natural agents. Antidotes or chelating agents are described in *Ayurveda* classics, which help to remove poison caused by metals. Some researchers have been done on various antidotes of *Ayurveda,* which clearly shows that they have potential to remove toxicity caused by metals from any source. These agents had already been practiced by ancient scholars. Some of those researches are described below.

11.7.1 Haritaki (Termenilia chebula)

Sarkar et al. (2012) revealed in their research that methyl extract of *Termenilia chebula* possess both reducing power and iron chelating activity. It has the ability to reduce the toxic level of iron in iron overload mice and hence protect liver from oxidative stress and fibrosis. Iron overload causes a signified increase of hydroxyproline, a marker of liver fibrosis and Ferritin. Extract significantly reduced the hydroxyproline content in iron intoxicated mice, thus signifying the hepatic fibrosis inhibit potency of fruit extract and also decreases the level of Ferritin because of its reductive release activity. It was concluded from the research that extract can reduce hepatic iron content in treated mice and supported its chelating potency.

11.7.2 Aragvadh (Cassia fistula)

Cassia fistula was evaluated for chelating effect (Dinis et al. 1994). The presence of chelating agents in the ethyl acetate extract of *C. auriculata, C. absus* and *C. fistula* disrupts the ferrozine—Fe^{2+} complex formation (Jayaraman et al. 2014).

11.7.3 Karvellaka (Momordica charantia)

In one of the studies, toxicity in rat was induced by lead, and the animals were treated with ethanolic extract of *Momordica charantia*. The oral administration of lead nitrate induced bone marrow injury. There was reduction in the serum erythrocyte count, total leukocyte count, lymphocyte count, mean corpuscular volume, and mean corpuscular hemoglobin concentration. The extract normalized all the above parameters with the neutrophils count was also decreased. Thus, this study showed that ethanolic extract of *M. charantia* has a satisfactory effect on toxicity induced by lead (Ehimigbai et al. 2015).

11.7.4 Lahsuna (Allium sativum)

The sulfhydryl-containing compounds have the ability to chelate metals. Garlic which has water-soluble organosulfur compounds, S-allylcysteine, and lipid soluble compounds like diallyl-sulfide, etc. shows supporting factors against heavy metal poisoning due to its possession of chemicals containing organosulfur groups, volatile oils, enzymes, carbohydrates, and amino acids; garlic was extensively exploited to treat the metal-induced toxicities. Recent studies support the fact that garlic contains compounds capable of detoxifying lead, cadmium, methylmercury, phenylmercury, and arsenic. The sulfur-containing amino acids methionine and cysteine, N-acetylcysteine, an acetylated analog of cysteine, the methionine metabolite S-adenosylmethionine, α-lipoic acid, and the tripeptide glutathione all contribute to the chelation and excretion of metals from the human body. The clastogenic effects of the heavy metals were also reduced by administration of garlic. Fatal effects caused by metal accumulation and mitochondrial injury were effectively reduced by garlic (Flora and Pachuari 2010).

11.7.5 Dhanyak (Coriandrum sativum)

It is a popular culinary and medicinal herb, gained attention when soup was reported to enhance mercury excretion following dental amalgam removal. In different research studies, it decreased the lead absorption into bone. It has the ability to remove toxicity caused by heavy metals like mercury. In particular, coriander seems to be the only chelating agent that can remove these metals from the central nervous system. It helps to remove mercury, lead, and other heavy metals. Coriander contains antioxidants, with the leaves having the highest levels (Sears 2013).

11.7.6 Mandukparni (Centella asiatica)

Saxena and Flora (2006) reported in their research study that extract of *C. asiatica* was administered with DMSA (meso 2,3 dimercaptosuccinic acid) against experimental lead intoxication in rats. It was found that combined administration was most effective in reducing biogenic amines, oxidation stress besides reducing body lead burden. Thus, supplementation of herb extract during chelation could be recommended for achieving optimum effects of chelation therapy.

11.7.7 Shigru (Moringa oliefera)

Efficacy of combined administration of *M. oliefera* powder extract with a thiol chelator monoisoamyl DMSA post-arsenic exposure in mice was studied. Arsenic exposure caused a significant decrease in blood glutathione with increase in the production of ROS in blood and soft tissues. Combined administration of MiADMSA with *M. oliefera* proved better than all other treatment in the recovery of most of the above parameters, accompanied by more pronounced depletion of Arsenic. The results suggest that concomitant administration of *M. oliefera* during chelation treatment with MiADMSA might be a better treatment option than monotherapy with the thiol chelators in chronic arsenic toxicity (Mishra et al. 2009).

11.7.8 Haridra (Curcuma longa)

Another interesting domain of investigation is curcumin metal chelation capacity, bearing probable correlation with its cytoprotective potency. In one of the studies, curcumin derivatives were investigated and designed as potential neuroprotective agents, acting as metal chelators with improved stability at physiological pH and increased cytotoxic activity with respect to curcumin (Ferrari et al. 2014). Thus, the skill of curcumin to chelate metal ions such as iron and copper could be a useful feature for detoxifying body from metal toxicity.

11.7.9 Nimbu (Citrus limon) and Antioxidant

Ascorbic acid (present in sour fruit viz., lemon, etc.) having antioxidant activity is used as chelator for metal toxicity (Kleszczewska 2001; Tamafo et al. 2017). The lemon juice (*Nimbu swarasa*) is used in *Ayurveda* for purification process of many metals (Table 11.2). These are presumed to play a key role in minimizing the damage from oxidative products, including free radicals. Vitamin C and other antioxidants including bioflavanoids also support metal binding induction of reactive oxygen species by metals, and subsequent depletion of antioxidant cell defenses can result in disruption of the antioxidant balance in tissues. This balance can be overcome by either reducing the metal interacts with biomolecules or inducing oxidative damage or by bolstering the cell's antioxidant defenses through endogenous supplementation of antioxidant molecules. These antioxidants when given either alone or in combination with a chelating agent proved to be effective in mobilizing metal from soft as well as hard tissues. Many studies on the effects of vitamin C on lead intoxication have been performed. Vitamin C attenuates the oxidative damage and histopathological changes induced by $CdCl_2$ in the lungs and brain of rats. It has been reported to act as chelating agents for lead, with a similar potency to that of EDTA (Kleszczewska 2001).

11.7.10 Tannins

Triphala is an *Ayurvedic* medicine used at many places in the purification process of metals. *Triphala* consisting of fruits of three herbs, viz., *Terminalia chebula, Terminalia bellerica, and Phyllanthus emblica.* The main phytoconstituent of *Triphala* is tannin, which is present in abundant amount in *Triphala*. Phenols can affect the biological availability or activity of metal ions by chelating the metal (Dinis et al. 1994). One of the research studies was designed to find out the chelating capacity of tannin for copper, iron, and zinc ions in which percentage of bound metal ions were calculated. The studies revealed that tannin was able to chelate these ions. Thus, it is recommended that tannins may also have high affinities for metals (Karamac 2009).

11.7.11 Glutathione (GSH)

GSH is a protein found in foods. Food rich in GSH is asparagus, walnuts, avocado, and raw milk of goat (Weirzbicka et al. 1989). GSH is another powerful chelator involved in cellular response, transport, and excretion of metal cations and is a biomarker for toxic metal overload (Heba 2017). The detoxifying processes naturally generate large amounts of free radicals, which combats by making antioxidant enzymes, glutathione-S-transferase (GST), glutathione peroxides (GPOX), and superoxide dismutase (SOD). These endogenous antioxidants are GSH and selenium-dependent. GSHs in the diet are precursors to these antioxidant enzymes (Sears 2013). GSH is able to bind, transport, and store several metals, thus affecting metal homeostasis in biological systems. GSH has been shown to protect against Hg^{2+}-mediated toxicity in isolated proximal tubule fragments from rabbits and proximal tubular cells from rats. The bile appears to be a main excretory pathway for some metal–GSH complexes. GSH can chelate metals and reduce their toxicity (Aseth et al. 2016). Goat milk is used in different purification processes of metals in *Ayurveda* as well as antidote in toxicity caused by improperly prepared *Bhasma* (Choube 2000).

11.7.12 Cow's Urine

This agent is used at many places in *Ayurvedic* classics for purification process of metals. In recent study, it was found that cow's urine exhibits antitoxic activity against cadmium chloride and can be used as a bioenhancer for zinc. Mature male mice, exposed to cadmium chloride only, showed 0% fertility rate. However, the animals given a combination of cadmium chloride, cow's urine, and zinc sulfate showed 90% fertility rate with 100% viability and lactation indices. Besides this, the fertility index was also found to be 88% in the group treated with cadmium chloride and cow's urine. This result showed the chelating capacity of cow's urine (Singla and Kaur 2016). Chelating action of cow's urine is quite possible because of its antioxidant activity. The antioxidant status of redistilled cow's urine is contributed mainly by volatile fatty acids (1500 mg/L) as revealed by the GC-MS studies. These fatty acids and other antioxidants might cause the observed protective effects.

11.7.13 Madhu (Honey)

Gluconic acid is the carboxylic acid formed by the oxidation of the first carbon of glucose with antiseptic and chelating properties. It is found in plant and honey. The gluconate ion chelates calcium, iron, and other heavy metals. Aqueous gluconic acid solution contains cyclic ester glucono delta lactone structure which chelates metal ions and forms very stable complexes (Paul et al. 2017). It has already been mentioned that in most of the toxicity cases of metals, viz., silver, arsenic honey is used with other herbs like cumin, cilantro, etc. to remove metal toxicity symptoms from the body.

11.7.14 Boron

A study published on boron in experimental and toxicology pathology showed that heavy metal treatments increased the frequencies of sister chromatid exchange micronuclei in the DNA of lymphocytes and the plasma malondialdehyde level, whereas the tested boron compounds significantly reduced the genotoxic effects induced by low doses of heavy metals (Turkez et al. 2012). Their results revealed that the protective roles of boron compounds occurred with the effectiveness of their antioxidant capacity. In conclusion, these compounds could be useful in the development of functional food and raw materials of medicine. In *Ayurvedic* literature also borax is used as antidote/chelating agent in toxicity caused by arsenic compounds (Table 11.2).

11.8 Conclusions

Toxicity is the degree to which a substance can damage an organism. *Ayurvedic* acharya's kept bird's eye on the use of these *Bhasma* on patients. The therapeutic action and the adverse effects are based on the keen observations, theories, beliefs, and experiences of the ancient *acharyas*. These concepts may also reply the needless hue and cry existing regarding the toxicity of the metallic *Bahamas*. A central concept of toxicology is that the effect of a toxin is dose-dependent. For example, in a very toxic substance such as snake venom, there is a dose below which there is no detectable toxic effect, which itself is used in snake poisoning. *Bhasmas* cause toxicity only when they are improperly prepared, with greater dose and duration level may cause various adverse effects.

The cations, anions, ligands, etc. are the basis of chelation therapy, which are used in contemporary science. However, these terms were not known/discovered at the classical treasure of *Ayurveda*. In spite of that, various methods and substances were used as antidotes, which played the dynamic role in removing the metal toxicity from the body. These natural antidotes may be considered as chelating agents of *Ayurveda*, which are not only helpful to remove the toxic effects of metal and minerals but also protect the loss of essential elements from the body without causing any side effects. *Bhasma*s have no serious dangerous effect on body function as a whole. However, caution should be taken while preparing these *Bhasma*s and calculating the dose and duration during clinical practice.

References

Angle CR (1996) Chelation therapies for metal intoxication: toxicology of metals. CRC Press, Boca Raton, FL, pp 487–504

Aseth J, Crisponi G, Anderson O (2016) Chelation therapy in the treatment of metal intoxication. Academic press, London

Chaudhary AK, Singh N (2010) Herbo mineral formulation (Rasaoushadhies) of Ayurveda an amazing inheritance of Ayurvedic pharmaceutics. Ancient Sci Life 30(1):18–26

Choube D (2000) Brihat Rasaraja Sundar. Chaukhambha Orientalia, Varanasi, India

Dinis T, Madeira VMC, Almeida LM (1994) Action of phenolic derivatives (acetoaminophen, salycilate and 5-aminosalycilate) as inhibitors of membrane lipid peroxidation and as peroxyl radical scavengers. Arch Pharmacal Res 315:161–169

Ehimigbai ROA, Grillo DB, Eze GI, Ezeuko VC (2015) Protective effects of ethanolic extract of Mormodica charantia leaf on lead nitrate-induced bone marrow toxicity. J Exp Clin Anat 14:13–17

Ferrari E, Benassi R, Sacchi S, Pignedoli F, Asti M, Saladini M (2014) Curcumin derivatives as metal—chelating agents with potential multifunctional activity for pharmaceutical applications. J Inorg Biochem 139:38–48

Flora SJ, Pachuari V (2010) Chelation in metal intoxication. Int J Environ Res Public Health 7:2745–2788

Galib Barve M, Meshru M, Jagtap C, Patgiri BJ, Prajapati PK (2011) Therapeutic potentials of metals in ancient India: a review through Charak Samhita. J Ayurveda Integr Med 2(2):55–63

Heba AY (2017) Food as method of heavy metal detoxification. Adv Clin Toxicol 2(1):000115

Jayaraman P, Sivaprakasam E, Rajesh V, Mathivanan K, Arumugam P (2014) Comparative analysis of antioxidant activity and phytochemical potential of *Cassia absus* Linn., *Cassia auriculata* Linn., *Cassia fistula* Linn. Indian J Drugs Dis 3(1):298–304

Jha CB (2000) Ayurvediya Rasashastra, Choukhamba Saurabharati Prakashan, Varanasi, India

Karamac M (2009) Chelation of Cu(II), Zn(II), Fe(II) by tannins constituents of selected edible nuts. Int J Mol Sci 10(12):5485–5497

Kleszczewska E (2001) Biological role of reactions of L-ascorbic acid with Metals. Postępy Higieny: Medycyny Doświadczalnej 55(1):81–94

Lemire JA, Harrison JJ, Turner RJ (2013) Antimicrobial activity of metals: mechanisms, molecular targets and applications. Nature 11:371–384

Mishra D, Gupta R, Pant SC, Kushwah P, Satish HT, Flora SJS (2009) Co-dminitration of monoisoamyl dimercaptosuccinic acid and *Moring oleifera* seed powder protects arsenic induced oxidative stress and metal distribution in mice. J Toxicol Mech Methods 19(2): 169–182

Pandey S, Chaudhary AK (2016) Chelation therapy and chelating agents of Ayurveda. Int J Green Pharm 10(3):143–150

Pathad YV, Lokhande JN (2014) Handbook of metallonutraceuticals. CRC Press, Boca Raton, FL

Paul S, Hossen S, Tanvir EM, Afroz R, Hossen D, Das S, Bhoumik NC, Karim N, Juliana FM, Gan SH, Khalil I (2017) Minerals, toxic heavy metals, and antioxidant properties of honeys from Bangladesh. J Chem 2017: Article ID 6101793. https://doi.org/10.1155/2017/6101793

Sarkar R, Hazra B, Mandal N (2012) Reducing power and iron chelating property of *Termenalia chebula* (Retz.) alleviates iron induced liver toxicity in mice. BMC Complementory Alternetive Med 212:144–167

Saxena G, Flora SJ (2006) Changes in brain biogenic amines and haem biosynthesis and their response to combined administration of succimers and *Centella asiatica* in lead poisoned rats. J Pharm Pharmacol 58:547–559

Sears ME (2013) Chelation harnessing and enhancing heavy metal detoxification: a review. Sci World J 2013. Article ID 219840, p 13. http://dx.doi.org/10.1155/2013/219840

Sharma S (1998) Rasa Tarangini, Motilal Banarasidas, New Delhi, India

Singla S, Kaur S (2016) Biological activities of cow urine: an Ayurvedic elixir. Eur J Pharm Med Res 3(4):118–124

Tamafo ADF, Ghogomu JN, Nkungli NK, Mama DB, Younang E (2017) Quantum chemical investigation on the antioxidant activity of neutral and anionic forms of Juglone: metal chelation and its effect on radical scavenging activity. J Chem 2017

Turkez H, Geyikoglu F, Tatar A, Keles MS, Kaplan I (2012) The effects of some boron compounds against heavy metal toxicity in human blood. Exp Toxicol Pathol 64:93–101

Upadhyay M (1994) Ayurved Prakash, Chaukhamba Bharati Academy, New Delhi, India

Weirzbicka GT, Hagen T, Tones DP (1989) Glutathione in food. J Food Compos Anal 2(4): 327–337

Chapter 12
The Flop Side of Using Heavy Metal(oids)s in the Traditional Medicine: Toxic Insults and Injury to Human Health

Jayanta Kumar Biswas, Mahendra Rai, Monojit Mondal and Avinash P. Ingle

Abstract Traditional medicine is the earliest healthcare system of humanity, which relies on the revered traditional legacy of healing powers hidden in the natural objects like medicinal plants, animals, etc. It encompasses the Indian Ayurveda, traditional Chinese medicine, Arabic Unani medicine, and other forms of indigenous medicine. The Ayurveda is the most commonly practised system of traditional medicine in the Indian subcontinent and has been carving niche in the Western countries. It is based on the Vedic hypothesis that there are some common cardinal premises underlying the harmony and homeostasis maintained in the microcosm (individual body) and macrocosm (nature/universe). Both man and the universe are composed of the same basic elements, and disease manifests when the balance is destabilized. Some heavy metal(oid)s are added intentionally in Ayurvedic products as it is thought that the equilibrium of lead, copper, gold, iron, mercury, silver, tin, zinc thallium, and arsenic is essential for normal functioning of the human body. Similarly, traditional Chinese medicine believes that the human body has an organic unity based on the opposing and complementary relationships of yin and yang. Such medicine also contains heavy metals which come from contaminated soil source or are deliberately added as ingredients for specific curative cause. Traditional medicine focuses on causes, not the symptoms, heal the "whole", not the "part" by only correcting the symptoms, like the modern medicine. These low-cost medicines are thought of treating diseases and disorders without posing any risk of side effects. But it is wrong in reality, raising human health concerns and

J. K. Biswas (✉) · M. Mondal
Pollution, Ecotoxicology and Ecotechnology Research Unit,
Department of Ecological Studies, University of Kalyani,
Kalyani, Nadia 741235, West Bengal, India
e-mail: biswajoy2008@gmail.com

J. K. Biswas
International Centre for Ecological Engineering, University of Kalyani,
Kalyani 741235, West Bengal, India

M. Rai · A. P. Ingle
Nanobiotechnology Laboratory, Department of Biotechnology,
SGB Amravati University, Amravati 444602, Maharashtra, India

M. Rai et al. (eds.), *Biomedical Applications of Metals*,
https://doi.org/10.1007/978-3-319-74814-6_12

side effects due to their pharmaceutically non-validated nature and indiscriminate and irrational use. The quality, safety, and toxicity of herbal medicines have become a major concern for public health, health authorities, and pharmaceutical industries. Herbal medicines and products may contain highly active pharmacological components or contaminants including several toxic metals and metaloids. The metal(oid) contaminants or additives may be introduced during different phases such as cultivation, harvesting, collecting, cleaning, and drying of the medicinal plants in contaminated environment and/or during the processing and formulation of the herbal products. The objective of the present chapter is to show how through traditional medicine humans may be exposed to a cocktail of heavy metal(oid)s—the nonbiodegradable toxic group of environmental chemicals. Citing selected priority heavy metal(oid)s like lead, cadmium, chromium, arsenic, and mercury, it presents the spectra of vast array of toxic insults and injuries inflicted by them, ranging from cell to system levels, as well as the unique biochemical/molecular fingerprints the toxicants leave on human body.

Keywords Traditional treatment · Herbal medicine · Heavy metal(oid)s
Human health risk · Toxicity · Oxidative stress · Carcinogenicity
Quality control

12.1 Introduction

Traditional medicine (TM) is the sum total of the knowledge, skill, and practices based on the theories, beliefs, and experiences indigenous to different cultures, whether explicable or not, used in the maintenance of health as well as in the prevention, diagnosis, improvement, or treatment of physical and mental illness (WHO 2013). It refers to the systems of Indian Ayurveda, traditional Chinese medicine (TCM), Arabic Unani medicine, and other forms of indigenous medicine. TM is the earliest healthcare system of humanity, which is based on the long tradition of healing powers associated with the Earth's natural systems entailing medicinal plants and animal species, clean air, spring water, or the natural scenery. The Ayurvedic system of medicine has great antiquity, dating back to about 5000 years B.C. It is the TM system of Hindu Vedic tradition. The Samhita of the Atharvaveda itself contains 114 hymns offering magical cure of diseases (Agarwal et al. 2012). Its pharmacopeia (Materia Medica) contains resources in the form of drugs and scores of medicinal formulations derived from leaves, herbs, roots, bark, animal, metal, and mineral sources found in nature for the treatment of different diseases (Gesler 1992). Today, the number of medicinal and aromatic plants used in the world is around 20,000 and 4000 of these drugs are still used widely in the world (Fakankun et al. 2014; Sharma and Kala 2017). Ayurvedic herbal medicine has been refined over thousands of years through its utilization and experience. In about 800 BC, the primary medical healing school was founded in India. Charaka, a renowned medical scholar, healer, and herbalist in his writings described 1500 medicinal plants in his book the “Charaka Samhita” (Nunn 2002). Bronze-Age China of Shang Dynasty used herbal medicines prepared from seeds. Huangdi Neijing, an early Chinese medical book mentioned hundreds of herbal drugs (Hong 2004). The earliest known Greek herbal medicines were those of Diocles of Carystus (third-century BC) and one more by Krateuas (first-century BC) (Robson and Baek 2009).

The TM systems like Ayurveda and TCM are by principle, holistic medicines focussing on the human systems rather than diseases. Traditional medicine concentrates on the causes, not the symptoms, heal the “whole” body, not the “parts”. They prevent the diseases and repair the damage rather than curing the disease. As a traditional legacy, these medicines are considered as a low-cost and risk-free (or low risk) prophylactic measure. They fundamentally intend to promote health and enhance the quality of life, with therapeutic strategies for treatment of specific diseases or symptoms in a holistic way (Patwardhan et al. 2005). TCM considers the human at the heart of the universe, as an antenna between celestial and earthly elements. Water, earth, metal, wood, and fire are the five elements of the material world. The world is a single unit and its movement gives rise to “yin” and “yang”, the two main antithetic aspects. Human body has an organic unity based on the opposing and complementary relationships of yin and yang. The four corporal humors (qi, blood, moisture, and essence) and internal organ systems (zang fu) play fundamental roles in balancing the yin and yang in human body. Proper formation, maintenance, and circulation of these energies are essential for physiological functions and sound health. When the two energies drop out of harmony, disease develops. Herbal medicines are used to correct this imbalance of yin–yang in the human body (Gibert 1998; Cheng 2000). Ayurveda considers that the universe is composed of permutations and combinations of the five elements (Pancha mahabhutas). These are akasha (ether), vayu (air), teja (fire), aap (water), and prithvi (earth). The five elements can be seen to exist in the material universe in both organic and inorganic objects at all scales of life. In humans, elements are coded into three forces, which govern all life processes. These three forces (kapha, pitta, and vata) are known as the three doshas (tridosha) which regulate every physiological process in human body. The interplay among them determines the qualities and conditions of the individual. A harmonious balance between them reflects the healthy state while their imbalance as a result of an excess (vriddhi) or deficiency (kshaya) manifests as signs or symptoms of disease (Lad 1985; Bahall 2017). Naturally, the traditional medicines often prescribe metals and minerals as an essential part of human health care.

Traditional medicines are low-cost medicines and are thought of treating all sorts of human diseases and disorders without posing any risk of side effects. But it is wrong in reality, raising human health concerns and side effects of natural medicines due to their indiscriminate and irrational use. Herbal medicines and products may contain highly active pharmacological components or contaminants including several toxic metals and metaloids (Ababneh 2017). The objective of the present chapter is to show how through traditional medicine, humans may be exposed to a cocktail of heavy metal(oid)s—the nonbiodegradable toxic group of environmental chemicals. By citing selected heavy metal(oid)s like lead, cadmium, chromium, arsenic, and mercury, it presents the spectra of vast array of toxic insults and injuries inflicted by them, ranging cell to system levels, as well as the unique biochemical/molecular fingerprints the toxicants leave on human body.

12.2 Heavy Metals and Metalloids Used in TM

Although, TM has been used since ages, the past few decades have witnessed remarkable global increase in TM usage. About 70–80% of the world population still primarily relies on nonconventional medications, mostly derived from herbal plants (WHO 2007). Indian Ayurveda has been gaining popularity in Western countries. In the United States, Ayurvedic remedies are now available from South Asian markets, ayurvedic practitioners, health food stores, and the Internet. Ayurveda is the most commonly practised system of traditional medicine in the Indian subcontinent; Unani, and Siddha are other traditional medicine systems in South Asia.

The Ayurveda is based on the Vedic hypothesis that there are common cardinal principles underlying the microcosm (individual) and macrocosm (universe) and that man and the universe are composed of the same basic elements and disease occurs when the balance is lost (Chopra and Doiphode 2002; Gogtay et al. 2002). The heavy metals (HMs) within Ayurvedic products are generally not present as contaminants but are added intentionally. The equilibrium of lead, copper, gold, iron, mercury, silver, tin, and zinc are seen in Ayurveda as essential for the normal functioning of the human body and sound health (Zhu 1998). Some products contain other HMs, such as thallium and arsenic (Chopra and Doiphode 2002; Gogtay et al. 2002). During the medieval period around the eighth century A.D., Rasashastra as an integral part of Ayurveda promoted use of certain HMs and minerals in therapeutics. Ayurvedic classics written before that time, like *Charaka Samhita*, and *Sushruta Samhita*, etc., contain descriptions of metals and minerals, their processing techniques and utilization in therapeutics, etc. The *Charaka Samhita* prescribed metals like gold, silver, iron, copper, lead, tin, etc., as well as some alloys were used to treat a wide range of diseases. Fine powders of these metals were prescribed for both internal and external applications: parada (mercury) for the treatment of skin disorders; swarna (gold) for rejuvenation, treating bleeding disorders, abscess, arthritis; rajata (silver) for rejuvenation, hiccup, respiratory distress, and protecting skin after burning wounds; tamra (copper) for hiccup, respiratory distress and arthritis treatment, skin disorders, and eye disorders; loha (iron) for rejuvenation, skin diseases, leukoderma, and anemia. There are also prescriptions in favor of lead, cadmium, chromium, arsenic, etc. Ayurvedic texts acknowledge that those HMs in Ayurvedic medicines could have some toxicity but that could be detoxified which has been dealt in a specific area within Ayurveda known as "Vishagarvajrodhika Tantra" (Thatte et al. 1993). These procedures include heating and cooling products in buttermilk, cow's urine, sesame oil, and the use of "mineral herbs" or other herbal products such as tamarind (Thatte et al. 1993; Chopra and Doiphode 2002). Although these processes may have some effect on the bioavailability of HMs, reports state that they would not have significant enough effect on detoxifying them (Ernst 2002a; Lynch and Braithwaite 2005).

Chinese herbal medicines are also often contaminated with HMs like arsenic, cadmium, chromium, lead, mercury, etc., sometimes even at toxic levels (Ernst 2002a; Lin et al. 2010). Several studies have also shown that potentially worrisome contamination in herbal medicines relates to patented or proprietary medicines (Ernst 2002a; Ang et al. 2003; Saper et al. 2004; Cooper et al. 2007; Martena et al. 2010). They are frequently a heterogeneous mixture of different substances of diverse origin (e.g., plant, mineral, and animal) in either pill or extract form, and therefore, differ from raw herbal extracts (Yee et al. 2005). Patented herbal medicines are reported to have intentionally added heavy metals, such as arsenic (Liu et al. 2008a), mercury (Liu et al. 2008b), and lead (Saper et al. 2008). HMs have also been found in raw Chinese herbal medicines (Han et al. 2008; Wu et al. 2008; Lu et al. 2009), and some related plant species are known to be HM hyper-accumulators (Lai and Chen 2005; Turan and Bringu 2007; Wei et al. 2008). The medical use of Au can be dated back to 2500 B.C. in China. In traditional Chinese medicine, mercury is included as an ingredient of preparations of "cinnabaris" (mercury sulfide), "calomel" (mercury chloride), or "hydrargyri oxydum rubrum" (mercury oxide) which are used as a tranquillizer, an antiepileptic, for ulcers or to treat insomnia (Koh and Woo 2000). Lead is used as "MiTuoSeng" (Lithargyrum) and arsenic as "Xiong Huang" (Realgar) in preparation of traditional medicines (Thatte et al. 1993). These constituents are thus not contaminants but ingredients deliberately added for specific curative purpose. Again, in Greece, silver was employed in the treatment of wounds and ulcers according to the Greek physician Hippocrates. The ancient Egyptians also knew how to sterilize water with copper.

12.3 Toxic Landscape of TM

The general conception among the people is that "natural" means "safe" and harmless and has no risk associated with its use. But it is wrong in reality, and hence arises human health concerns and side effects of natural medicines due to its indiscriminate and irrational use. Most of the herbal products are not validated according to the recommended pharmaceutical guidelines (Chan 2003; WHO 2013). The safety and quality of medicinal herbal products have become a major concern for health authorities, pharmaceutical industries, and the general public (WHO 2007). Parallel to the increasing interest in the therapeutic benefits of herbal products, there has been an increasing concern over the safety and toxicity of traditional/natural herbal formulations available on the market. Herbal medicines and products may contain highly active pharmacological components or contaminants including minerals, toxic metals and metaloids like lead, cadmium, chromium, arsenic, and mercury (Fabricant and Farnsworth 2001; Martena et al. 2010;

Saeed et al. 2010; Adepoju-Bello et al. 2012). It has been shown that herbal remedies incorporated in Asian traditional herbal preparation for therapeutic purposes caused intoxications in users (Robert et al. 2008; Martena et al. 2010). Generally, the geography, geochemical soil characteristics, contaminants in the soil, water and air, and other growth, transport, and storage conditions can significantly affect the properties and the quality of the herbs and their formulations (Ernst 2002b; Saad et al. 2006). The HM contamination in TM may be introduced during different phases such as cultivation, harvesting, collecting, cleaning, and drying of the medicinal plants. It occurs due to contaminated environment in which the medicinal plants grow, the polluted conditions in which the plants are dried and processed, the storage conditions, or during manufacturing of the final form (Saeed et al. 2010). HMs may also come from irrigation water as a result of the industrial waste disposal, mining activities, and the usage of certain types of fertilizers and pesticides (Dghaim et al. 2015). The other possibility is the accidental contamination during the manufacturing process such as grinding, mixing, and the exposure to HMs from metal-releasing equipment (Chan 2003). The intentional addition of HMs during the preparation as part of the ingredients for a curative purpose constitutes another source (Ernst 2002a).

12.4 Toxic Effects of Heavy Metal(oid)s on Humans Health

Although, we require about 25 key elements for proper health. However, the elemental hexagon of life is composed of six elements, i.e., carbon hydrogen, oxygen, nitrogen, phosphorus, and sulfur, the first four elements accounting for 99% of the total human body weight. Different metal ions which are required for a vast array of physiological and biochemical processes in human body are included in the list of essential elements for human life. They include iron, zinc, copper, manganese, sodium, potassium, calcium, and magnesium, and also metals formerly thought of only as poisons, such as selenium, molybdenum, nickel, silicon, vanadium, and, possibly, arsenic (Thompson and Orvig 2003). Metals such as zinc, copper, iron, manganese, and chromium are essential nutrients. In small amounts, they are required for maintaining good health but on excess beyond certain levels, they can become toxic. Imbalance of metal homeostasis and of metal bioavailability, and/or metal toxicity are responsible for a multitude of human diseases (Korfali et al. 2013). Of the 35 metals that are of concern for us, 23 are HMs: antimony, arsenic, bismuth, cadmium, cerium, chromium, cobalt, copper, gallium, gold, iron, lead, manganese, mercury, nickel, platinum, silver, tellurium, thallium, tin, uranium, vanadium, and zinc (Mosby et al. 1996). HMs are the ubiquitous and non-biodegradable group of environmental chemicals with a density generally greater than about 5 g/cm^3 and an atomic mass greater than that of calcium. Majority are extremely toxic because as ions or in certain compound forms, they are water soluble, and can therefore, be easily absorbed into tissues of plants and animals including humans. After absorption, these metals tend to bind to biomolecules like proteins and nucleic acids, impairing biochemical functions. HM toxicity can lower energy levels and damage the functioning of the brain, lungs, kidney, liver, blood composition, and other important organs. Long-term exposure can lead to gradually progressing physical, muscular, and neurodegenerative processes that imitate diseases such as multiple sclerosis, Parkinson's disease, Alzheimer's disease, and muscular dystrophy. Repeated long-term exposure of some metals and their compounds may even cause cancer (Jarup 2003).

Humans may be exposed to a cocktail of HMs mingled in medicine. Their toxicity depends on several factors including the dose, route of exposure, and chemical species, as well as the age, gender, genetics, and nutritional status of exposed individuals. Because of their high degree of toxicity, lead, cadmium, chromium, mercury, and arsenic rank among the priority metals that are of public health significance (Tchounwou et al. 2012). The toxic effects and actions of the most important HMs and priority metals present in TMs are discussed below.

12.4.1 Lead

Exposure to lead can cause a variety of health problems. Studies show that there are no "safe" levels (Lanphear et al. 2005). The primary target organ of lead is the central nervous system. It can cause permanent damage to the brain and nervous system manifested in the form of behavioral changes, particularly impairment of cognitive and behavioral development as well as learning deficits (ATSDR 2007). Acute exposure can cause loss of appetite, headache, hypertension, abdominal pain, renal dysfunction, fatigue, sleeplessness, arthritis, hallucinations, and vertigo. Chronic exposure of lead can result in mental retardation, birth defects, psychosis, autism, allergies, dyslexia, weight loss, hyperactivity, paralysis, muscular weakness, brain damage, kidney damage, and may even cause death (Martin and Griswold 2009). Prolonged exposure to lead poses dangers to the normal functioning of the kidneys and nervous system, for example, leading to dysfunction or hypertension in adults and delays in children's physical and mental development including decreased intelligence quotient. Lead is known as systemic poisons because, once reached into the blood circulation, it is distributed throughout the body, where it affects the organs and tissues. Lead exposure may have an adverse effect on the blood, nervous, immune, renal, skeletal, muscular, reproductive, and cardiovascular systems causing poor muscle coordination, gastrointestinal symptoms, brain and kidneys damage, hearing and vision impairments, and reproductive defects. It inhibits hematopoiesis as it interferes with heme synthesis which may lead to anemia. It also affects the kidneys inducing renal tubular dysfunction. Its effects on gastrointestinal (GI) tract may be manifested in nausea, anorexia, and severe abdominal cramps. Other effects of lead poisoning are muscle pain, joint ache, skeletal growth inhibition, and immuno inhibition. It can cross the placental barrier and may affect the fetus resulting in miscarriage, abortion, and stillbirth.

Lead distribution in the body initially depends on the blood flow into various tissues and almost 95% of lead is deposited in the form of insoluble phosphate in bones (Papanikolaou et al. 2005).

Lead can complex with various biomolecules and adversely affect their functions. As a electropositive metal, lead has a high affinity to the -SH group. The enzymes that depend on -SH group like adenyl cyclase and aminotransferase can be inhibited by lead. Adenyl cyclase catalyzes the conversion of ATP to cAMP needed in brain neurotransmission. Aminotransferase is involved in transamination and thus plays significant role in protein metabolism. As a chemical mimic of Ca^{2+}, it can exert a competitive action in mitochondrial respiration and neurological processes. The main biochemical processes responsible for inducing lead toxicity include potential of lead to inhibit calcium actions and its ability to react with proteins (ATSDR 2007). Once inside the body, lead gets bound into minerals in place of calcium. It then interacts with biological molecules thereby interfering with their normal actions.

Lead diminishes the activities of diverse enzymes by causing changes in their structure such as sulfhydryl and amide enzymes. It inhibits enzyme activity by competing with essential cations for binding sites (Flora et al. 2007). Lead-induced oxidative stress is a key mechanism responsible for its toxicity (Fig. 12.1). Lead exerts toxicity in the cells by some ionic mechanism and oxidative stress (Pizzino et al. 2014). Many researchers have shown that oxidative stress in living cells is caused by the imbalance between the production of free radicals and the generation of antioxidants to detoxify the reactive intermediates or to repair oxidative damage. Antioxidants, such as glutathione, present in the cell protect it from free radicals such as H_2O_2. Subject to lead stress, the level of the ROS increases and the level of antioxidants decreases. Since glutathione exists both in reduced (GSH) and oxidized (GSSG) state, the reduced form of glutathione gives its reducing equivalents ($H^+ + e^-$) from its thiol groups of cysteine to ROS in order to make them stable. In the presence of the enzyme glutathione peroxidase, reduced glutathione readily binds with another molecule of glutathione after donating the electron and forms glutathione disulfide (GSSG). The reduced form (GSH) of glutathione accounts for 90% of the total glutathione content and the oxidized form (GSSG) accounts for 10% under normal conditions. Under oxidative stress, the concentration of GSSG exceeds the concentration of GSH. The other biomarker for oxidative stress is lipid peroxidation, since the free radical collects electron from lipid molecules of the cell membrane, which eventually causes lipid peroxidation (Wadhwa et al. 2012). In case of severe oxidative shock in presence of very high lead concentrations, ROS may destroy structural integrity of the cells, proteins, nucleic acid, membranes, and lipids (Mathew et al. 2011). The ionic mechanism of lead toxicity occurs mainly due to the ability of lead metal ions to replace other bivalent cations like Ca^{2+}, Mg^{2+}, Fe^{2+}, and monovalent cations like Na^+, which ultimately disturbs the biological metabolism of the cell. It results in significant changes in various biological processes such as cell adhesion, intra- and intercellular signaling, protein folding, maturation, apoptosis, ionic transportation, enzyme regulation, and release of neurotransmitters. Lead can substitute Ca even in very low (picomolar) concentration affecting protein kinase C, which regulates neural excitation and memory.

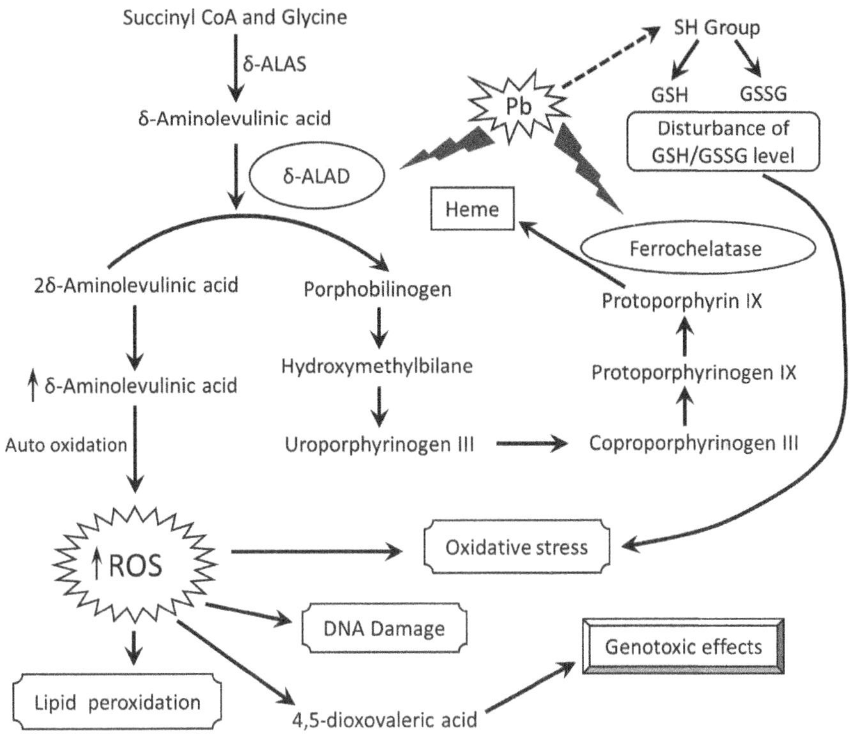

Fig. 12.1 Biochemical toxic activities of lead (Pb) in the form of inhibition of heme synthesis, imbalance in antioxidant homeostasis, oxidative stress, and genotoxicity

As lead induces oxidative damage as a result of imbalance in antioxidants system of body's defense against oxidative stress, the imbalance of Glutathione (GSH) and glutathione disulfide (GSSG) is resulted since Pb has high binding affinity for sulfhydryl rich proteins like GSH. Reduction in glutathione reductase levels leads to decrease in the level of glutathione, the body's main antioxidant. This results because of the ability of lead to bind directly with thiol groups.

The most familiar biochemical action of lead is the inhibition of δ-aminolevulinic acid dehydratase (ALA-D) and ferrochelatase, the key enzymes involved in heme synthesis (Fig. 12.1). ALA-D is responsible for converting δ-aminolevulinic acid into porphobilinogen, whereas ferrochelatase catalyzes the incorporation of Fe^{2+} into protoporphyrin IX to synthesize heme. Lead inhibits δ-aminolevulinic acid dehydratase (δ-ALA-D) enzyme thus leading to increased levels of δ-aminolevulinic acid (δ-ALA) in blood. This increased blood levels of δ-aminolevulinic acid (δ-ALA) contribute in increasing the ROS level following lead assault. Another pathway of heme interference by lead includes inhibition of enzyme ferrochelatase and thus reducing the incorporation of iron (Fe) into heme. Thus, inhibition of these important enzymes by lead can severely impair heme synthesis.

12.4.2 Cadmium

Cadmium and its compounds are classified as Group 1 carcinogens for humans by the International Agency for Research on Cancer (Henson and Chedrese 2004). Cadmium can cause both acute and chronic intoxications (Chakraborty et al. 2013). Cadmium is highly toxic to the kidney and it accumulates in the proximal tubular cells in higher concentrations (Fig. 12.2). It can cause bone mineralization either through bone damage or by renal dysfunction. Osteoporosis (skeletal damage) is a critical effect of cadmium exposure along with disturbances in calcium metabolism, formation of renal stones and hypercalciuria. If cadmium is ingested in high amounts, it can lead to stomach irritation and result in vomiting and diarrhea. On chronic exposure, it can be deposited in the kidneys, resulting in morphopathological changes, and finally kidney disease and fragile bones (Bernard 2008). Premature birth and reduced birth weights of the neonate may be resulted in case of high cadmium exposure during human pregnancy (Henson and Chedrese 2004). CNS is one of the sensitive parts of biological system that can become easily damaged during the early phase of neonatal development. Cadmium can cross the placental barrier and reach fetal tissue exerting harmful effects including neurotoxicity.

Cadmium has also been recognized as a major causative factor for neurodegenerative disorders including Parkinson's disease and Alzheimer's disease (Jiang et al. 2007). Figure 12.2 explains human body's interaction with cadmium and mechanism of its toxicity. Once cadmium enters into the blood, it is transported by proteins such as albumin and metallothionein (MT) in a bound form. Reaching

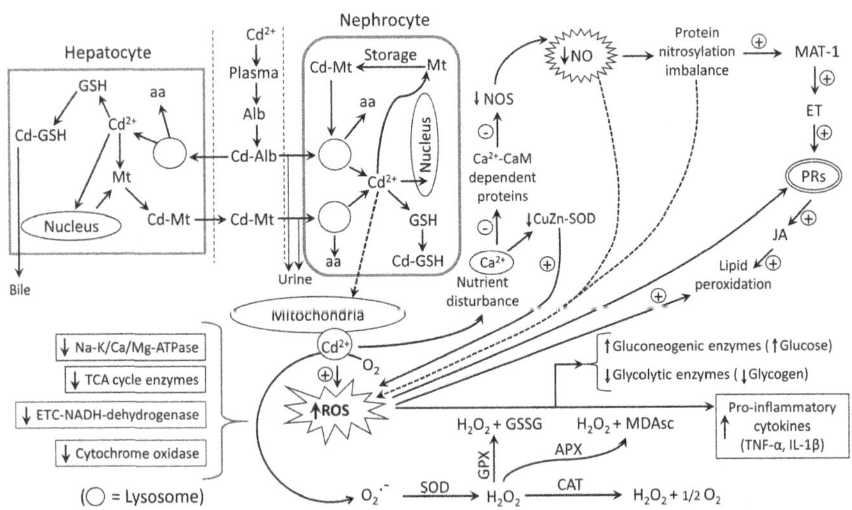

Fig. 12.2 Toxic links of cadmium, oxidative stress, and carcinogenesis. Chronic Cd (II) exposure can induce expression of metallothionin (MT) and triggers adaptive mechanisms toward oxidative stress, limiting ROS-induced carcinogenesis

gastrointestinal tract, cadmium enters liver where it initiates the production of metallothionein and cadmium metallothionein is released into sinusoidal blood. Cadmium concentration increases by 3000 fold when it binds to cysteine-rich protein such as metallothionein. Cadmium may enter the hepatic cycle as cadmium-glutathione conjugates after being secreted into the biliary tract. Whereas, in biliary tract, these cadmium conjugates are broken into cadmium-cysteine complexes and cadmium can again enter into the small intestine (Zalups and Ahmad 2003). Moreover, it has been observed that cadmium can be stored for a long time in kidney which can lead toward tubular necrosis (Orlowski and Piotrowski 2003). Cadmium(II) is sequestered by metallothionin, it accumulates in liver and kidney and the biological half-life of renal cadmium is up to 30 years. In the liver, the cysteine-metallothionein complex causes hepatotoxicity and then it circulates to the kidney and gets accumulated in the renal tissue causing nephrotoxicity. Proximal tubule cells are the main cellular targets of cadmium-mediated nephrotoxicity. Cadmium has the capability to bind with cysteine, glutamate, histidine, and aspartate ligands and can lead to the deficiency of iron (Castagnetto et al. 2002). Cadmium and zinc have the same oxidation states and hence cadmium can replace zinc present in metallothionein, thereby inhibiting it from acting as a free radical scavenger within the cell.

Cadmium(II) is a classified carcinogen triggering tumors in lung, kidney, and prostate (Waalkes 2003). The actual mechanisms of carcinogenesis are not clearly revealed, but might involve the replacement of essential metals in various biomolecules and enzymes. For example, replacement of zinc in zinc finger structures has been proposed as molecular basis for the inactivation of DNA repair enzymes, including XPA (Asmuss et al. 2000). Cadmium inhibits base excision repair at concentrations that are not enough to induce ROS (Dally and Hartwig 1997). Mechanisms contributing in DNA repair are sensitive targets for cadmium and regarded as major target for cadmium-induced carcinogenesis (Giaginis et al. 2006).

Studies have demonstrated that cadmium can affect cellular redox homeostasis (Waisberg et al. 2003). Increased cellular levels of superoxide anion radical and hydrogen peroxide appear concomitant with the upregulation of proto-oncogenes, especially c-fos, c-jun, and c-myc. Cadmium-induced ROS can also trigger genotoxicity, including DNA double-strand breaks in mammalian cells (Liu and Jan 2000). ROS generation could thus contribute to the carcinogenic potency of cadmium, but, nevertheless also trigger additional effects, including apoptosis (Hart et al. 1999).

Since cadmium(II) is not redox-active, replacement of iron and copper ions from intracellular depots, especially ferritin and apoferritin, has been discussed as indirect source for oxidative stress. In addition, cadmium was shown to inhibit complex III of the mitochondrial respiratory chain (Fig. 12.2). This alternative route of ROS generation leads to the accumulation of semiubiquinones and the formation of superoxide anion radical (Wang et al. 2004; Nair et al. 2013). Another aspect comes from the suppression of the cellular antioxidant system by cadmium, as an indirect trigger of oxidative stress (Fig. 12.2). For example, cadmium inhibits expression of antioxidant enzymes such as superoxide dismutase and catalase (Casalino et al. 2002), thereby contributing to augmented levels of $O_2^{\bullet-}$ and H_2O_2 and subsequent lipid peroxidation. In addition, ROS can be generated via cytokines, because of pro-inflammatory effects of cadmium(II) in liver tissue (Kayama et al. 1995). ROS are implicated in the toxicology of cadmium, mainly via the peroxidation of lipids. Inhibition of DNA repair, epigenetic alterations of DNA methylation and resistance toward apoptosis have been proposed as dominant mechanisms in cadmium-mediated carcinogenesis. The reason for the limited impact of ROS might lie in the adaptation of long-term cadmium-exposed cells by upregulation of antioxidant proteins. Elevated levels of GSH, as well as antioxidant enzymes and metallothionein have been observed (Klaassen et al. 1999).

12.4.3 Chromium

Chromium(VI) compounds (e.g., CrO_4^{2-}) have been classified as human carcinogens by the IARC (Proctor et al. 2016). In contrast to chromium(III), negatively charged chromate ions (CrO_4^{2-}) can easily and efficiently penetrate anionic channels in cell membranes, followed by intracellular reduction to chromium(V) and chromium(III) compounds (Fig. 12.3). These sequential reductions occur after chromium(VI) is bound by GSH (O'Brien et al. 2003), but GSH can be replaced by other cellular reductants, as for example ascorbate. In contrast to chromium(VI), chromium(V) and chromium(III) compounds can directly interact with DNA, thereby forming binary chromium-DNA adducts, or cross-links between DNA and proteins, ascorbate or gluthathione, respectively (Zhitkovich 2005). Although, chromium(III) is not considered a human carcinogen, it plays an apparent key role in the carcinogenesis triggered by hexavalent chromium (Tavakkoli et al. 2017). Figure 12.3 shows that besides DNA adduct formation via chromium(III), exposure to chromium(VI) can also trigger the generation of ROS and oxidative stress leading to chromium-induced DNA damage (Molyneux and Davies 1995). Different mechanisms have been suggested (Fig. 12.3). For example, reduction of chromium(VI) generates gluthathione-thiyl radicals that can reduce molecular oxygen to superoxide anion radicals (Wetterhahn et al. 1989). Both chromium(IV) and chromium(III) can also participate in Fenton-type reactions that generate hydroxy radicals. Notably, these Fenton reactions occur in parallel to the reduction of chromium and reconvert the compound into higher oxidation states. Chromium-mediated generation of hydroxy radicals can furthermore occur by Haber–Weiss reactions, which depend on endogenous superoxide anion radical and H_2O_2 (Shi et al. 1998).

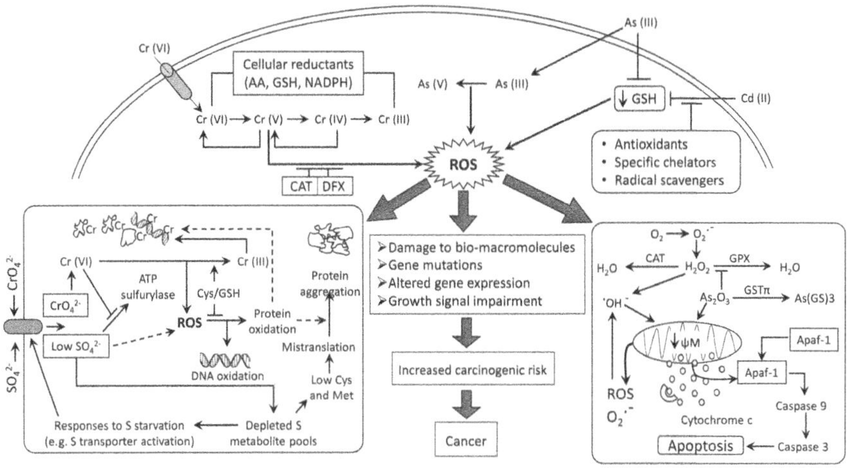

Fig. 12.3 Conceptual scheme showing carcinogenic risk induced by chromium and arsenic through free radical formation

12.4.4 Arsenic

The inorganic forms of arsenic such as arsenite and arsenate are found to be more dangerous to human health. They are highly carcinogenic and can cause cancer of lungs, liver, bladder, and skin. Arsenic toxicity can be either acute or chronic and chronic arsenic toxicity is termed as arsenicosis. Pigmentation and keratosis (called as "raindrops on a dusty road") are the specific skin lesions that indicate chronic arsenic toxicity (Martin and Griswold 2009). Lower levels of arsenic exposure can cause nausea and vomiting, reduced production of erythrocytes and leukocytes, abnormal heartbeat, pricking sensation in hands and legs, and damage to blood vessels. Long-term chronic exposure can lead to the formation of skin lesions, internal cancers, neurological problems, pulmonary disease, peripheral vascular disease, hypertension and cardiovascular disease, and diabetes mellitus (Smith et al. 2000). Chronic arsenicosis results in many irreversible changes in the vital organs and the mortality rate is higher. In spite of the magnitude of this potentially lethal toxicity, there is no effective treatment for this disease.

Multiple mechanisms have been suggested to explain arsenic-induced carcinogenesis (Fig. 12.3). Besides, its recognized capacity to induce oxidative stress (Piatek et al. 2008), arsenic also interacts with cellular targets such as the thiol groups of various proteins. In fact, *S*-adenosyl methionine (SAM) and glutathione (GSH) are required at several stages for metabolic conversion of both arsenite [As(III)] and arsenate [As(V)]. The capacity of trivalent arsenic to bind thiol groups has been suggested as trigger for inactivation of various zinc finger proteins (Piatek et al. 2008). Potential targets include DNA repair enzymes such as XPA and XPD (Piatek et al. 2008). Arsenic also inhibits nuclear excision repair (NER) of DNA adducts caused by other genotoxins, for example, benzo[*a*]pyrene and to act as cocarcinogen in concert with other mutagens (Waalkes et al. 2004). Although, no arsenic compound has been shown to directly form covalent DNA adducts, accumulation of DNA damage triggered by oxidative stress might be enhanced through concomitant inhibition of repair pathways. Inorganic arsenic compounds are also known to interact with methyl transferses and are substrates of arsenite methyltransferase AS(III)MT. In fact, chronic exposure to inorganic arsenic has been proposed to cause hypomethylation of DNA, thereby enhancing the expression of estrogen receptor and cyclin D1 (Chen et al. 2004). Both proteins promote cell cycle progression and might thus contribute to an increased oncogenic risk. Methylation of arsenite could possibly lead to depletion of SAM and therefore, account for activation of another set of genes involved in C1 (methyl) metabolism. DNA hypermethylation has also been shown to inhibit expression of tumor suppressor proteins, especially p53 and the cyclin-dependent kinase inhibitor p16Ink4a (Franco et al. 2008).

Figure 12.3 gives a possible induction of oxidative stress proposed as a major mode of action in arsenic-induced carcinogenesis (Kitchin and Conolly 2009). Although, precise mechanisms of ROS generation have not yet been revealed. It might involve formation of hydroxy radicals. Mitochondria are the primary target. Arsenic triggers rapid morphologic changes in this organelle and leads to inactivation of mitochondrial enzymes and loss of mitochondrial membrane potential. Arsenite constitutes a bypass for electrons from the respiratory chain, thereby facilitating the formation of superoxide anion radical. Additional proposed mechanisms include the reduction of oxygen by arsenic(III), thereby leading directly to the generation of H_2O_2 and/or formation of arsenic peroxyl radicals as central mediators of DNA damage.

12.4.5 Mercury

Mercury is considered as a highly hazardous metal owing to its toxicity. Due to the excess health effects associated with exposure to mercury, the present standard for drinking water has been set at lower levels of 0.002 mg/L and 0.001 mg/L by the Environmental Protection Act and World Health Organization (WHO 2004). The nervous system is very sensitive to all types of mercury (Bellanger et al. 2013). Increased exposure of mercury can alter brain functions and lead to shyness, tremors, memory problems, irritability, and changes in vision or hearing. Symptoms of organic mercury poisoning include depression, memory problems, tremors, fatigue, headache, hair loss, etc. Since these symptoms are common also in other conditions, it may be difficult to diagnose such cases (Martin and Griswold 2009). Methylmercury is a neurotoxic compound which is responsible for microtubule destruction, mitochondrial damage, lipid peroxidation, and accumulation of neurotoxic molecules such as serotonin, aspartate, and glutamate (Patrick 2002). Brain is the main target organ for mercury, yet it can impair any organ and lead to malfunctioning of nerves, kidneys, and muscles. It can cause disruption to the membrane potential and interrupt with intracellular calcium homeostasis. Mercury binds to freely available thiols as the stability constants are high (Patrick 2002). Mercury plays a key role in damaging the tertiary and quaternary protein structure and alters the cellular function by attaching to the selenohydryl and sulfhydryl groups which undergo reaction with methyl mercury and hamper the cellular structure. It also intervenes with the process of transcription and translation resulting in the disappearance of ribosomes and eradication of endoplasmic reticulum and the activity of natural killer cells. The cellular integrity is also affected causing free radical formation. The basis for HM chelation is that even though the mercury sulfhydryl bond is stable and divided to surrounding sulfhydryl consisting ligands, it also contributes free sulfhydryl groups to promote metal mobility within the ligands. EPA has declared that mercuric chloride and methyl mercury are highly carcinogenic. The toxic effects of mercury arise from its inhibition of different enzymatic activities and cellular damage. It shows selective affinity to react with -SH group. It affects the metabolism of mineral elements like sodium and potassium by increasing their permeability. It inhibits the active transport mechanism through dissipation of normal cation gradient, destroys mitochondrial apparatus, and causes cell lysis and mutagenesis.

12.5 Conclusions

Toxic heavy metals present in traditional herbal medicines pose potential health risks to the consumers. The toxicity level of a few heavy metals can be just above the background concentrations present naturally in the environment. Further, studies are required to determine the presence of toxic metals and to assess their long-term cumulative risk on consumer health. The presence of heavy metals in these medications could expose the consumers to different adverse health effects. There is a need for imparting culturally appropriate education to inform the public about potential toxicity associated with such herbal products. Therefore, proper sensitization and general awareness should be generated among the consumers and producers to minimize this risk. Hence, thorough knowledge of heavy metals in medicines is urgently required for taking proper mitigatory and defensive measures. To safeguard the public health, the need of the hour is to initiate and operationalize effective monitoring and control system as well as quality assessment and assurance of herbal products. It is essential to strengthen the quality assurance, safety, appropriate use, and effectiveness of TMs by regulating products, practices, and practitioners through education and training, skills development, capacity building, and therapies. Monitoring the exposure and timely intervention for reducing additional exposure to heavy metals in the environment and in humans can become a momentous step toward prevention of heavy metal hazard. National as well as international cooperation is vital for framing appropriate strategies to prevent heavy metal contamination in traditional medicines. There is need for continuous monitoring of herbal drugs sold in the market to make sure wholesome and safe drugs are sold for human consumption. In the line of conventional drugs, herbal products should be subjected to adequate quality control requirements as per recommendation of WHO, to ensure their efficacy, potency, and safety. Otherwise the traditional medicines which are intended to safeguard human life may even appear as "natural" threat in disguise to human life!

References

Ababneh FA (2017) The hazard content of cadmium, lead, and other trace elements in some medicinal herbs and their water infusions. Intern J Anal Chem 2017. Article ID 6971916. https://doi.org/10.1155/2017/6971916

Adepoju-Bello AA, Isa OA, Oguntibeju OO, Ayoola GA, Adejumo OO (2012) Analysis of some selected toxic metals in registered herbal products manufactured in Nigeria. Afr J Biotech 11 (26):6918–6922

Agarwal P, Fatima A, Singhm PP (2012) Herbal medicine scenario in India and European Countries. J Pharmacognosy Phytochem 1:4105–4117

Agency for Toxic Substances and Disease Registry (ATSDR) (2007) Toxicological profile for lead (update), Public Health Service. Department of Health and Human Services, Atlanta, GA, USA, US

Ang HH, Lee EL, Matsumoto K (2003) Analysis of lead content in herbal preparations in Malaysia. Hum Exp Toxicol 22:445–451

Asmuss M, Mullenders LH, Hartwig A (2000) Interference by toxic metal compounds with isolated zinc finger DNA repair proteins. Toxicol Lett 112–113:227–231

Bahall M (2017) Use of complementary and alternative medicine by patients with end-stage renal disease on haemodialysis in Trinidad: a descriptive study. BMC Complement Altern Med 17:250. https://doi.org/10.1186/s12906-017-1755-7

Bellanger M, Pichery C, Aerts D, Berglund M, Castaño A, Čejchanová M et al (2013) Economic benefits of methylmercury exposure control in Europe: monetary value of neurotoxicity prevention. Environ Health 12:3. https://doi.org/10.1186/1476-069X-12-3

Bernard A (2008) Cadmium & its adverse effects on human health. Indian J Med Res 128(4): 557–564

Casalino E, Calzaretti G, Sblano C, Landriscina C (2002) Molecular inhibitory mechanisms of antioxidant enzymes in rat liver and kidney by cadmium. Toxicology 179:37–50

Castagnetto JM, Hennessy SW, Roberts VA, Getzoff ED, Tainer JA, Pique ME (2002) MDB: the metalloprotein database and browser at the Scripps Research Institute. Nucleic Acids Res 30 (1):379–382

Chakraborty S, Dutta AR, Sural S, Gupta D, Sen S (2013) Ailing bones and failing kidneys: a case of chronic cadmium toxicity. Ann Clin Biochem 50(5):492–495

Chan K (2003) Some aspects of toxic contaminants in herbal medicines. Chemosphere 52(9):1361–1371

Chen H, Li S, Liu J, Diwan BA, Barrett JC, Waalkes MP (2004) Chronic inorganic arsenic exposure induces hepatic global and individual gene hypomethylation: implications for arsenic hepatocarcinogenesis. Carcinogenesis 25:1779–1786

Cheng JT (2000) Review: drug therapy in Chinese traditional medicine. J Clin Pharmacol 40: 445–450

Chopra A, Doiphode VV (2002) Ayurvedic medicine. Core concept therapeutic principles and current relevance. Med Clin North Am 86:75–89

Cooper K, Noller B, Connell D, Yu J, Sadler R, Olszowy H et al (2007) Public health risks from heavy metals and metalloids present in traditional Chinese medicines. J Toxicol Environ Health A70:1694–1699

Dally H, Hartwig A (1997) Induction and repair inhibition of oxidative DNA damage by nickel(II) and cadmium(II) in mammalian cells. Carcinogenesis 18:1021–1026

Dghaim RS, AlKhatib HR, Khan MA (2015) Determination of heavy metals concentration in traditional herbs commonly consumed in the United Arab Emirates. J Environ Public Health 2015. Article ID 973878. http://dx.doi.org/10.1155/2015/973878

Ernst E (2002a) Toxic heavy metals and undeclared drugs in Asian herbal medicines. Trends Pharmacol Sci 23(3):136–139

Ernst E (2002b) Heavy metals in traditional Indian remedies. Eur J Clin Pharmacol 57:891–896

Fabricant DS, Farnsworth NR (2001) The value of plants used in traditional medicine for drug discovery. Environ Health Perspect 109(1):69–75

Fakankun OA, Babayemi JO, Utiaruk JJ (2014) Variations in the mineral composition and heavy metals content of *Moringa oleifera*. African J Environ Sci Technol 7(6):372–379

Flora S, Saxena G, Gautam P, Kaur P, Gill KD (2007) Response of lead-induced oxidative stress and alterations in biogenic amines in different rat brain regions to combined administration of DMSA and MiADMSA. Chem Biol Interact 170:209–220

Franco R, Schoneveld O, Georgakilas AG, Panayiotidis MI (2008) Oxidative stress DNA methylation and carcinogenesis. Cancer Lett 266:6–11

Gesler WM (1992) Therapeutic landscapes: medical issues in light of the new cultural geography. Soc Sci Med 34(7):735–746

Giaginis C, Gatzidou E, Theocharis S (2006) DNA repair systems as targets of cadmium toxicity. Toxicol Appl Pharmacol 213:282–290

Gibert TF (1998) Reflections on traditional Chinese medicine and its pharmacopoeia. Annales Pharmaceutiques Françaises 56:282–285

Gogtay NJ, Bhatt HA, Dalvi SS, Kshirsagar NA (2002) The use and safety of nonallopathic Indian medicines. Drug Saf 25:1005–1019

Han XL, Zhang XB, Guo LP, Huang LQ, Li MJ, Sun YZ et al (2008) Statistical analysis of residues of heavy metals in Chinese crude drugs. China J Chin Mater Med 33:2041–2048

Hart BA, Lee CH, Shukla GS, Shukla A, Osier M, Eneman JD, Chiu JF (1999) Characterization of cadmium-induced apoptosis in rat lung epithelial cells: evidence for the participation of oxidant stress. Toxicology 133:43–58

Henson MC, Chedrese PJ (2004) Endocrine disruption by cadmium a common environmental toxicant with paradoxical effects on reproduction. Exp Biol Med (Maywood) 229(5):383–392

Hong FF (2004) History of medicine in China. McGill J Med 8:7984

Jarup L (2003) Hazards of heavy metal contamination. Br Med Bull 68(1):167–182

Jiang LF, Yao TM, Zhu ZL, Wang C, Ji LN (2007) Impacts of Cd (II) on the conformation and self-aggregation of Alzheimer's tau fragment corresponding to the third repeat of microtubule-binding domain. Biochem Biophys Acta 1774:1414–1421

Kayama F, Yoshida T, Elwell MR, Luster MI (1995) Role of tumor necrosis factor-alpha in cadmium-induced hepatotoxicity. Toxicol Appl Pharmacol 131:224–234

Kitchin KT, Conolly R (2009) Arsenic-induced carcinogenesis-oxidative stress as a possible mode of action and future research needs for more biologically based risk assessment. Chem Res Toxicol 23:327–335

Klaassen CD, Liu J, Choudhuri S (1999) Metallothionein: an intracellular protein to protect against cadmium toxicity. Annu Rev Pharmacol Toxicol 39:267–294

Koh HL, Woo SO (2000) Chinese proprietary medicine in Singapore regulatory control of toxic heavy metals and undeclared drugs. Drug Saf 23:351–362

Korfali SI, Mroueh M, Al-Zein M, Salem R (2013) Metal concentration in commonly used medicinal herbs and infusion by Lebanese population: health impact. J Food Res 2(2):70–80

Lad V (1985) The human constitution. Ayurveda: the science of self-healing. Lotus Press, Wilmot, pp 26–36

Lai HY, Chen ZS (2005) The EDTA effect on phytoextraction of single and combined metals contaminated soils using rainbow pink (*Dianthus chinensis*). Chemosphere 60:1062–1071
Lanphear BP, Hornung R, Khoury J, Yolton K, Baghurst P, Bellinger DC et al (2005) Low-level environmental lead exposure and children's intellectual function: an international pooled analysis. Environ Health Perspect 113:894–899
Lin CG, Schaider LA, Brabander DJ, Woolf AD (2010) Pediatric lead exposure from imported Indian spices and cultural powders. Pediatrics 125:E828–E835
Liu F, Jan KY (2000) DNA damage in arsenite and cadmium-treated bovine aortic endothelial cells. Free Radic Biol Med 28:55–63
Liu J, Lu YF, Wu Q, Goyer R, Waalkes MP (2008a) Mineral arsenicals in traditional medicines: orpiment realgar and arsenolite. J Pharmacol Exp Ther 326:363–368
Liu J, Shi JZ, Yu LM, Goyer RA, Waalkes MP (2008b) Mercury in traditional medicines: is cinnabar toxicologically similar to common mercurials? Exp Biol Med 233:810–817
Lu FL, Chen YH, Tseng MC, Lo CF, Lin JH (2009) Survey on heavy metals in raw material of traditional Chinese medicine (V). Annual report BFDA Taiwan ROC 27:51–64
Lynch E, Braithwaite R (2005) A review of the clinical and toxicological aspects of "traditional" (herbal) medicines adulterated with heavy metals. Expert Opin Drug Saf 4:769–778
Martena MJ, Van Der Wielen JC, Rietjens IM, Klerx WN, De Groot HN, Konings EJ (2010) Monitoring of mercury arsenic and lead in traditional Asian herbal preparations on the Dutch market and estimation of associated risks. U.S. National Library Med Control Expo Risk 27:190–205
Martin S and Griswold W (2009) Human health effects of heavy metals. Environ Sci Technol Briefs Cit 15:1–6. Center for Hazardous Substance Research Manhattan Kan, USA
Mathew BB, Tiwari A, Jatawa SK (2011) Free radicals and antioxidants: a review. J Pharm Res 4 (12):4340–4343
Molyneux MJ, Davies MJ (1995) Direct evidence for the hydroxyl radical-induced damage to nucleic acids by chromium(VI)-derived species: implications for chromium carcinogenesis. Carcinogenesis 16:875–882
Mosby CV, Glanze WD, Anderson KN (1996) Mosby medical encyclopedia the signet: revised edition. St. Louis
Nair AR, DeGheselle O, Smeets K, Van Kerkhove E, Cuypers A (2013) Cadmium-induced pathologies: where is the oxidative balance lost (or not)? Int J Mol Sci 14(3):6116–6143
Nunn FJ (2002) Ancient Egyptian medicine. University of Oklahoma Press, p 151
O'Brien TJ, Ceryak S, Patierno SR (2003) Complexities of chromium carcinogenesis: role of cellular response repair and recovery mechanisms. Mutat Res 533:3–36
Orlowski C, Piotrowski JK (2003) Biological levels of cadmium and zinc in the small intestine of non-occupationally exposed human subjects. Hum Exp Toxicol 22:57–63
Papanikolaou NC, Hatzidaki EG, Belivanis S, Tzanakakis GN, Tsatsakis AM (2005) Lead toxicity update. A brief review. Med Sci Monit 11(10):RA329
Patrick L (2002) Mercury toxicity and antioxidants: part 1: role of glutathione and alpha-lipoic acid in the treatment of mercury toxicity. Altern Med Rev 7(6):456–471
Patwardhan B, Warude D, Pushpangadan P, Bhatt N (2005) Ayurveda and traditional chinese medicine: a comparative overview. eCAM 2(4):465–473
Piatek K, Schwerdtle T, Hartwig A, Bal W (2008) Monomethylarsenous acid destroys a tetrathiolate zinc finger much more efficiently than inorganic arsenite: mechanistic considerations and consequences for DNA repair inhibition. Chem Res Toxicol 21:600–606
Pizzino G, Bitto A, Interdonato M, Galfo F, Irrera N, Mecchio A, Squadrito F (2014) Oxidative stress and DNA repair and detoxification gene expression in adoles-cents exposed to heavy metals living in the milazzo-valle del Mela area (Sicily Italy). Redox Biol J 2:686–693
Proctor DM, Suh M, Mittal L, Hirsch S, Valdes Salgado R, Bartlett C, van Landingham C, Rohr A, Crump K (2016) Inhalation cancer risk assessment of hexavalent chromium based on updated mortality for painesville chromate production workers. J Eposure Sci Environ Epidemiol 26:224–231

Robert BS, Russel SP, Awusha S, Nadia K, Roger BD, Janet P, Venkatesh T, De Stefano T (2008) Lead mercury and arsenic in US and Indian-manufactured ayurvedic medicines sold via the internet. JAMA 300(8):915–923

Robson B, Baek OK (2009) The engines of hippocrates: from the dawn of medicine to medical and pharmaceutical informatics. Wiley, p 50

Saad B, Azaizeh H, Abu-Hijleh G, Said O (2006) Safety of traditional Arab herbal medicine. Evid-Based Complem Altern Med 3(4):433–439

Saeed M, Muhammed N, Khan H, Khan SA (2010) Analysis of toxic heavy metals in branded Pakistani herbal products. J Chem Soc Pak 32(4):471–475

Saper RB, Kales SN, Paquin J, Burns MJ, Eisenberg DM, Davis RB et al (2004) Heavy metal content of ayurvedic herbal medicine products. JAMA 292:2868–2873

Saper RB, Phillips RS, Sehgal A, Khouri N, Davis RB, Paquin J et al (2008) Lead mercury andarsenic in US- and Indian-manufactured ayurvedic medicines sold via the internet. JAMA 300:915–923

Sharma N, Kala CP (2017) Harvesting and management of medicinal and aromatic plants in the Himalaya. J Appl Res Med Aromat Plants. https://doi.org/10.1016/j.jarmap.2017.09.003

Shi X, Leonard SS, Liu KJ, Zang L, Gannett PM, Rojanasakul Y, Castranova V, Vallyathan V (1998) Cr(III)-mediated hydroxyl radical generation *via* Haber-Weiss cycle. J Inorg Biochem 69:263–268

Smith AH, Lingas EO, Rahman M (2000) Contamination of drinking-water by arsenic in Bangladesh: a public health emergency. Bulletin World Health Organization 78(9):1093–1103

Tavakkoli L, Nasab ZZ, Khanjani N (2017) Environmental and occupational exposure to chromium in Iran: a systematic review. J Epidemiol Res 3:31–39

Tchounwou PB, Yedjou CG, Patlolla AK, Sutton DJ (2012) Heavy metal toxicity & the environment. EXS 101:133–164

Thatte UM, Rege NN, Phatak SD, Dahanukar SA (1993) The flip side of ayurveda. J Postgrad Med 39:179–182

Thompson KH, Orvig C (2003) Boon and bane of metal ions in medicine. Science 300(5621):936–939

Turan M, Bringu A (2007) Phytoremediation based on canola (*Brassica napus* L.) and Indian mustard (*Brassica juncea* L.) planted on spiked soil by aliquot amount of Cd Cu Pb and Zn. Plant Soil Environ 53:7–15

Waalkes MP (2003) Cadmium carcinogenesis. Mutat Res 533:107–120

Waalkes MP, Liu J, Ward JM, Diwan BA (2004) Animal models for arsenic carcinogenesis: inorganic arsenic is a transplacental carcinogen in mice. Toxicol Appl Pharmacol 198:377–384

Wadhwa N, Mathew BB, Jatawa S, Tiwari A (2012) Lipid peroxidation: mechanism models and significance. Intern J Current Sci 3:29–38

Waisberg M, Joseph P, Hale B, Beyersmann D (2003) Molecular and cellular mechanisms of cadmium carcinogenesis. Toxicology 192:95–117

Wang Y, Fang J, Leonard SS, Rao KM (2004) Cadmium inhibits the electron transfer chain and induces reactive oxygen species. Free Radic Biol Med 36:1434–1443

Wei S, Zhou Q, Mathews S (2008) A newly found cadmium accumulator *Taraxacum mongolicum*. J Hazard Mater 159:544–547

Wetterhahn KE, Hamilton JW, Aiyar J, Borges KM, Floyd R (1989) Mechanism of chromium(VI) carcinogenesis. Reactive intermediates and effect on gene expression. Biol Trace Elem Res 21:405–411

World Health Organisation (WHO) (2004) Guidelines for drinking-water quality. Sixty-first meeting Rome 10–19 June 2003. Joint FAO/WHO expert committee on food additives. Available from www.ftp.fao.org/es/esn/jecfa/jecfa61sc.pdf

World Health Organisation (WHO) (2007) Guidelines for assessing quality of herbal medicines with reference to contaminants and residues. Geneva Switzerland

World Health Organisation (WHO) (2013) WHO traditional medicine strategy: 2014–2023. WHO Press, Geneva Switzerland, p 78

Wu J, Zou Y, Zhan X, Chen S, Lu G, Lai F (2008) Survey of heavy metal pollution in four Chinese crude drugs and their cultivated soils. Bull Environ Contam Toxicol 81:571–573

Yee SK, Chu SS, Xu YM, Choo PL (2005) Regulatory control of Chinese proprietary medicines in Singapore. Health Policy 71:133–149

Zalups RK, Ahmad S (2003) Molecular handling of cadmium in transporting epithelia. Toxicol Appl Pharmacol 186:163–188

Zhitkovich A (2005) Importance of chromium-DNA adducts in mutagenicity and toxicity of chromium(VI). Chem Res Toxicol 18:3–11

Zhu YP (1998) Chinese materia medica: chemistry pharmacology and applications. Harwood Academic Publishers

Chapter 13
Impact of Heavy Metal Carcinogens on Human Health

Sanjay Mishra, Amit Kumar Mani Tiwari and Abbas Ali Mahdi

Abstract During the development of human activities, it has been noticed that such activities contribute to the discharge of toxic chemicals like metals and metalloids into the atmosphere. These toxic metals are accumulated in the dietary articles of human beings. Food chain polluted with toxic metals and metalloids is a significant path of human exposure and thus may cause a number of hazardous effects on human health. Nevertheless, cancer is a leading cause of morbidity, mortality, and premature death worldwide. Certain approaches like less exposure to carcinogenic factors can reduce the risk of most cancer types in human. Epigenetic variations in the etiology of cancer have led to increasing of cancer research studies in the recent years. Although epigenetic effects of these elements have more prominent role than their genetic effects, these elements are able to alter the pattern of cancer-related genes' expression profiles. Hence, an understanding of the principal epigenetically mechanisms of these trace elements and the compounds that could reduce their toxicities or the number of cancer cases is necessary. Conceivably, the toxic effects of these elements in many regions are anticipated but antioxidant supplements may eradicate the reactive oxygen species as foremost effects of these elements. In this chapter, we tried to focus on various studies dealing with epigenetic effects of carcinogens on human health.

Keywords Bioavailability · Cancer prevention · Stem cell · Epigenetic effects of carcinogens · Heavy metals and metal toxicity

S. Mishra (✉) · A. K. M. Tiwari
Laboratory of Biochemistry, Department of Biotechnology,
IFTM University, Delhi Road (NH 24), Moradabad 244102, Uttar Pradesh, India
e-mail: sanjaymishra@iftmuniversity.ac.in; sanjaymishra66@gmail.com

A. A. Mahdi
Department of Biochemistry, King George's Medical University,
Lucknow 226003, Uttar Pradesh, India

M. Rai et al. (eds.), *Biomedical Applications of Metals*,
https://doi.org/10.1007/978-3-319-74814-6_13

13.1 Introduction

Almost thirty chemical elements are constantly found in bio-organisms, participating in fundamental biochemical and physiological functions, and documented as necessary elements for life (Barnham and Bush 2014). Greater part of the identified metals and metalloids are very toxic to bio-organisms and even those measured as crucial can be toxic if present in excess (Mudgal et al. 2010; Jaishankar et al. 2014) as a consequence of human activities. They can perturb significant biochemical processes, constituting an important threat for the health of plants and animal systems, including human beings (Mudgal et al. 2010; Tiwari et al. 2017). Plants and animals take up these elements from soils, sediments, and water by contact with their external surfaces, through ingestion and inhalation of airborne particles and vaporized metals. The assimilation of an element (i.e., the bioavailable fraction) depends on a number of physicochemical factors such as chemical speciation, solubility in organic medium, pH, etc. (Namieśnika and Rabajczyk 2010). In soils, metals and metalloids can arise in both solid and aqueous phases. In solution, these elements can exist either as free ions or as various complexes associated with organic or inorganic ligands or as suspended colloidal particles. In the solid phase, they can be adsorbed or absorbed on organic and inorganic soil components (Track 2010). In general, ions in solution are more available for plant uptake and entering into the food chain. Metal ions present in the solid phase available under certain biological and physicochemical conditions, such as exudation of special chelators, desorption, redox, and pH changes. Animals are exposed to these toxicants through respiratory, the skin, and digestive systems (Prashanth et al. 2015). After entering the body, the metal deposited in nasopharyngeal, tracheobronchial, or pulmonary compartments may be transported by mucociliary action to the gastrointestinal tract. Macrophages phagocyted the wandering metals. Food is the most important route for entering essential and toxic elements. Some elements like mercury (Hg) are biologically magnified at higher trophic level. The dietary contribution for toxic metal intake has been extensively studied by Santos et al. (2004). If the body is deficient in minerals and trace elements, it will absorb heavy metals in their place. Every cell membrane breaks down and rebuilds every two weeks but does not release the heavy metals if essential fats are not ingested or if bad fats are ingested. The liver, which performs detoxification 100% of the time, cannot perform this important task without all the essential nutrients.

Chemical elements present as free ions and those readily ionized are almost completely absorbed by the body. Transition metals readily form stable covalent complexes and usually interact as parts of macromolecules (proteins, enzymes, hormones, etc.) according to their chemical characteristics including oxidation state (Mudgal et al. 2010; Tchounwou et al. 2012; Sharma et al. 2014). These metals are complexed with amino acids (glutathione (GSH), cysteine, and histidine) and proteins (metallothioneins, transferrin, ferritin, lactoferrin, hemosiderin, ceruloplasmin, and melanotransferrin) (Table 13.1). Health damage triggered by toxic metals may be less (irritation) or acute (teratogenic, mutagenic, and carcinogenic).

Table 13.1 Major toxic metals and their reactive forms

Metal	Toxicity
Cd	All forms are toxic and need attention
Pb	Organic forms are more toxic and easily absorbed by the gastrointestinal tract
As	Inorganic arsenate [As(+5)] or [As(+3)] is more toxic
Hg	Hg(II) organomercurials mainly methylmercury, biologically magnified

These reactive elements of food present as complexes with fiber have a low solubility within the intestinal lumen and are poorly absorbed (Table 13.2). Absorption of these minerals promotes by low concentration of fiber and absence of phytates, oxalates in the diet (Hazell 1985; Tiwari et al. 2012). Micronutrients can interact with toxic metals at several points in the body like absorption, transport, binding to target proteins, metabolism, sequestration, excretion of toxic metals and finally, in secondary symptoms of toxicity such as oxidative stress (Jan et al. 2015). Thus, a diet poor in micronutrients can have an important influence on the toxicity. In biological fluids and tissues, most metals and metalloids are not present as free cations. In blood, they are usually bound to red cells or to plasma proteins. Lead (Pb) and cadmium (Cd) are almost completely bound to red blood cells. The chemical elements bound to plasma proteins constitute the fraction available for transport into and out of the tissues (Silva et al. 2005).

Albumin, a plasma protein, has a pronounced capacity to bind several metals. In order to avoid undesirable health effects as resulted from "excessive" intake of toxicants (including toxic metals), international and national scientific organizations such as FAO/WHO, FDA, European Union, etc. have used the safety guidelines for establishing acceptable or tolerable intakes of substances that exhibit threshold toxicity. The acceptable daily intake (ADI) or tolerable daily intake (TDI) or provisional tolerable weekly intakes (PTWI) are used to describe "safe" levels of intake for several toxicants including toxic metals (Kroes and Kozianowski 2002; Oforka et al. 2012). For majority of toxicity, it is thought that there is a dose below the recommended level that has no adverse effect. For chemicals that give rise to such toxic effects, a TDI, i.e., an estimate of the amount of a substance in food, is expressed on a body weight basis (mg kg^{-1} or mg kg^{-1} of body weight) that can be ingested over a lifetime without appreciable health risk.

Table 13.2 Food sources of toxic metals

Metal	Food source
Cd	Egg, fish, mushroom, garlic, spinach, wheat, rice, oat, corn, soybean, peanuts, mushroom
Pb	Egg, cocoa powder, rice, wheat, potato, calcium supplement, smoked food, wine, beer, milk, carrot, raisins
As	Green papaya, rice, tomato, carrot, seafood, Indian mustard, bovine and chicken meat, wine, milk
Hg	Egg, mushroom, seafood, fish oil

Exposure greater than the TDI value for short period should not have deleterious effects upon health. However, acute effects may occur if the TDI is substantially exceeded even for short periods of time. Additionally, contaminants possessing very long half-lives can be accumulated in the body and chronic effects are most often observed when critical concentrations are reached in target tissues, ultimately resulting in cancer that is a foremost reason of morbidity, mortality, and premature death worldwide (Kanavos 2006; Thun et al. 2010; Santos et al. 2013).

13.2 Heavy Metals Versus Cancer

This continual and emergent burden of cancer in the world's populations' warrants finely tuned public health awareness. Prevention, early detection, and therapy have all established parameters in checking certain types of cancer and in thus dropping down the burden of premature death and advanced disease (Mishra et al. 2010; Mudgal et al. 2010; Rebecca et al. 2017). The occurrence and mortality as a result of multifactorial polygenic diseases such as varieties of cancer diverge depending upon genetic susceptibility and environmental precursors as they have certain mendelian subsets. Speedy alterations in diet and lifestyle may affect heritability of the variant phenotypes, which are dependent on the nutraceutical supplementation for their expression (Mishra et al. 2010; Mudgal et al. 2010). It is likely to distinguish the interaction of specific nutraceuticals, with the genetic code possessed by all nucleated cells (Mudgal et al. 2010). In many countries, though, these well-recognized approaches to cancer check have not been applied to their complete potential and in many countries are not applied at all. In addition, immense disparities still exist in cancer check in reference to gender, race, ethnicity, and socioeconomic status.

A variety of carcinogens have already been recognized, and the pertinent information regarding these agents is accessible, although humans make use of many food and beverage items, assuming that they are harmless. One example is the potentially harmful presence of heavy metals, which can cause serious health problems (Mudgal et al. 2010). People may be exposed to heavy metals during the course of their lifetime. The heavy metals in drinking water create the greatest threat to public health in this context. This necessitates setting appropriate quality control measures. The major source of heavy metals in drinking water is contamination of surface and ground waters by industrial sewage and agricultural runoff (Karavoltsos et al. 2008; Hariprasad and Dayananda 2013). In the areas where water delivery network is made of alloys containing heavy metals, some people may not afford bottled or mineral water with restricted heavy metal concentrations and thus consumes tap water; therefore, the likelihood of contamination of drinking water with heavy metals increases to a great extent (Leivadara et al. 2008). According to some WHO information, the concentration of these elements in groundwater is elevated in several countries including Bangladesh, India, and Argentina (WHO 1987, 2003). Heavy metals in drinking water are toxic and can easily penetrate the body.

The genetic and epigenetic impacts of these elements are coupled with an increased risk of varieties of cancer (Bower et al. 2005; Caffo et al. 2014; Jaishankar et al. 2014).

Epigenetic mechanisms play a significant role than genetic events in carcinogenesis. These effects take place most often during the early stages of tumor development. Epigenetic events consist of reversible alteration of histone proteins and CpG islands of gene promoters, which affect not only gene expression of germ and somatic cells but also cause indirect gene sequence alterations (Jones and Baylin 2002; Vaziri Gohar et al. 2007). CpG islands (5′-CG-3′ sequence) subsist in about 40% of mammalian genes. Hypermethylation or hypomethylation of C5 position of the cytosine base is implicated in the inhibition of expression of tumor suppressor genes or the raise of the oncogene expression, both of which contribute to cancer development as well as progression (Ehrlich 2009; Jin et al. 2011; Subramaniam et al. 2014). Gene silencing can also occur through methylation of lysine 9 in histone-H3 (H3-K9) that results in a cascade of clustering of a number of proteins including HP1 protein, SUV39H1 histone methyltransferase, histone deacetylases, DNA methyltransferases, and lastly methyl-C binding proteins (MBD) (Jackson et al. 2002; Tamaru and Selker 2001; Vogelstein and Kinzler 2004). Methylated cytosine may be spontaneously deaminated to create a thymine, leading to a specific transition mutation in CpG islands, for example, in the TP_{53} tumor suppressor gene as a protector of genome. Besides, hypermethylation of histone proteins results in alterations in the chromatin configuration, predisposing cells to allelic loss at a specific locus in the chromosomes (Egger et al. 2004). Such genetic and epigenetic changes in growth-control genes such as DNA repair genes, tumor suppressor genes, oncogenes, and apoptotic genes come close together to determine the cellular phenotype and demarcation (Vaziri Gohar et al. 2007; Mohammadi et al. 2008).

As far as ranking the carcinogens is concerned, heavy metals have been classified by the International Agency for Research on Cancer (IARC) and Environmental Protection Agency (EPA) as the first group, excepting selenium, which has been listed within group 3 (not carcinogen to humans) of the IARC classification (Mishra et al. 2010). The main aim of this chapter is to focus on comparison of the epigenetic effects caused by various heavy metals in cancer-concerned genes in biological systems, including human. In addition, it was also discussed that incidence of cancer can be reduced by adopting prevention behavior especially in terms of drinking water considering the following elements concomitant with their conjugative.

13.2.1 Lead (Pb)

Pb is used in storage batteries, cable coverings, plumbing, ammunition, manufacturing of tetraethyl Pb, sound absorbers, radiation shields around X-ray equipment, nuclear reactors, and paints, while the oxide is used in producing fine "crystal glass" and “flint glass” with a high refractive index for achromatic lenses, solder, and insecticides (Chidananda and Jagadeesh 2015). Pb enters the human body in many ways. It can be inhaled in dust from lead paints or waste gases from leaded gasoline. It is found in trace amounts in various foods, notably fish, which are heavily subjected to industrial pollution plants that can absorb Pb from soils and from a $PbEt_4$ traffic-induced air pollution (90% of total Pb emissions into the atmosphere). Pb can contaminate water and consequently enter the aquatic food chains (Kaste et al. 2003; Verma and Dwivedi 2013; Weber et al. 2013). Pb is a toxic metal and most people and animals receive the largest portion of their daily Pb intake via food. Pb can enter food during storage and manufacture, e.g., in canned food and in alcoholic drinks (Eticha and Hymete 2014). Cosmetics are also an important source of Pb contamination. The amount of Pb absorbed depends on age and the extent to which Pb particles are dissolved in the stomach. The proportion of Pb absorbed from the gastrointestinal tract is about 10% in adults, whereas levels of 40–50% have been reported for infants. Milk, fasting, low levels of calcium, vitamin D, and iron have been shown to increase Pb absorption in laboratory animals (WHO 2001). Children under 6 years are especially susceptible to the adverse effects of Pb, as the blood–brain barrier is not yet fully developed in young children; hematological and neurological adverse effects of Pb occur at lower threshold levels than in adults. Pb has effects on erythropoiesis and heme biosynthesis. Chronic Pb intoxication in adults resulted in anemia, some types of cancer, reproductive harm in males while in young children hormonal imbalance of metabolite of vitamin D, namely 1,25-dihydroxy-vitamin D, and drop in IQ (Siddiqui et al. 2002; Tandon et al. 2001; Tiwari et al. 2012).

13.2.2 Cadmium (Cd)

Compounds of Cd are highly toxic to humans. Cd is used in several industrial processes such as protective coatings (electroplating) for metals like iron, preparation of Cd–Ni batteries, control rods, and shields within nuclear reactors (Malik et al. 2014). Some compounds are used as stabilizers for PVC. For nonsmoking population, the major exposure pathway is through food. Cd is readily taken up by plants. Potential source of Cd toxicity is the use of commercial sludge to fertilize agricultural fields. Some root crops (carrots and parsnip) and some leafy crops (lettuce and spinach) are able to accumulate more Cd than other plant foods. Grain crops like rice and wheat can accumulate relatively high amounts of Cd (Kibria et al. 2006).

Its absorption is increased by calcium, protein, and vitamin D. Internal organs of mammals such as liver and kidneys may also contain high amounts of Cd. The dietary Cd absorption rate in humans has been estimated at 5% of its total intake. The metal transporter protein Nramp2, known also as DMT1, seems to be involved in Cd absorption (Tallkvist et al. 2001). The daily intake of Cd was estimated as 25–60 μg for a 70 kg person from uncontaminated areas but values may rise up to

10–61 μg day^{-1}. Cd is a normal constituent of tobacco, because *Nicotiana* species is able to concentrate Cd independent of soil Cd content. The Cd content in tobacco ranged between 1 and 2 μg g^{-1} dry weight, equivalent to 0.5–1 μg $cigarette^{-1}$ (Hui et al. 2015). Approximately, 10% of the inhaled Cd oxide is deposited in lung tissues, and another 30–40% is absorbed into systemic blood circulation of smokers. Smokers have 4–5 times higher Cd levels in blood and 2–3 times greater amounts of Cd in their kidneys than do nonsmokers. Itai–Itai disease was caused by large amounts of Cd in the village's water supply of Toyama city, Japan, from 1939 to 1954 (Oudeh et al. 2002; Bishak et al. 2015).

Cd is a cumulative toxicant that affects kidneys, produce various toxic effects in the body, and disturbed bone metabolism and the reproductive system, endocrine system, and also carcinogenic (Rachdaoui and Sarkar 2013). It develops several morphopathological changes in the kidneys due to long-term exposure to Cd. Increasing intakes of zinc can reduce the renal toxicity of Cd. Cd exposure increases calcium excretion, thus causing skeletal demineralization, which may lead to increase in bone fragility and risk of fractures (Wu et al. 2001). Cd and its compounds are currently classified by IARC as a Group 1 carcinogen for humans. Occupational human exposure has been linked to lung cancer. Cd exposure, during human pregnancy, led to reduced birth weights and premature birth (Henson and Chedrese 2004; Jaishankar et al. 2014; Rengarajan et al. 2015). Besides, Kippler et al. (2012) found evidence of a sex difference in the association between maternal Cd exposure and birth size that was noticeable only in girls. Outcomes add support for the need to reduce Cd pollution to improve public health.

13.2.3 Aluminum (Al)

The certain specific compounds of Al have been used in wide range of applications in different industries including cosmetics and food additives (Darbre 2005; Stahl et al. 2017). Al-mediated carcinogenesis is due to its binding ability to the estrogen receptor and imitates estrogen functions, thus named metallo-estrogen. Metallo estrogen triggers the expression of genes found in estrogen-responsive elements (EREs). There is evidence that definite salts of Al such as those found in anti-aspirants can remain in applied regions of axillae and mammary glands for prolonged periods if not washed properly thus providing the probability for continuous exposure to Al and enhancement of risk of breast cancer due to increasing replication errors in cancer related genes (Sun et al. 2007). It has been demonstrated that if antiperspirants containing Al applied on the skin around the underarm and breast areas, it is not washed off completely, some Al salts remain in the area. This results in continuous exposure and ultimately increases the risk of breast cancer (Stellman et al. 2000). There are two different groups of estrogen receptors (ER). The first group exists in cytosol/nucleus (ER-α and ER-β) and acts as transcription factors by directly binding to ERE, whereas the second one exists in plasma membrane as transmembrane G-protein coupled receptors. These ERs can also control gene expression by means of interaction with other transcription factors, without binding directly to ERE. Plasma membrane located ER46 is involved in endothelial nitric oxide synthase (eNOS) phosphorylation and rapid nitric oxide (NO) release through phosphatidylinositol 3-kinase in endothelial cells. Another plasma membrane located ER family called ER66 manages reporter gene expression (Darbre 2005). Al can bind to both nuclear and membrane of ERs, and ERE; as a consequence, it can trigger both ER signal transductions. Consequently, as expected, Al^{3+} treatment assists in intracellular NO generation (Satoh et al. 2007; Joshi et al. 2013). Al may produce pro-oxidant effect in rats and could be of interest for understanding the controversial role of Al in assessing toxicity (Joshi et al. 2013).

In addition to breast carcinogenesis, estrogen can activate telomerase gene expression as a gene containing ERE, in ER-α-positive cell, but not in ER-negative cells, these results in endometrial cancer (Harley 2008). The epigenetic effects of Al take place through the binding of trivalent (Al^{3+}) to the phosphate groups of double-stranded DNA under physiologic pH, thus changing DNA topology from B to Z in $(CCG)_{12}$ repeat regions (Zhang et al. 2002). The expansion of the triplet repeats is named as "dynamic mutation", and may be localized in both coding and noncoding regions. A minimum of 5–10 triplet repeats increases the probability of hairpin formations, principally in the lagging strand. Movement of DNA polymerase along the hairpin structure leads to the replication slippage and genomic instability, causing deletion mutations. Expansion of more than 200 copies of these repeats leads to excessive methylation of cytosines in the promoter of FMR1 gene that results in fragile X syndrome (Lukusa and Fryns 2008).

13.2.4 Arsenic (As)

Arsenic is generally known as an epigenetic carcinogen metalloid when in the form of an inorganic compound. In the environment, arsenic is usually found combined with other elements as inorganic and organic forms. Inorganic arsenic is more poisonous than organic one (Hughes et al. 2011). Arsenic trioxide (As_2O_3) is the most common inorganic form of arsenic found in air, while arsenates (AsO_4^{-3}) or arsenites (AsO_2) occur in water, soil, or food. Arsenic may be also necessary ultra-trace element for red algae, chickens, rats, goats, and pigs and its deficiency inhibited growth (Pimparkar and Bhave 2010). Arsenic concentration is high in marine food. In fishes, arsenic ranged between 5 and 100 μg g^{-1} and reach up to 100–250 μg g^{-1} in species at the top of the food chain (Hughes et al. 2011).

Trivalent arsenite (As^{+3}) has more carcinogenic properties than the pentavalent arsenate (As^{+5}) (Patterson et al. 2003; Alkahtani 2009). Trivalent arsenic can bind with high affinity to thiol groups of proteins and reduced glutathione (GSH) (Suzuki et al. 2004). Longtime uptake of drinking water containing low levels of arsenite induces carcinogenesis in skin, lung, bladder, and kidney tissues, resulting from alteration in multiple signaling pathways. The risk of bladder cancer is more in people who drink water with an arsenic level above 100 ppb, and it increases the risk by more than 15 times compared with people living in areas with less than 10 ppb. Arsenic is methylated for detoxification and excretion from the body. This reaction gives rise to the carcinogenic properties of arsenic through the epigenetic transformations. This is contrary to the general belief about methylation, which is considered important way for detoxification. The toxicity of monomethyl arsenic (MMAs) and dimethyl arsenic (DMAs) is more than arsenite (Patterson et al. 2003; Suzuki et al. 2004). Arsenic methylation generally occurs by Glutathione S-transferase (GST), arsenic III methyltransferase (AS3MT), and S-adenosyl methionine (SAM). These enzymes compete with DNA methyltransferase (DNMT) for DNA methylation, hence inhibiting DNA methyltransferase indirectly and inducing the reactivation of silenced tumor suppressor genes (Huang 2002). Interaction with arsenic induces the ROS formation (through its reduction) as an inescapable reaction of regular cell metabolism (Galanis et al. 2008). ROS, acting as a second messenger, is involved in the activation of PI3 K/Akt pathway and the succeeding stimulation of transcription factor hypoxia-inducible factor-1 (HIF-1α) but not HIF-1β and vascular endothelial growth factor (VEGF) stimulation (Gao et al. 2004; Sharma et al. 2009). An additional essential mechanism of arsenic-induced carcinogenesis is through enhancing the genotoxicity of other carcinogens, together with ultraviolet radiation (UVR), ionizing radiation, alkylating agents, or oxidants. UVR induces nonmelanoma skin cancer. Strands of DNA exposed to photons of UVA and UVB break, and cyclobutane pyrimidine dimers (CPDs) are produced (Ravanat et al. 2001; Melnikova and Ananthaswamy 2005; Ramasamy et al. 2017). UVRs can trigger a zinc-finger protein family, poly (ADP-ribose) polymerase (PARP), and predominantly one member of this family, named PARP-1, has a vital role in the regulation of nucleotide excision repair (NER). CPDs have been recognized in p53 and PTCH tumor suppressor genes and ras oncogenes. Arsenite stimulates inducible nitric oxide synthase (iNOS) expression and NO production via mammalian mitogen-activated protein kinases p38 and activation of nuclear transcription factor-kappa B (NF-κB) (Ding et al. 2008; Ramasamy et al. 2017). Between 40 and 60% of arsenic intake is excreted into the urine (Fujihara et al. 2009). A foremost proportion (60–80%) of urinary arsenic is composed of dimethylated arsenic (Vahter 2000).

In humans, arsenic toxicity has been occured due to ingestion of As-containing powders or solutions accidentally, for suicide, homicide, or consumption of contaminated food or drinking water. Arsenic has been associated with hypertension and has serious effects on the cardiovascular system, and at high doses it causes hepatic damage (Lee et al. 2003; Yoshida et al. 2004). It has a suppressive effect on spermatogenesis and gonadotrophin and testosterone release in rats (Sarkar et al. 2003). There is correlation between arsenic exposure and diabetes mellitus (type II) (Walton et al. 2004). Different dermal effects are caused by inorganic arsenic ingestion like hyperkeratosis (formation of hyperkeratotic warts on the palms and soles), hyperpigmentation and hypopigmentation periorbital swellings, the occurrence of spontaneous abortion, and damage of nervous system (at high doses).

With advances in technology and the recent development of animal models for arsenic carcinogenicity, understanding of the toxicology of arsenic will continue to improve (Martine et al. 2011).

13.2.5 Chromium (Cr)

Trivalent chromium is an epigenetic carcinogen factor since it can form stable compounds with macromolecules such as DNA and cysteine residue of proteins and glutathione (Zhitkovich et al. 1995). The trivalent form of chromium cannot pass the cell membrane; however, the hexavalent salts are able to enter the cell and are converted to the trivalent form. Therefore, depending on the situation, reducing agents can affect carcinogenic properties of chromium inside the cell, and chromium (VI) can be converted to a carcinogen. During Cr (VI) reduction, many compounds such as oxygen radicals, DNA interstrand cross-links (ICLs), and single-strand breaks (SSBs) may form. ICLs act as physical barriers to DNA replication and transcription events, consequently, inducing apoptosis (Schnekenburger et al. 2007). The chromium carcinogenicity, particularly in lung epithelial cells and fibroblasts, is imposed through hypermethylation of CYP1a1 promoter. Chromium recruits histone deacetylase 1 (HDAC1) and DNMT1, especially to CYP1a1 promoter, and this assembly recruits BP1 and inhibits CYP1a1 gene expression (Wei et al. 2004). CYP1A1 is essential in the metabolism of carcinogens such as polycyclic aromatic hydrocarbons (PAHs) and heterocyclic amines, which are extensively distributed widely in the environment via automobile exhausts, cigarette smoke, charcoal-broiled cooking, and industrial waste. Contrary to other cytochrome P450, enzymes such as epoxide hydrolase and dihydrodiol dehydrogenase, which are involved in PAH- and Benzo(a)pyrene-induced carcinogenesis, CYP1A1 inhibits PAH carcinogenesis. Hence, inhibition of CYP1A1 by chromium leads to the production of a PAH (Wu et al. 2009). PAHs have a significant role in the activation of cytosolic ligand-activated transcription factor named aromatic hydrocarbon receptor (AhR) (Nebert et al. 2000). After formation, the PAH–AhR complex is transferred into the nucleus. In the nucleus, PAH is detached from the complex and AhR binds to its nuclear partner, Arnt. This new complex acts as a transcription factor and interacts with DRE of CYP1A1 gene, leading to the activation of CYP1A1 gene expression, consequently causing bioactivation of exogenous procarcinogens of both hepatocellular and lung carcinomas (Li et al. 2009).

It is appealing that PAH through binding to transcription factor AhR activates CYP1a1 gene expression, and CYP1A1 inhibits PAH carcinogenesis, but in the presence of Cr, the promoter of CYP1a1 is inactivated and PAH can act as carcinogens. Benzo(α) pyrene is also a member of polycyclic aromatic hydrocarbon (PAHs) family that is metabolically transformed from its pro-carcinogenic status to the carcinogenic metabolite (BP-7,8-dihydrodiol-9,10-epoxide (BPDE)), which can bind covalently to DNA and form BPDE–DNA adducts and reactive oxygen species. BPDE activates apoptosis through p53-independent and p53-dependent manner (Drukteinis et al. 2005). P53-dependent Cr-induced apoptosis occurs as a consequence ofincreasing p53 phosphorylation at serine, as well as up-regulation of proapoptotic gene bcl-XS, and caspase-7, and down-regulation of several anti-apoptotic genes from Bcl2 family (bcl-W and bcl-XL), and bax. These apoptotic events result in the destruction of the mitochondria and release of cytochrome c (Carlisle et al. 2000; Ha et al. 2003; Ceryak et al. 2004). Moreover, Cr induces the ATM protein production that phosphorylates and activates Chk_2 protein. The phosphorylated Chk2 in turn phosphorylates and activates p53. The phosphorylated p53 does not bind to MDM2 protein (Ha et al. 2003). Cr exposure at very high concentrations activates all subclasses of MAPK through phosphorylation; thus, Cr acts as a MAPK kinase and enhances survival/proliferation in a dose-dependent manner. This function is connected with its capability in ROS generation (Gao et al. 2002).

13.2.6 Nickel (Ni)

Water-insoluble nickel compounds including nickel sulfides, disulfides, and oxides readily enter the cell and are very potent carcinogens (Gao et al. 2002). In contrast, water-soluble nickel compounds including acetate, chloride, nitrate, and sulfate do not enter the cells as readily as water-insoluble nickel compounds (Ke et al. 2008). The increase in the usage of nickel compounds and the spread of nickel due to its dissolution from nickel ore-bearing rocks are the main causes of nickel presence in the environment. The primary source of nickel in drinking water is the leaching of metals in water network. However, food is the major source of nickel exposure in the nonsmoking, non-occupationally exposed population, but nickel absorption from water was considerably higher than absorption of nickel from beverages like tea, coffee, or orange juice and milk (Ke et al. 2008). Ni^{2+} induces carcinogenesis through several processes including DNA hypermethylation (H3K9 mono- and dimethylation), DNMT inhibition, DNA mutation, ROS generation, inhibiting histone H2A, H2B, H3, and H4 acetylation, converting the tumor suppressor genes to the heterochromatin, and considerable enhancements of the ubiquitination of H2A and H2B (Gao et al. 2002). Hence, nickel plays a pivotal role in the suppression or silencing of genes (Gao et al. 2002; Ke et al. 2008).

Nickel has been observed to bind to DNA in different positions. It binds to phosphate backbone of DNA in place of Mg and promotes the conversion of suppressor genes to the heterochromatin (Cangul et al. 2002). Moreover, its binding to histone H4 leads to the inhibition of lysine acetylation, and subsequently DNA hypermethylation (Broday et al. 2000). These events play an important role in silencing of tumor suppressor genes and the other genes that are involved in carcinogenesis pathways.

13.2.7 Selenium (Se)

Selenium is an essential trace element with a narrow range between toxic and therapeutic doses; its activity for that reason is highly dose-dependent. Enzymes containing selenium such as glutathione peroxidase, like other antioxidant elements, can protect body from oxidative damage and reduce the risk of cancer incidence and mortality through several pathways such as apoptosis and alteration of some collagen types (Rayman 2000).

Since selenium, like arsenic, is detoxified by methylation through S-adenosylmethionine pathway, competition between arsenic, selenium, and DNMT1 for methyl donated by S-adenosylmethionine leads to DNA hypomethylation, and an increase in arsenic retention in tissues (Xiang et al. 2008). Organic selenium compounds such as selenomethionine, Se-methyl-selenocysteine (Se-MSC), and particularly selenocystine (SeC) have shown more anticarcinogenic activity than inorganic compounds in lung cancer model systems. However, in contrast to selenomethionine, selenocystine decreases cellular reduced thiol agents like *N*-acetylcysteine (NAC) and GSH, thus increasing the ROS formation (Zou et al. 2008).

Selenium-containing proteins can induce apoptosis pathway through caspase activation. But, selenite, SeC, and selenomethionine mostly activate apoptosis by caspase-independent pathways through p53 activation and antiapoptotic inactivation and release of cytochrome c from mitochondria as follows. First, these compounds increase production of reactive oxygen species. ROS-mediated modified products such as DSBs are detected by ATM and ATR proteins, which in turn can activate p53 in MCF-7 human breast cancer cells and human prostate cancer. These DSBs can even synergistically increase the intracellular ROS production. Second, they induce p53 phosphorylation at Ser_{15}, Ser_{20}, and Ser_{392} residues, thus decreasing p53-MDM2 protein interaction and p53 stability (Chen and Wong 2008).

The Se-MSC shows its anticarcinogenic activity through down-regulation of some extracellular matrix proteins such as collagen type I alpha 1 (COL_1A1), COL_1A_2, and COL_7A_1, and up-regulation of COL_6A_1 and COL_4A_5 genes in human prostate cell line (Evans 2008; Hurst et al.2008).

13.2.8 Mercury (Hg)

Hg and its compounds are highly toxic, wide dispersion through the atmosphere. It is biomagnified through the food chain (Mendola et al. 2002). Hg is commonly used in dental amalgams, thermometers, barometers, and the development of large-scale industrial processes (e.g., chlor-alkali plants and PVC production) and release into the environment. Hg occurs in nature in mineral, cinnabar, metacinnabar, and hypercinnabar. Diet can be the main source of inorganic and organomercury compounds especially seafood, while dental amalgams are the main exposure source to elemental Hg. Mercury is organomercurial in the form of methylmercury which has toxicological characteristics. Minamata disease name given for the cause of methylmercury in seafood in Minamata and Niigata in Japan in the 1950–1960s resulting in the death of thousands of people (Costa et al. 2004). There are a number of key neurological symptoms of high-dose exposure to methylmercury in adults. As there is no specific medical test for the diagnosis of Minamata disease, a combination of these salient symptoms is used to identify cases. The principal effects are noticed to include motor disturbances, such as ataxia and tremors, as well as signs of sensory dysfunction, such as impaired vision (Gopinath et al. 2013). The predominant neuropathological feature is the degenerative changes in the cerebellum, which is likely to be the mechanism involved in many of the motor dysfunctions. The microscopical examination of the brain of patients that died in Minamata showed entire regions devoid of neurons, granular cells in the cerebellum, Golgi cells, and Purkinje cells. The most common clinical symptoms observed in adults in Minamata were paresthesia, ataxia, sensory disturbances, tremors, impairment of hearing, and difficulty in walking. Children showed similar symptoms but with a higher incidence and at lower Hg exposure levels. On the other hand, the predominant symptom in adults in Iraq was paresthesia, which usually occurred after a latent period. Children showed cerebral palsy, altered muscle tone, and deep tendon reflex, as well as delayed developmental stages. In humans, disruptions of higher functions have also been noted, as evidenced by depression and irritability (Sarkar et al. 2003; Costa et al. 2004). Some studies suggest that even minor increases in methylmercury exposures can cause harmful effects on the cardiovascular system, blisters in the upper gastrointestinal tract, vomiting, abdominal pain, constipation, and gastritis. Renal toxicity of organic forms is expressed by glomerulonephritis with proteinuria (glomerular and tubular) and nephritic syndrome (Pazhayattil and Shirali 2014).

Elemental Hg can be oxidized to Hg^{2+}, which accumulates preferentially in the kidneys. The increased excretion of low molecular weight proteins is demonstrated at low-level exposure and related to damage to the renal tubes. It is a potent neurotoxin to human due to their ability to cross the blood–brain barrier. It is absorbed in the gastrointestinal track, immediately entering the bloodstream. It readily passes the placental barrier affecting the developing nervous system of the fetus. Continuous exposure conditions to elemental Hg can lead to its accumulation in the thyroid. The acute exposure to elemental Hg vapors can cause "pink disease" or acrodynia (Bernhoft 2012).

13.3 Conclusions

Conclusively, the heavy metals play important role in the production of ROS and NF-kB, also human genetic differences through polymorphisms in GST, metallothioneins and heavy metal methyltransferase genes induce carcinogenesis. Noticeably, heavy metals are epigenetic carcinogen, solely responsible for tumors presentation and progression. Taken together, the data presented herein and the ongoing research provides new insights and biochemical and molecular mechanisms involved in the development of pathological conditions in human.

References

Alkahtani S (2009) Antioxidation and hypomethylation effects on genotoxicity and programmed cell death induced in mice somatic cells by arsenic trioxide. J Biol Sci 9:721–729

Barnham KJ, Bush AI (2014) Biological metals and metal-targeting compounds in major neurodegenerative diseases. Chem Soc Rev 43:6727–6749

Bernhoft RA (2012) Mercury toxicity and treatment: a review of the literature. J Environ Public Health 2012:1–10

Bishak YK, Payahoo L, Osatdrahimi A, Nourazarian A (2015) Mechanisms of cadmium carcinogenicity in the gastrointestinal tract. Asian Pac J Cancer Prev 16:9–21

Bower JJ, Leonard SS, Shi X (2005) Conference overview: molecular mechanisms of metal toxicity and carcinogenesis. Mol Cell Biochem 279:3–15

Broday L, Peng W, Kuo MH, Salnikow M, Zoroddu M, Costa M (2000) Nickel compounds are novel inhibitors of histone H_4 acetylation. Can Res 60:238–241

Caffo M, Caruso G, Fata GL, Barresi V, Visalli M, Venza M, Venza I (2014) Heavy metals and epigenetic alterations in brain tumors. Curr Genomics 15(6):457–463

Cangul H, Broday L, Salnikow K, Sutherland J, Peng W, Zhang Q, Poltaratsky V, Yee H, Zoroddu MA, Costa M (2002) Molecular mechanisms of nickel carcinogenesis. Toxicol Lett 127:69–75

Carlisle DL, Pritchard DE, Singh J, Owens BM, Blankenship LJ, Orenstein JM, Patierno SR (2000) Apoptosis and P53 induction in human lung fibroblasts exposed to chromium(VI): effect of ascorbate and tocopherol. Toxicol Sci 55(1):60–68

Ceryak S, Zingariello C, O'Brien T, Patierno SR (2004) Induction of pro-apoptotic and cell cycle-inhabiting gene in chromium (VI)-treated human lung fibroblasts: lack of effect of ERK. Mol Cell Biochem 255:139–149

Chen T, Wong YS (2008) Selenocystine induces caspase-independent apoptosis in MCF-7 human breast carcinoma cells with involvement of p53 phosphorylation and reactive oxygen species generation. Int J Biochem Cell Biol 41(3):666–676

Chidananda KN, Jagadeesh K (2015) Metal poisoning: a brief overview (2014). Intern J Pharm Pharm Res 2(4):165–174

Costa LG, Aschner M, Vitalone A, Syversen T, Soldin OP (2004) Developmental neuropathology of environmental agents. Annu Rev Pharmacol Toxicol 44:87–110

Darbre PD (2005) Aluminium, antiperspirants and breast cancer. J Inorg Biochem 99:1912–1919

Ding W, Hudso LG, Sun X, Feng C, Liu KJ (2008) As (III) inhibits ultraviolet radiation-induced cyclobutane pyrimidine dimer repair via generation of nitric oxide in human keratinocytes. Free Radic Biol Med 45:1065–1072

Drukteinis JS, Medrano T, Ablordeppey EA, Kitzman JM, Shiverick KT (2005) Benzo[a]pyrene, but not 2,3,7,8-TCDD, induces G2/M cell cycle arrest, p21CIP1 and p53 phosphorylation in human choriocarcinoma JEG-3 Cells: a distinct signaling pathway. Placenta 26:S87–S95

Egger G, Liang G, Aparicio A, Jones PA (2004) Epigenetics in human disease and prospects for epigenetic therapy. Nature 429:457–463

Ehrlich M (2009) DNA hypomethylation in cancer cells. Epigenomics 1(2):239–259

Eticha T, Hymete A (2014) Health risk assessment of heavy metals in locally produced beer to the population in Ethiopia. J Bioanalysis Biomed 6(6):065–068

Evans J (2008) Antioxidant supplements to prevent or slow down the progression of AMD: a systematic review and meta-analysis. Eye 22:751–760

Fujihara J, Fujii Y, Agusa T (2009) Ethnic differences in five intronic polymorphisms associated with arsenic metabolism within human arsenic (+3 oxidation state) methyltransferase (AS3MT) gene. Toxicol Appl Pharmacol 234(1):41–46

Galanis A, Karapetsas A, Sandaltzopoulos R (2008) Metal induced carcinogenesis, oxidative stress and hypoxia signaling. Mutat Res 674(1–2):31–35

Gao N, Jiang BH, Leonard SS, Corum L, Zhang Z, Roberts JR, Antonini J, Zheng JZ, Flynn DC, Castranova V, Shi X (2002) p38 signaling-mediated hypoxia-inducible factor 1α and vascular endothelial growth factor induction by Cr (VI) in DU145 human prostate carcinoma cells. J Biol Chem 277:45041–45048

Gao N, Shen L, Zhang Z, Leonard SS, He H, Zhang XG, Shi X, Jiang BH (2004) Arsenite induces HIF-1α and VEGF through PI3 K, Akt and reactive oxygen species in DU145 human prostate carcinoma cells. Mol Cell Biochem 255(1–2):33–45

Gopinath B, Schneider J, McMahon CM, Burlutsky G, Leeder SR, Mitchell P (2013) Dual sensory impairment in older adults increases the risk of mortality: a population-based study. PLoS One 8(3):e55054

Ha L, Ceryak S, Patierno SR (2003) Chromium (VI) activates ATM: requirement of ATM for both apoptosis and recovery from terminal growth arrest. J Biol Chem 278:17885–17894

Hariprasad NV, Dayananda HS (2013) Environmental impact due to agricultural runoff containing heavy metals—a review. Intern J Sci Res Publ 3(5):1–6

Harley B (2008) Telomerase and cancer therapeutics. Nat Rev Cancer 8:167–179

Hazell T (1985) Minerals in food: dietary sources, chemical forms, interactions, bioavailability. World Rev Nutr Diet 46:1–123

Henson MC, Chedrese PJ (2004) Endocrine disruption by cadmium, a common environmental toxicant with paradoxical effects on reproduction. Exp Biol Med 229:383–392

Huang S (2002) Histone methyltransferases, diet nutrients and tumour suppressors. Nat Rev Cancer 2:469–476

Hughes MF, Barbara D. Beck BD, Chen Y, Lewis AS, Thomas DJ (2011) Arsenic exposure and toxicology: a historical perspective. Toxicol Sci 123 (2):305–332

Hui F, Liu J, Gao Q, Lou B (2015) *Piriformospora indica* confers cadmium tolerance in *Nicotiana tabacum*. J Environ Sci 37:184–191

Hurst R, Elliott RM, Goldson AJ, Fairweather-Tait SJ (2008) Se-methylselenocysteine alters collagen gene and protein expression in human prostate cells. Cancer Lett 269(1):117–126

Jackson JP, Lindroth AM, Cao X, Jacobsen SE (2002) Control of CpNpG DNA methylation by the kryptonite histone H3 methyltransferase. Nature 416:556–560

Jaishankar M, Tseten T, Anbalagan N, Mathew BB, Beeregowda KN (2014) Toxicity, mechanism and health effects of some heavy metals. Interdisc Toxicol 7(2):60–72

Jan AT, Azam M, Siddiqui K, Ali A, Choi I, Haq QMR (2015) Heavy metals and human health: Mechanistic insight into toxicity and counter defense system of antioxidants. Int J Mol Sci 16:29592–29630

Jin B, Li Y, Robertson KD (2011) DNA methylation-superior or subordinate in the epigenetic hierarchy? Genes Cancer 2(6):607–617

Jones PA, Baylin SB (2002) The fundamental role of epigenetic events in cancer. Nat Rev Genet 3:415–428

Joshi DK, Choudhary M, Tripathi S, Negi MPS, Mahdi AA (2013) Age dependent relative risk of aluminium toxicity: Levels of metal and enzymic and non enzymic antioxidants status in liver, kidney and brain of aluminum treated young and old rats. Intern J Biol Pharm Res 4(3):176–185

Kanavos P (2006) The rising burden of cancer in the developing world. Annals of Oncology 17 (Suppl 8):viii15–viii23

Karavoltsos S, Sakellari A, Mihopoulos N, Dassenakis M, Scoullos MJ (2008) Evaluation of the quality of drinking-water in regions of Greece. Desalinations 224:317–329

Kaste JM, Friedland AJ, Sturup S (2003) Using stable and radioactive isotopes to trace atmospherically deposited Pb in montane forest soils. Environ Sci Technol 37:3560–3567

Ke Q, Ellen TP, Costa M (2008) Nickel compounds induce histone ubiquitination by inhibiting histone deubiquitinating enzyme activity. Toxicol Appl Pharmacol 228:190–199

Kibria MG, Osman KT, Ahmed MJ (2006) Cadmium and lead uptake by rice (*Oryza sativa* L.) grown in three different textured soils. Soil Environ 25(2):70–77

Kippler M, Tofail F, Gardner R, Rahman A, Hamadani JD, Bottai M, Vahter M (2012) Maternal cadmium exposure during pregnancy and size at birth: a prospective cohort study. Environ Health Perspect 120(2):284–289

Kroes R, Kozianowski G (2002) Threshold of toxicological concern in food safety assessment. Toxicol Lett 127:43–46

Lee MY, Jung BI, Chung SM, Bae ON, Lee JY, Park JD, Yang JS, Lee H, Chung JH (2003) Arsenic-induced dysfunction in relaxation of blood vessels. Environ Health Perspect 111:513–517

Leivadara SV, Nikolaou AD, Lekkas TD (2008) Determination of organic compounds in bottled waters. Food Chem 108:277–286

Li R, Shugart YY, Zhou W, An Y, Yang Y, Zhou Y, Zhang B, Lu D, Wang H, Qian J, Jin L (2009) Common genetic variations of the cytochrome P450 1A1 gene and risk of hepatocellular carcinoma in a Chinese population. Eur J Cancer 45:1239–1247

Lukusa T, Fryns JP (2008) Human chromosome fragility. Biochimica Biophysica Acta 1779:3–16

Malik D, Singh S, Thakur J, Singh RK, Kaur A, Nijhawan S (2014) heavy metal pollution of the Yamuna river: An introspection. Intern J Current Microbiol Appl Sci 3(10):856–863

Martine VD, Vucic EA, Becker-Santos DD, Gil L, Lam WL (2011) Arsenic exposure and the induction of human cancers. J Toxicol 2011:431287. https://doi.org/10.1155/2011/431287

Melnikova VO, Ananthaswamy HN (2005) Cellular and molecular events leading to the development of skin cancer. Mutat Res 571:91–106

Mendola P, Selevan SG, Gutter S, Rice D (2002) Environmental factors associated with a spectrum of neuro-developmental deficits. Mental Retard Develop Disabil 8:188–197

Mishra S, Dwivedi SP, Singh RB (2010) A review on epigenetic effect of heavy metal carcinogens on human health. Open Nutraceutical J 3:188–193

Mohammadi A, Vaziri-Gohar A, Shakibaie MR (2008) Mutations in tumor suppressor TP53 gene in formalin- fixed, paraffin embedded tissues of squamous cell carcinoma (SCC) of lung cancer. Am J Biochem Biotechnol 4(1):1–6

Mudgal V, Madaan N, Mudgal A, Singh RB (2010) Effect of toxic metals on human health. Open Nutraceutical J 3:94–99

Namieśnika J, Rabajczyk A (2010) The speciation and physico-chemical forms of metals in surface waters and sediments. Chem Speciat Bioavailab 22(1):1–24

Nebert DW, Roe AL, Dieter MZ, Solis WA, Yang Y, Dalton TP (2000) Role of the aromatic hydrocarbon receptor and [Ah] gene battery in the oxidative stress response, cell cycle control and apoptosis. Biochem Pharmacol 59:65–85

Oforka NC, Osuji LC, Onwuachu UI (2012) Estimation of dietary intake of cadmium, lead, manganese, zinc and nickel due to consumption of chicken meat by inhabitants of Port-Harcourt Metropolis. Nigeria. Arch Appl Sci Res 4(1):675–684

Oudeh M, Khan M, Scullion J (2002) Plant accumulation of potentially toxic elements in sewage sludge as affected by soil organic matter level and mycorrhizal fungi. Environ Pollut 116:293–300

Patterson TJ, Ngo M, Aronov PA, Reznikova TV, Green PG, Rice RH (2003) Biological activity of inorganic arsenic and antimony reflects oxidation state in cultured human keratinocytes. Chem Res Toxicol 16:1624–1631

Pazhayattil GS, Shirali AC (2014) Drug-induced impairment of renal function. Intern J Nephrol Renovascular Dis 7:457–468

Pimparkar BD, Bhave A (2010) Arsenicosis: review of recent advances. JAPI 58:617–629

Prashanth L, Kattapagari KK, Chitturi RT, Baddam VR, Prasad LK (2015) A review on role of essential trace elements in health and disease. J NTR Univ Health Sci 4:75–85

Rachdaoui N, Sarkar DK (2013) Effects of alcohol on the endocrine system. Endocrinol Metab Clin North America 42(3):593–615

Ramasamy K, Shanmugam M, Balupillai A, Govindhasamy K, Gunaseelan S, Muthusamy G, Robert BM, Nagarajan RP (2017) Ultraviolet radiation-induced carcinogenesis: mechanisms and experimental models. J Radiat Cancer Res 8(1):4–19

Ravanat JL, Douki T, Cadet J (2001) Direct and indirect effects of UV radiation on DNA and its components. J Photochem Photobiol 63:88–102

Rayman MP (2000) The importance of selenium to human health. Lancet 356:233–241

Rebecca LS, Kimberly DM, Ahmedin Jemal DVM (2017). Cancer statistics-2017. CA Cancer J Clin 67:7–30

Rengarajan T, Rajendran P, Nandakumar N, Lokeshkumar B, Rajendran P, Nishigaki I (2015) Exposure to polycyclic aromatic hydrocarbons with special focus on cancer. Asian Pacific J Trop Biomed 5(3):182–189

Santos EE, Lauria DC, Porto da Silveira CL (2004) Assessment of daily intake of trace elements due to consumption of foodstuffs by adult inhabitants of Rio de Janeiro city. Sci Total Environ 327:69–79

Santos SS, Melo LR, Koifman RJ, Koifman S (2013) Cancer incidence, hospital morbidity, and mortality in young adults in Brazil. Cad Saúde Pública, Rio de Janeiro 29(5):1029–1040

Sarkar M, Chaudhuri GR, Chattopadhyay A, Biswas NM (2003) Effect of sodium arsenite on spermatogenesis, plasma gonadotrophins and testosterone in rats. Asian J Androl 5:27–31

Satoh E, Yasuda I, Yamada T, Suzuki Y, Ohyashiki T (2007) Involvement of NO generation in aluminum-induced cell death. Biol Pharm Bull 30:1390–1394

Schnekenburger M, Peng L, Puga A (2007) HDAC1 bound to the Cyp1a1 promoter blocks histone acetylation associated with Ah receptor-mediated trans-activation. Biochimica Biophysica Acta 1769:569–578

Sharma V, Kalim S, Sivastava MK, Nanda S, Mishra S (2009) Oxidative stress and coxsackievirus infections as mediators of beta cell damage: a review. Sci Res Essay 4(2):042–058

Sharma B, Singh S, Siddiqi NJ (2014). Biomedical implications of heavy metals induced imbalances in redox systems. BioMed Res Intern 2014:640754. https://doi.org/10.1155/2014/640754

Siddiqui MK, Srivastava S, Mehrotra PK (2002) Environmental exposure to lead as a risk for prostate cancer. Biomed Environ Sci 15:298–305

Silva ALO, Barrocas PRG, Jacob SDC, Moreira JC (2005) Dietary intake and health effects of selected toxic elements. Braz J Plant Physiol 17(1):79–93

Stahl T, Falk S, Rohrbeck A, Georgii S, Herzog C, Wiegand A, Hotz S, Boschek B, Zorn H, Brunn H (2017) Migration of aluminum from food contact materials to food-a health risk for consumers? Part I of III: exposure to aluminum, release of aluminum, tolerable weekly intake (TWI), toxicological effects of aluminum, study design, and methods. Environ Sci Europe 29:19

Stellman SD, Djordjevic MV, Britton JA, Muscat JE, Citron ML, Kemeny M, Busch E, Gong L (2000) Breast cancer risk in relation to adipose concentrations of organochlorine pesticides and polychlorinated biphenyls in Long Island, New York. Cancer Epidemiol Biomark Prev 9:1241–1249

Subramaniam D, Thombre R, Dhar A, Anant S (2014) DNA methyltransferases: a novel target for prevention and therapy. Frontiers in Oncology 4(80):1–13

Sun X, Fontaine JM, Bartl I, Behnam B, Welsh MJ, Benndorf R (2007) Induction of Hsp22 (HspB8) by estrogen and the metallo-estrogen cadmium in estrogen receptor-positive breast cancer cells. Cell Stress Chaperones 2:307–319

Suzuki KT, Katagiri A, Sakuma Y, Ogra Y, Ohmichi M (2004) Distributions and chemical forms of arsenic after intravenous administration of dimethylarsinic andmonomethylarsonic acids to rats. Toxicol Appl Pharmacol 198:336–344

Tallkvist J, Bowlus CL, Lonnerdal B (2001) DMT1 gene expression and cadmium absorption in human absorptive enterocytes. Toxicol Lett 122:171–177
Tamaru H, Selker EU (2001) A histone H3 methyltransferase controls DNA methylation in Neurospora crassa. Nature 414:277–283
Tandon SK, Chatterjee M, Bhargava A, Shukla V, Bihari V (2001) Lead poisoning in Indian silver refiners. Sci Total Environ 281:177–182
Tchounwou PB, Yedjou CG, Patlolla AK, Sutton DJ (2012) Heavy metals toxicity and the environment. NIH Public Access 101:133–164
Thun MJ, DeLancey JO, Center MM, Jemal A, Ward EM (2010) The global burden of cancer: priorities for prevention. Carcinogenesis 31(1):100–110
Tiwari AKM, Mahdi AA, Mishra S (2017) Study on impact of iron and folic acid on the plasma trace minerals in pregnant anemic women. Indian J Clin Biochem First Online: 24 May 2017 https://doi.org/10.1007/s12291-017-0653-6
Tiwari AKM, Mahdi AA, Zahra F, Sharma S, Negi MPS (2012) Evaluation of low blood lead levels and its association with oxidative stress in pregnant anemic women: a comparative prospective study. Indian J Clin Biochem 27(3):246–252
Track FMG (2010) Trace elements: general soil chemistry, principles and processes. In: Hooda PS (ed) Trace elements in soils. Blackwell Publishing Ltd, pp. 9–37
Vahter M (2000) Genetic polymorphism in the biotransformation of inorganic and its role in toxicity. Toxicol Lett 112–113:209–217
Vaziri Gohar A, Mohammadi A, Heidari M (2007) Molecular genetics of cancer. Samer, Tehran, Iran. ISBN 978-964-91351-0-6
Verma R, Dwivedi P (2013) Heavy metal water pollution—a case study. Recent Res Sci Technol 5 (5):98–99
Vogelstein B, Kinzler KW (2004) Cancer genes and the pathways they control. Nat Med 10:789–799
Walton FS, Harmon AW, Paul DS, Drobna Z, Patel YM, Styblo M (2004) Inhibition of insulin-dependent glucose uptake by trivalent arsenicals: possible mechanism of arsenic-induced diabetes. Toxicol Appl Pharmacol 198:424–433
Weber P, RodolfoBehr E, De LellisKnorr C, Vendruscolo DS, Flores EMM, Dressler VL, Baldisserotto B (2013) Metals in the water, sediment, and tissues of two fish species from different trophic levels in a subtropical Brazilian river. Microchem J 106:61–66
Wei YD, Tepperman K, Huang MY, Sartor MA, Puga A (2004) Chromium inhibits transcription from polycyclic aromatic hydrocarbon-inducible promoters by blocking the release of histone deacetylase and preventing the binding of p300 to chromatin. J Biol Chem 279:4110–4119
WHO (1987) World Health Organization, Geneva. Environ Health Criteria 1987, No. 58
WHO (2001) Air quality guidelines—second edition. WHO Regional Office for Europe, Copenhagen, Denmark, 2001
WHO (2003) Arsenic in Drinking-water. Background document for development of WHO Guidelines for Drinking-water Quality, 2003
Wu X, Jin T, Wang Z, Ye T, Kong Q, Nordberg G (2001) Urinary calcium as a biomarker of renal dysfunction in a general population exposed to cadmium. J Occup Environ Med 43:898–904
Wu JP, Chang LP, Yao HT, Chang H, Tsai HT, Tsai MH, Yeh TK, Lin P (2009) Involvement of oxidative stress and activation of aryl hydrocarbon receptor in elevation of CYP1A1 expression and activity in lung cells and tissues by arsenic: an in vitro and in vivo study. Toxicol Sci 107:385–393
Xiang N, Zhao R, Song G, Zhong W (2008) Selenite reactivates silenced genes by modifying DNA methylation and histones in prostate cancer cells. Carcinogenesis 29:2175–2181
Yoshida T, Yamauchi H, Fan Sun G (2004) Chronic health effects in people exposed to arsenic via the drinking water: dose-response relationships in review. Toxicol Appl Pharmacol 198:243–252

Zhang RY, Lui Y, Pang DW, Cai RX, Qi YP (2002) Spectroscopic and voltammetric study on the binding of aluminium (III) to DNA. Anal Sci 18:761–767

Zhitkovich A, Voitkun V, Costa M (1995) Glutathione and free amino acids form stable complexes with DNA following exposure of intact mammalian cells to chromate. Carcinogenesis 16:907–913

Zou Y, Niu P, Yang J, Yuan J, Wu T, Chen X (2008) The JNK signaling pathway is involved in sodium-selenite-induced apoptosis mediated by reactive oxygen in HepG2 cells. Cancer Biol Ther 7:689–696

Chapter 14
Biochemical and Molecular Targets of Heavy Metals and Their Actions

Abhishek Kumar, Nitika Singh, Rukmani Pandey, Vivek Kumar Gupta and Bechan Sharma

Abstract Heavy metals belong to the groups of transition elements and are defined in terms of their chemical properties, atomic weight, density, or specific gravity as compared to water. Heavy metals could be metalloids, lanthanides, and actinides. The heavy metals reach into humans and animals through contaminated air and water as well as food stuffs especially from fish, chicken, vegetables, vaccinations, dental fillings, and deodorants. Most of the heavy metals, when accumulated in excess, induce toxicity by damaging the central nervous system (CNS), energy metabolism, ion-transporters, cardiovascular systems, respiratory systems, reproductory systems, and vital organs such as lungs, liver, and brain leading to the physical, physiological, and behavioral disorders. Arsenic (As) has been shown to generate skin diseases and cancer; lead (Pb) poisoning induces infertility and neurotoxicity/neurodegeneration; and mercury (Hg) intake causes harmful effects in lactating mothers, fetuses, and children. Cadmium (Cd), considered to act like both an occupational and non-occupational toxicant, has been reported to be one of the carcinogens. The strategies to combat heavy metals toxicity include appropriate intake of antioxidants, phytochemicals, and minerals. The present chapter is an endeavor to illustrate an updated account of various aspects of heavy metals toxicity with a particular reference to their biomedical implications as well as the use of phytochemicals and minerals toward the treatment of their adverse effects.

Keywords Heavy metals · Cadmium · Lead · Arsenic · Mercury
Zinc · Mechanisms · Toxicity

A. Kumar · N. Singh · V. K. Gupta · B. Sharma (✉)
Department of Biochemistry, University of Allahabad, Allahabad 211002, Uttar Pradesh, India
e-mail: bechansharma@gmail.com

R. Pandey
Developmental Toxicology Laboratory, Systems Toxicology and Health Risk Assessment Group, CSIR-Indian Institute of Toxicology Research (CSIR-IITR), Vishvigyan Bhavan, 31-Mahatma Gandhi Marg, Lucknow 226001, Uttar Pradesh, India

M. Rai et al. (eds.), *Biomedical Applications of Metals*,
https://doi.org/10.1007/978-3-319-74814-6_14

14.1 Introduction

Heavy metals are the inorganic elements with relatively high density, high specific gravity (five times more as compared to water), and high atomic number and weight. It is naturally present in the earth crust, and anthropogenic activities of human beings lead to their accumulation in the environment above their permissible limit (Sharma et al. 2014).

Exposure of these heavy metals is a common phenomenon due to their environmental pervasiveness. The widely known consequence of these heavy metals intoxication includes the development of neurotoxicity, genotoxicity, and carcinogenicity (Fergusson 1990). Heavy metals also affect most of the organ systems including central nervous system (CNS), peripheral nervous systems (PNS), gastrointestinal (GI) systems, cardiovascular systems, hematopoietic systems, renal systems, and reproductive system. However, the mechanism and effect of this toxicant vary with dose, duration, mode of action, chemical, their valence, and the age of the individual.

There are some heavy metals which are required for the normal biological functioning of cells like selenium, manganese, zinc, and copper which participates in regulating various metabolic and signaling pathways. These metals possess coordination chemistry and redox properties which provides them an extra advantage by which these metals could escape out of the control mechanism such as transport, homeostasis, compartmentalization, and binding to designated cell constituents. While the biggest disadvantage lies in their ability to replace other metals normally present in the binding sites, this nature of heavy metals makes them toxic and ultimately leading to malfunctioning effect. Sometimes, these metals bind with nuclear proteins and DNA causing oxidative deterioration of these biological macromolecules (Leonard et al. 2004; Flora et al. 2008).

Among all the heavy metals, arsenic, lead, cadmium, and mercury are reported to cause serious health complications in humans (Flora et al. 2008). It has been reported by various workers that the exposure of an organism to a higher level of these metals may cause the production of free radicals such as reactive oxygen species (ROS) and reactive nitrogen species (RNS) which may result in oxidative stress (Leonard et al. 2004; ATSDR 2007). Oxidative stress is considered to be one of the major mechanisms of heavy metal toxicity (Manke et al. 2013). For example, arsenic exposure induces productions of reactive oxygen species (ROS) followed by increased oxidative stress (Shi et al. 2004), and this oxidative stress is often found to be associated with the development of tumors in lung, skin, liver, bladder, and kidney (Waalkes et al. 2004). Lead is known to induce a broad range of physiological, biochemical, and behavioral dysfunctions in laboratory animals and humans (Goyer 1996; Flora et al. 2008) including central and peripheral nervous systems, haemopoietic system, cardiovascular system (Lanphear et al. 2000), kidneys (Damek-Poprawa and Sawicka-Kapusta 2004), liver (Sharma and Street 1980), and the reproductive systems of males and females (Ronis et al. 1998). Cadmium exposure also induces ROS production and thereby mutagenesis (Filipic et al. 2006).

Similarly, the intoxication of mercury affects different organ systems as well as mitochondrial function (Lund et al. 1993; Sharma et al. 2014; Gupta and Sharma 2015).

The present chapter covers the overview of the source, mechanisms, biochemical, and molecular targets as well as the phytochemicals against toxic metals such as Pb, Cd, As, and Hg. The current knowledge of toxic effects of metal-induced oxidative stress suggests that possible measures should be taken to reduce their toxic effects and to achieve physiological recoveries. This chapter also illustrates the role of essential trace metals such as Zn, Cu, and the Se in proper biological maintenance and also the toxicity induced by them when used in excess.

14.2 Sources of Heavy Metals in Environment

Heavy metals are naturally and ubiquitously present in earth's crust. These elements are the most ancient toxins against humans, having been utilized for several years. Several natural and anthropogenic processes are involved in providing entry of heavy metals into the environment (VanDam et al. 1995; Pacyna 1996; Shallari et al. 1998; Bradl 2002; Waalkes et al. 2007; Strater et al. 2010). The most noteworthy natural sources are erosion, weathering of minerals, and volcanic action, while anthropogenic sources include smelting, mining, electroplating, utilization of pesticides, fertilizers and also biosolids in farming, sludge dumping, industrial release, atmospheric fixation, etc. (Modaihsh et al. 2004; Chehregani and Malayeri 2007; Fulekar et al. 2009; Wuana and Okieimen 2011). The anthropogenic sources of heavy metals are summarized in Table 14.1.

Use of cadmium is common in various industrial activities, and major application of cadmium includes pigments, alloy, and batteries (Wilson 1988). Other sources of cadmium include emissions from mining, industrial activities, smelting,

Table 14.1 Heavy metals and their sources

Heavy metals	Sources	References
Cadmium	Electroplating, phosphate fertilizers, batteries, paints and pigments, and plastic stabilizers	Salem et al. (2000), Pulford and Watson (2003)
Arsenic	Wood preservatives and pesticides	Thangavel and Subbhuraam (2004)
Lead	Use of herbicides and insecticides, gaseous emission from combustion of lead blended fuels, and battery manufacture	Thangavel and Subbhuraam (2004), Wuana and Okieimen (2011)
Mercury	Medical wastes and use of pesticides, fish and dental amalgam	Memon et al. (2001), Wuana and Okieimen (2011), Rodrigues et al. (2012)

and manufacturing of batteries, pigments, stabilizers, and alloys (ATSDR 2008). Foodstuffs are also contributing as a major source of cadmium exposure such as leafy vegetables, grain and seeds, potatoes and molluscs, and crustaceans (Satarug et al. 2003).

Volcanic eruptions and soil erosions are the natural phenomena, and these natural activities increase the environmental pollution of arsenic (ATSDR 2000). Arsenic is also used in several industrial manufactured products such as wood preservatives, agricultural application products, and dyestuffs. Mercury is highly utilized in electrical industry and used in making electric appliances such as batteries, switches, and thermostats. Also, it is used in dentistry, in the production of caustic soda and as solvents for various precious metals (Tchounwou et al. 2003a, b).

14.3 Role in Biological Functions

Mostly heavy metals are nonessential for living organisms. Some of the heavy metals serve as cofactors in several enzymes. The only known favorable biological function of cadmium is observed in diatoms (*Thalassiosira weissflogii*). The marine diatoms use cadmium as cofactors for their enzymes. Arsenic is used as drug for treatment of many veterinary diseases. Drugs based on Arsenic are useful and very effective against some tropical diseases such as amoebic dysentery and sleeping sickness (African). It is also used in treatment of parasitic diseases including filariasis in animals (Centeno et al. 2005). Recently, arsenic trioxide has been approved by the Food and Drug Administration (FDA) as an anticancer agent in the treatment of acute promyelocytic leukaemia. Its therapeutic action has been attributed to the induction of programmed cell death (apoptosis) in leukaemia cells (Yedjou and Tchounwou 2007). Lead and mercury have no any beneficial biological functions.

14.4 Biochemical Targets for Heavy Metals Toxicity

14.4.1 Cadmium

Cadmium is a naturally occurring metal and it is situated in between zinc (Zn) and mercury (Hg) in periodic table. Its chemical behavior is similar to Zn and it forms divalent cation complexes with other elements. Cadmium toxicity is well reported in various organs and tissues. The most prominent targets of cadmium are nervous system, cardiovascular system, respiratory system, excretory, and reproductive system.

This metal has no known useful biological role in mammals and prolongs encounter with this metal show harmful consequences (Zadorozhnaja et al. 2000).

The excretion rate of Cd from the body is inadequate which enhance the biological half-life around 15–30 years (Varga et al. 1993; Bhattacharyya et al. 2000; Henson and Anderson 2000). Due to the long biological half-life of Cd, it accumulates in various parts of an organism such as liver, kidney, as well as in the reproductive organs including testis, ovaries, and placenta (Paksy et al. 1997; Zadorozhnaja et al. 2000; Brohi et al. 2017). Moreover, the human exposed to this metal are more prone to health complications like renal disease, osteoporosis, hypertension, and leukaemia, as well as cancers of the lung, urinary bladder, kidney, pancreas, prostate, and breast (Satoh et al. 2002). Humans are mainly exposed to cadmium via inhalation or cigarette smoke and through ingestion of contaminated food. The blood and urine cadmium content is higher in cigarette smoker and lower in non-smokers (Becker et al. 2002; Mannino et al. 2004). The foodstuffs that are rich in cadmium such as mushroom, seaweeds, shellfish, mussels and cocoa powder can build up more accumulation in human bodies. The U.S. National Toxicology Program and International Agency for Research on Cancer (IARC 1993) have concluded that there is satisfactory validation that cadmium is a human cancer-causing agent. Other target tissues of cadmium carcinogenesis in humans are liver, testicles, adrenals, and the hemopoietic system (IARC 1993; Waalkes et al. 1996). Some studies also reported that environmental and occupational cadmium exposure is also associated with progression and induction of cancers in kidney, prostate, and stomach (Waalkes et al. 1996).

Cadmium is a serious gastrointestinal and pulmonary irritant, which can be lethal if ingested or inhaled. Ingestion of high amount of cadmium induces several symptoms such as muscle cramps, abdominal pain, nausea, burning sensation, vomiting, salivation, shock, vertigo, loss of consciousness, and convulsions usually appear within 15–30 min (Baselt and Cravey 1995). In fact, several years before, Friberg (1948, 1950) had reported that damage to lungs and kidneys might be the earliest effects on workers exposed to cadmium. Later on, it was found that acute ingestion of cadmium can cause gastrointestinal tract erosion, pulmonary, renal or hepatic injury, and coma (Baselt and Cravey 1995; Baselt 2000). Chronic exposure to cadmium has a depressive effect on levels of several neurotransmitters such as acetylcholine, serotonin, and norepinephrine (Singhal et al. 1976). Experiments performed on rodents also explain that chronic inhalation of cadmium causes pulmonary adenocarcinomas (Waalkes and Berthan 1995; Waalkes et al. 1996) and proliferative prostatic lesions after systemic or direct exposure (Waalkes and Rehm 1992). Cadmium can also bind to E-cadherin (a cell–cell adhesion glycoprotein) at Ca (II)-binding region, disrupting cell-to-cell adhesion (Pearson and Prozialeck 2001). Toxicity of cadmium also led to an alteration in the activities of certain enzymes in the mammalian systems. The cadmium administration to rats significantly influences the activity of antioxidant enzymes such as Cu, Zn-superoxide dismutase (SOD), glutathione peroxidase (GPx), catalase (CAT), glutathione reductase (GR), and glutathione-S-transferase (GST), and increases the lipid peroxidation, and thereby causes oxidative stress (Ognjanovic et al. 2003).

14.4.2 Arsenic

Arsenic is a ubiquitous element and present in at low concentrations in all environmental conditions (NRCC 1978; ATSDR 2000). Nearly, 200 million people are affected globally by arsenic exposure, whereas about 70 million people are suffering in India. The trivalent arsenite and pentavalent arsenate are the major forms of inorganic arsenic. The report based on extensive surveys explained that several millions of peoples throughout the world are exposed to arsenic chronically. Peoples living in countries like India, Mexico, Taiwan, Bangladesh, and Uruguay, where the groundwater is extensively contaminated with arsenic, are mostly exposed. The arsenic exposure occurs through dermal contact, inhalation, and parental route to some extent (Tchounwou et al. 1999; ATSDR 2000). The dissolve arsenic compounds are absorbed with high efficiency than the lower solubility compounds such as lead arsenide, arsenic selenide, and gallium arsenide, whereas high acute dermal contact with inorganic arsenic solutions results in systemic skin toxicity (Smith et al. 1992). Arsenic contamination affects all organ systems, and its major targets include the renal, nervous, respiratory, gastrointestinal nervous, dermatologic, and cardiovascular systems (Tchounwou et al. 2003a, b). Research has also pointed to significantly higher standardized mortality rates for cancers of the bladder, kidney, skin, and liver in many areas of arsenic pollution. The severity of adverse health effects is related to the chemical form of arsenic, and is also time- and dose-dependent (Tchounwou et al. 2002; Yedjou et al. 2006). The evidence from studies strongly supports the carcinogenicity of arsenic in humans, but the mechanism of tumor progression in humans is not completely understood (Chappell et al. 1997). Several epidemiological studies have validated the strong association between arsenic toxicity and adverse effects on human health and increased risks of tumor formation.

One of the known adverse effects of arsenic is the reactive oxygen species (ROS) production which causes oxidative stress (Shi et al. 2004). The interaction between these reactive species and biomolecules results in alteration and loss of regulatory mechanism of the cell, which may lead to cell death. Several studies indicate that oxidative stress created by arsenic toxicity influence the antioxidant enzyme such as catalase (CAT), superoxide dismutase (SOD), glutathione peroxidase (GPx), as well as nonenzymatic factors, for example, sulfhydryl group containing peptides (Shi et al. 2004). The oxidative stress is also associated with physiological changes which cause late complications in diabetes mellitus (Parthiban et al. 1995; Rin et al. 1995). Some of the researchers are proposing that it may play a major role in vascular and neurological complications in diabetic patients (Baynes 1991; Kolb and Kolb-Bachofen 1992; Giugliano et al. 1996; Yamanaka et al. 2001; Singh et al. 2017). Arsenic also increases the rate of lipid peroxidation (LPO) , and high level of these lipid peroxides has been indicated in diabetic patients (Lyons 1991; Inada et al. 1995; Borcea et al. 1999). Arsenic may affect the central nervous system (CNS) and cause significant alterations in the behavioral pattern of exposed animals. Arsenic causes biomethylation in the brain which results in the development of neurotoxicity.

14.4.3 Lead

Lead is a potent occupational toxin which is non-biodegradable. It persists in the environment for a long time. In the human body, most of the absorbed lead is accumulated in kidney, followed by liver and other tissues such as brain and heart, but the skeleton represents the major fraction of overall lead content in the human body (Flora et al. 2006). The most susceptible target for lead poisoning is nervous system, and the poor attention spam, headache, loss of memory, dullness, and irritability are the early symptoms of lead exposure on the central nervous system (ATSDR 1999; CDC 2001). The major target of lead toxicity includes liver, central nervous system, reproductive system, hematopoietic system, and endocrine system (ATSDR 1999). It is most hazardous for pregnant women. The absorbed lead can readily transfer to developing embryo (Ong et al. 1985). It may cause early birth, reduce body weight and neuro development, and reproductive disability in offspring (Andrews et al. 1994).

Lead produces toxicity on most of the organ system and induces a broad range of physiological, biochemical, and genetical dysfunctions, because it is one of the most clinically significant heavy metals. The most sensitive target of lead exposure is the central nervous system. Pb causes neurotoxicity but significantly decreases pediatric cognitive functions. Lead toxicity interferes with enzymatic steps in the heme pathway and reduces the body's capacity for formation of hemoglobin. In severe cases of lead poisoning, children or adults may present with severe cramping abdominal pain, which may be mistaken for an acute abdomen or appendicitis. Cardiovascular hypertension is a complex condition with many different causes and risk factors, including age, weight, diet, and exercise habits. Lead poisoning effects as examined in the literature include low sperm count, fertility, and pregnancy outcomes. Williams et al. (2010) have reported that the higher blood lead was associated with later pubertal onset in this prospective study of peri-pubertal Russian boys. Studies on the effects of lead on the endocrine system are mainly based on occupationally lead-exposed workers and experimental animal models. Although evidence is conflicting, it has been reported that accumulation of lead affects the majority of the endocrine glands. In particular, it appears to affect the hypothalamic–pituitary axis causing blunted TSH, GH, and FSH/LH responses to TRH, GHRH, and GnRH stimulation, respectively.

Some of the key metabolic enzymes are major target for lead toxicity. Lead can mimic the essential mineral ions such as iron, zinc, and calcium which play an important role of cofactors with several enzymes. Thus, replacement of these metals with lead will interfere with enzyme function. Lead is well known for its involvement in ROS production. The ROS-mediated damage of cell membrane and DNA damage are common in lead toxicity. Lead also interferes with antioxidant enzymes such as SOD, GPx, and CAT and nonenzymatic antioxidant molecules (Valko et al. 2005; Flora et al. 2008; Sharma et al. 2014).

14.4.4 Mercury

In nature, mercury is available in different physical and chemical forms, and all forms of mercury can produce toxic effects. The various forms of mercury are mercurous (Hg I), elemental mercury vapor (Hg), and mercuric (Hg II) and organic mercuric compounds (Rubino 2015). All forms of mercury are toxic to humans and have toxic effects in different organs such as kidney, brain, and lung (Fitzgerald and Clarkson 1991; Zalups and Koropatnik 2000). Exposure to mercury can induce several diseases such as Minamata disease, acrodynia (pink disease), and Hunter-Russell syndrome. The organic and elemental mercury show wide range of toxicity including gastrointestinal toxicity, neurotoxicity, and nephrotoxicity (Zalups 2002). The mercurous and mercuric ions create toxicity generally by interacting with the thiol group of essential molecules and protein such as GSH and metallothionein (MT) (Hultberg et al. 2001). Some of the researchers have reported that mammals exposed to mercuric chloride result in alterations in several antioxidants enzymes such as SOD, GPX, CAT, and GR. Exposure to mercury also causes the change in the rate of lipid peroxidation in comparison to non-contaminated groups (Yee and Choi 1996; Mahboob et al. 2001). Mercury also affects the numbers of the stress of protein including heat shock proteins and glucose-regulated proteins (Goering et al. 2000; Papaconstantinou et al. 2003). The action and targets of different chemical forms of mercury are given in Fig. 14.1. Some of the hypotheses supported that the injuries in the central nervous system caused by methylmercury are due to ROS production (Zhang et al. 2009). Studies demonstrated that methylmercury inhibits the cell division and migration in both in vivo and in vitro conditions (Grandjean et al. 1997; Graeme and Pollack 1998; Grandjean et al. 1999). Another researcher also reported that mercury intoxication is related to the increased risk of myocardial infarction, hypertension, coronary dysfunction, atherosclerosis, and increased risk of cardiovascular disease (Rhee and Choi 1989; Guallar et al. 2002; Yoshizawa et al. 2002).

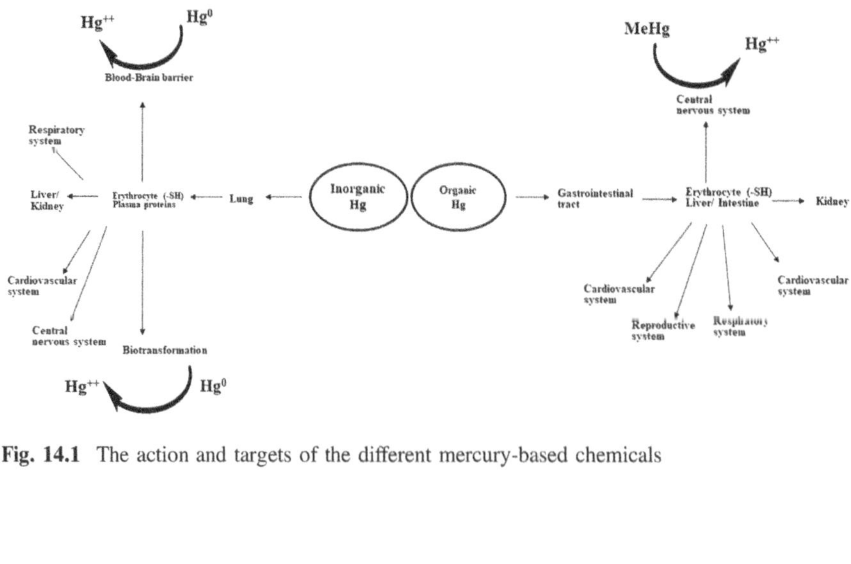

Fig. 14.1 The action and targets of the different mercury-based chemicals

14.5 Molecular Mechanism of Heavy Metals Toxicity

14.5.1 Cadmium

The mechanism of action of cadmium is not well understood. The main action of cadmium in mutagenesis is generation of ROS (Filipic et al. 2006). Due to rise in ROS level, various physiological perturbations develop such as increased permeability of blood–brain barrier and alteration in synaptic transmission. Cadmium is a non-redox active metal and cannot initiated by itself Fenton reactions (Casalino et al. 1997). Therefore, it induces oxidative stress via indirect process. Some of the known mechanism through which it act are (1) Cd combines with thiol groups of enzymes involved in antioxidant mechanisms, such as glutathione peroxidase (GPx), SOD, and catalase, and inhibits their activities (Wang et al. 2004); (2) Cd decreases in the intracellular GSH content; (3) Cd inhibits GPx activity by forming cadmium–selenium complexes; and (4) Cd inhibits complex III of the mitochondrial electronic transport chain and increases the production of ROS (Wang et al. 2004) which may trigger the apoptosis pathways.

14.5.2 Arsenic

Arsenic interacts with thiol group or sulfhydryl groups of protein and can inactivate around 200 enzymes, a principal mechanism of arsenic toxicity. As(V) can also replace the phosphate molecules which are actively involved in several biochemical pathways, and thereby affect that pathways (Goyer 2001; Hughes 2002). Arsenic exposure may impair the cellular respiration by inhibiting the various mitochondrial enzymes and uncoupling the oxidative phosphorylation. Several metabolic pathways may cause methylation of arsenic leading to the formation of methyl metabolites of arsenic that are more toxic than arsenite (Tchounwou et al. 2003a, b). Further, comet assay pointed out the role of arsenic trioxide in the induction of DNA damage in human lymphocytes (Anderson et al. 1994). While some of its compounds can also trigger the gene amplification, inhibit DNA repair system, and arrest cells in mitosis, it also induces the expression of the c-fos gene and oxidative stress protein heme oxygenase, and also acts as a promoter for various toxic agents (Barrett et al. 1989; Hartmann and Peit 1994; Saleha-Banu et al. 2001). Several mechanisms are reported for arsenic-induced carcinogenesis but the available information is not fulfilled to understand the actual mechanism of its action. Some of the reported mechanisms are hypoxia inducing both genetic and epigenetic changes (Salnikow and Zhitkovich 2008), modulation of gene expression (Huang et al. 2004), enhanced cell proliferation (Simeonova et al. 2000), and induction of oxidative stress (Shi et al. 2004). The regulation and mechanism of action of arsenic are given in Fig. 14.2. Arsenic can also interfere with the signaling pathways (p53 signaling pathway) that are involved in promotion and progression of several

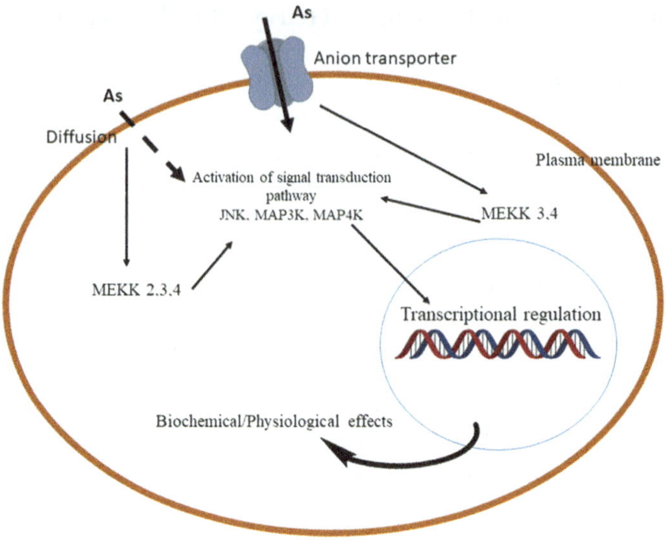

Fig. 14.2 Mechanism of action of arsenic in signaling pathway

tumors in mammals (Porter et al. 1999; Vogt and Rossman 2001). A recent review discusses nine different possible modes of action of arsenic carcinogenesis: oxidative stress, induced chromosomal abnormalities, altered DNA methylation patterns, altered DNA repair, altered growth factors, suppression of p53, enhanced cell proliferation, promotion/progression, and gene amplification (Miller et al. 2002). Three modes (oxidative stress, chromosomal abnormality, and altered growth factors) of arsenic carcinogenesis have shown a degree of positive evidence, both in experimental systems (animal and human cells) and in human tissues. However, the other mechanisms do not have much evidence especially from in vivo studies.

14.5.3 Lead

The mechanisms which involve lead-induced toxicity primarily damage to the cell membrane and DNA as well as damage to the enzymatic antioxidant molecule such as catalase, glucose-6-phosphate dehydrogenase (G6PD), GPx, and SOD and nonenzymatic antioxidants such as GSH of animals and human systems. Several kinds of literature indicate that lead-induced toxicity might be involved in the multifactorial mechanism of action. This multifactorial mechanism can be oxidative stress, enzyme inhibition, DNA damage, change in gene expression, and adventitious like mimicry. In all mechanism, reactive oxygen species induced by lead is a well-known mechanism. The lead has electron-sharing affinities that can result in formation of covalent attachment with sulphydryl groups of cellular components. Lead is known to adversely influence the metabolism of glutathione and cause toxicity. Several mechanisms are proposed for lead-induced oxidative stress: (1) Direct effect of lead on cell membranes, (2) lead–hemoglobin interaction, (3) δ-aminolevulinic acid (δ-ALA)-induced generation of ROS, and (4) effect of lead on the antioxidant defense system of cells.

14.5.4 Mercury

The molecular mechanisms of toxicity of mercury are basically through the production of oxidative stress (Sharma et al. 2014). After absorption, it forms complexes with cysteine residues of proteins and diminishes the cellular antioxidants. Inorganic mercury has been reported to cause a defect in electron transport and oxidative phosphorylation at ubiquinone-cytochrome b5 step by producing ROS and creating oxidative stress (Marnett 2000). The oxidative stress also involved in the disruption of calcium homoeostasis. Both types of mercury, organic and inorganic, disrupt the calcium homoeostasis but their action of mechanisms is different. Organic mercury is supposed to increase the intracellular calcium by stimulating the influx of extracellular calcium and mobilizing intracellular stores, whereas inorganic mercury disrupts the homoeostasis by accelerating the influx of extracellular calcium (Kim et al. 2010). The link between mercury intoxication and carcinogenesis is not much clear. Some studies have confirmed the genotoxic potential of mercury, whereas others have not shown any connection between mercury exposure and its genotoxicity (Valko et al. 2004). Generation of oxidative stress and ROS production during mercury toxicity has been reported to be associated with DNA damage, which can lead to the initiation of carcinogenic process (Ogura et al. 1996; Valko et al. 2006). The free radical production may also induce the conformational changes in enzymes and other proteins that are actively involved in cell cycle regulation such as chromosomal segregation, mitotic spindle, and DNA repair (Valko et al. 2006).

14.6 Phytochemicals in Alleviation of Heavy Metal Toxicity

The plants are rich in antioxidant potentials such as polyphenols and flavonoids. However, plants may also have the ameliorative effect against the heavy metal toxicity. Several researchers also reported the heavy metal scavenging activity of phytochemicals. The oral administrations of soya bean supplementation and *Arthrospira maxima* reduce the cadmium-induced genotoxic and cardiovascular implications (Brochin et al. 2008; Argüelles et al. 2013). Many phytochemicals such as phycocyanobilin, carotenes, vitamin C, and vitamin E obtained from cyanobacterial species such as *Chlorella* and *Spirulina* have shown their protective effects against lead- and cadmium-induced toxicity (Amin et al. 2006; Shim et al. 2008; Shim and Om 2008; Yun et al. 2011; Gupta et al. 2015). Several research works provide strong evidence for antiapoptotic activity of garlic extract and its inhibitory effect on mitochondrial injury caused by cadmium and lead. Garlic is rich in phytochemical, allicin (Shahsavani et al. 2011; Sadeghi et al. 2013).

Leaf extracts of *Annona muricata* and *Hippophae rhamnoides* have been beneficial against arsenic-induced toxicity. Both are rich in vitamins, carotenoids, and organic acids which give positive effects in antidote against arsenic toxicity (Jomova et al. 2011; Gupta and Flora 2005, 2006; George et al. 2015). Some of the researchers have also shown that phytochemicals not only ameliorate the toxicity of heavy metals but also reduce the body burden of accumulated heavy metals. Tomato extracts have potential to reduce bioaccumulation of heavy metals, in particular against lead- and cadmium-induced intoxication (Nwokocha et al. 2012). An overview of some phytochemicals active against heavy metal toxicity is presented in Table 14.2.

14.7 Role of Essential Mineral Ions in Mitigation of Heavy Metals Toxicity

14.7.1 Zinc

Zinc, a ubiquitous trace element essential as a catalytic, structural, and regulatory ion, is indispensable for growth and development of the microorganisms, plants, and animals (Mocchegiani and Muzzioli 2000). Average human intake of zinc ranges between 2.5 and 10 mg/day (Letavayova et al. 2006). It is well known for its role as a cofactor for superoxide dismutase (SOD), and it protects biological structures from damage caused by free radicals by maintaining adequate levels of SOD and metallothionein, as well as preventing interaction between chemical groups with iron. It is a part of the zinc-dependent thymic hormone that is essential for thymic functions such as T-cell maturation and differentiation (Mocchegiani and Muzzioli 2000). Its antioxidant function is attributed to its function of blocking the negatively charged sites, thereby preventing lipid peroxidation. Its deficiency has mostly been associated with an increase in the levels of lipid peroxidation of mitochondrial and microsomal membranes along with osmotic fragility of the erythrocyte membrane. Zinc-binding proteins such as metallothioneins (MTs) are present in virtually all living organisms. These proteins play a significant role in zinc uptake, distribution, storage, and release, and are protective in situations of stress (exposure to oxyradicals), exposure to toxic metals, and low Zn nutrition (Vasak and Hasler 2000; Coyle et al. 2002). Zn as a part of MTs improves excretion of metals such as Pb, As, etc. from the body. In a study, Jamieson et al. (2006)

Table 14.2 Phytochemicals active against heavy metals toxicity

S. No.	Source	Phytochemical	Biological function/property
1.	Black cumin (*Nigella sativa*)	β-Carotenes, vit. B1, vit. B6, vit. C, and vit. E	Antioxidative property
2.	Cyanobacteria (*Spirulina* and *Chlorella*)	Phycocyanobilin	Act as antioxidant
3.	Coriander, fruits, vegetables, green and black tea, red wine	Phenolics	Antioxidative property
4.	Red wine, tea, onion, tomato, radish, and olive oil	Quercetin	The expression of some enzymes such as cyclooxygenase-2 (COX-2) endothelial nitric oxide synthase (eNOS) and inducible nitric oxide synthase are induced by quercetin Quercetin modulation of signaling pathway including mitogen-activated protein kinases (MAPKs) and nuclear factor kappa B (NF-κB) and formation of an excretable complex with Pb hydroxyl and superoxide groups scavenge radicals, whereas the phenolic groups act as possible chelating sites.
5.	Citrus mainly Orange, grapefruit, and tomatoes	Naringenin	Enzyme activity recovers by antioxidant property of Naringenin by scavenging free radicals and chelating Cd
6.	Rice (*Oryza sativa*)	γ-Oryzanol	Testicular Cd level decrease by γ-Oryzanol and its increases δ-aminolevulinic acid dehydratase (ALAD) activity, and reduces lipid peroxidation
7.	Cherry, grapefruit, and berries	Anthocyanin/ flavonoids	Cd-induced oxidative stress protected by anthocyanin. It also reduces the Pb-induced oxidative stress
8.	Garlic	Allicin	Allicin decreases arsenic-induced oxidative stress by forming a complex
9.	*Pueraria mirifica* plant	Puerarin	Phosphoinositide-3-kinase (PI3K), protein kinase B (Akt), and endothelial nitric oxide synthase (eNOS) pathways are regulated by puerarin. It also protects DNA damage (apoptosis) from oxidative stress
10.	Turmeric	Curcumin	Curcumin forms a complex by binding with Pb and decreases the lipid peroxidation, neurotoxicity, and nephrotoxicity

found that marginal Zn deficiency enhances accumulation of Pb in bone, while its supplementation reduces its absorption and, as such, its accumulation in rats. Co-administration of zinc and lead, which compete for similar binding sites on enzymes, results in the reverse inhibition of aminolevulinic acid dehydrogenase in male Wistar rats, suggesting that administration of zinc suppresses the toxic effects of lead (Flora et al. 1989, 1999). In a similar study, supplementation of Zn was found to be associated with a reduction in the effects of $HgCl_2$ (Franciscato et al. 2011). Possessing significant potential to displace Zn from Zn-metalloproteinases, it eliminates the effect of $HgCl_2$ on neural development (Guzzi and Laporta 2008). Zn along with Se has been associated with a reduction in MeHg-induced toxicity. All this indicates that it plays a protective role against the damage of different metals through reduction in absorption, competing for binding to enzymes and through induction of molecules such as MTs. Besides having positive effects, supplementation of Zn has also been found associated with displacement of essential metals to substitute normal physiological activities (Briner 2014). On one side, where the supplementation of Zn seems to protect against oxidative damage of iron in the instance of iron supplementation, long-term or higher dosage treatment of Zn has been associated with the depletion of copper (Suzuki 1997; Maret and Sandstead 2006). As such, a balanced approach to the supplementation of these metal ions is necessary to prevent unwanted complications. The action of Zn in amelioration of heavy metal-induced toxicity is illustrated in Fig. 14.3.

14.7.2 Copper

Copper, an essential trace metal, acts as a cofactor for a variety of proteins and enzymes required for maturation of cytoplasmic cuproproteins and assembly of enzymes in different cell organelles (ceruloplasmin and tyrosinase in the case of

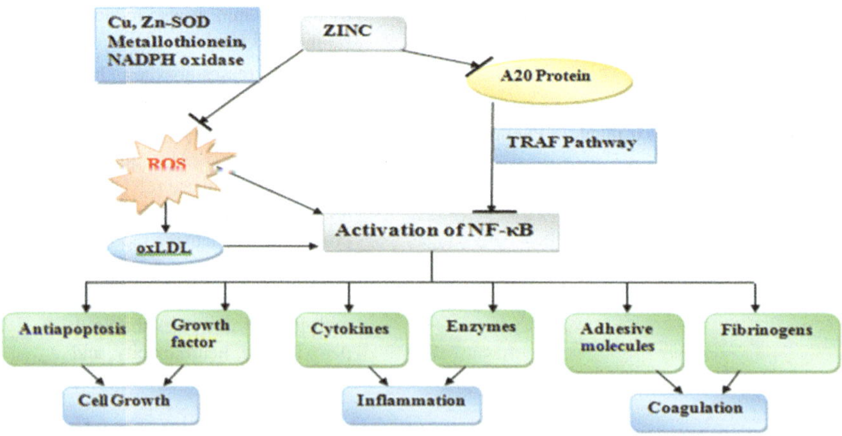

Fig. 14.3 Protective effect of zinc against heavy metal-induced toxicity

Golgi apparatus and cytochrome c oxidase concerning mitochondria). Copper uptake occurs in a tightly regulated process through specific high-affinity plasma membrane copper transporters or low-affinity permeases (DeFeo et al. 2007; Kim et al. 2008). Binding to chaperone proteins results in the transfer of copper to its final destination or any intermediate location from which its transport to other cell compartments or efflux out of cells can occur in cases in which concentration exceeds the optimum level. It acts as a cofactor for a broad range of metal-binding enzymes, and it fluctuates between the oxidized Cu (II) and reduced Cu (I) forms. In humans, its average intake varies between 260 and 700 g/day. Although adequate intake of copper protects lead, higher consumption has been associated with increased lead absorption (Flora et al. 1982). Its presence in excess amounts led to its involvement in the generation of highly reactive oxidative species (such as hydroxyl radicals), well known for their devastating effects on cells, particularly DNA damage and oxidation of proteins and lipids (Halliwell and Gutteridge 1990). Cu (I) and Cu (II) that hold high affinity for protein sites having cysteine, methionine, and histidine side chains act as potential ligands that led to the displacement of essential metal ions from their active sites, thereby resulting in the misfolding of proteins. As such, its uptake, followed by distribution and utilization, and finally, excretion from the body, needs to be tightly regulated (O'Halloran and Culotta 2000).

14.7.3 Selenium

Selenium (Se) is an essential trace element found in humans, animals, and some bacteria. In humans, its sources include meat, cereal grains, and fish. Average intake required for normal body functioning varies according to the age group: from 17 g/day (children) to 45 g/day (Adults). As selenoproteins, it contributes significantly to the maintenance of essential biological functions. It exists in two forms: organic, as selenomethionine (SeMet), selenocysteine (SeCys), and methylselenocysteine (MeSeCys); and inorganic, as selenite and selenate (Letavayova et al. 2006). It has been found to play an important role in at least 25 human selenoproteins by being part of the primary amino acid sequence as selenocysteine (SeCys) (Kryukov et al. 2003; Foster et al. 2006). Among the series of selenoproteins, thioredoxin reductase and glutathione peroxidase representing selenoenzyme play critical roles in the maintenance of cellular redox homoeostasis (Rayman 2000). By acting as an antimutagenic agent, it prevents malignant transformation of normal cells. As a part of glutathione peroxidases (GSH-Pxs) and thioredoxin reductase, it is primarily associated with protecting DNA and other cellular components from oxidative damage (Trueba et al. 2004). It increases the antioxidant capacity of cells by enhancing the activity of superoxide dismutase associated with the scavenging of superoxide radicals, increasing glutathione reductase activity and, as such, glutathione content as part of its protection against heavy metals. Having the ability to enhance the levels of glutathione and metallothioneins (MTs), its supplementation has been found to be associated with reversing the effect of different metals (Abdulla and Chmielnicka 1990; Sharma et al. 2014). Its interaction with heavy metals such as mercury counteracts their adverse consequences via the formation of insoluble complexes that prevent them from exerting toxic effects on the body (Whagner 1992; Suzuki 1997). Se administration was found to have a positive effect in reducing the Pb and As toxicities through increased production of selenoproteins, competition at key enzymes, and through the formation of inert Se–metal complexes (Kalia and Flora 2005). In addition to its antioxidant property, it plays an important role in thyroid hormone metabolism and redox reactions (Cano et al. 2007; Combs et al. 2009). Bronzetti et al. (2001) have reported that within certain limits, Se may have anticarcinogenic effects. However, at concentrations higher than those necessary for nutrition, it can have adverse effects by acting as a genotoxin and a carcinogen. Besides being toxic in itself at higher concentrations, it has been found to enhance the toxicity imposed by Pb (Kalia and Flora 2005). With greater chances to cause selenosis, higher intake to combat toxicity associated with metals such as mercury does not make it an excellent choice for therapy.

14.8 Conclusions

Heavy metals have been exhaustively studied by different workers, and they have presented different mechanisms of their toxic effects on cardiovascular system, kidney, neurons, and brain of animals and humans. In humans, the treatment of heavy metal poisoning involved application of chelating agents, though the side effects of chelating agents are the issues associated with it. On the other hand, some transition elements such as vanadium, manganese, iron, cobalt, copper, zinc, selenium, strontium, and molybdenum in small quantities are required for good human health. It has been observed that the deficiency of these essential metals may increase susceptibility to heavy metal poisoning. Selenium inhibits accumulation of mercury and increases excretion of arsenic and mercury. High concentration of folic acid in blood of pregnant woman helps in reducing the blood levels of mercury and cadmium. The uses of antioxidants such as vitamin C, garlic, alpha-lipoic acid, and glutathione help to reduce the adverse effects induced by Pb, Cd, and Cu. The roles of various plant-based principles in alleviating the heavy metals toxicity in humans are significant. However, still extensive research is needed to understand the targets of actions of heavy metals and to investigate the appropriate, cost-effective and safe therapeutics to overcome their toxic effects.

Acknowledgements AK, NS, and VKG are grateful to University Grants Commission-New Delhi for providing financial support in the form of research fellowships. RP acknowledges UGC-New Delhi for providing financial support. The work is supported by DST-FIST and UGC-SAP programs in the department.

References

Abdulla M, Chmielnicka J (1990) New aspects on the distribution and metabolism of essential trace elements after dietary exposure to toxic metals. Biol Trace Elem Res 23:25–53

Agency for Toxic Substances and Disease Registry (ATSDR) (1999) Public Health Service. U.S. Department of Health and Human Services; Toxicological Profile for Lead, Atlanta

Agency for Toxic Substances and Disease Registry (ATSDR) (2000) Toxicological profile for arsenic TP-92/09. Center for Disease Control, Atlanta, Georgia

Agency for Toxic Substances and Disease Registry (ATSDR) (2008) Draft toxicological profile for cadmium, Atlanta, GA

Amin A, Hamza A, Daoud S (2006) Spirulina protects against cadmium-induced hepatotoxicity in rats. Am J Pharmacol Toxicol 1:21–25

Anderson D, Yu TW, Phillips BJ, Schemezer P (1994) The effect of various antioxidants and other modifying agents on oxygen-radical-generated DNA damage in human lymphocytes in the comet assay. Mutat Res 307:261–271

Andrews KW, Savitz DA, Hertz-Picciotto I (1994) Prenatal lead exposure in relation to gestational age and birth weight: a review of epidemiologic studies. Am J Ind Med 26:13–32

Argüelles VJ, González IA, Madrigal BE, Germán CC (2013) Amelioration of cadmium-produced teratogenicity and genotoxicity in mice given *Arthrospira maxima* (Spirulina) treatment. Evidence-Based Complementary and Alternative Medicine 2013: Article ID 604535. http://dx.doi.org/10.1155/2013/604535

Barrett JC, Lamb PW, Wang TC, Lee TC (1989) Mechanisms of arsenic-induced cell transformation. Biol Trace Elem Res 21:421–429

Baselt RC (2000) Disposition of toxic drugs and chemicals in man, 5th edn. Chemical Toxicology Institute, Foster City, CA

Baselt RC, Cravey RH (1995) Disposition of toxic drugs and chemicals in man, 4th edn. Year Book Medical Publishers, Chicago, IL, pp 105–107

Baynes JW (1991) Role of oxidative stress in development of complications in diabetes. Diabetes 40:405–412

Becker K, Kaus S, Krause C, Lepom P, Schulz C, Seiwert M et al (2002) German Environmental Survey 1998 (GerES III): environmental pollutants in blood of the German population. Int J Hyg Environ Health 205:297–308

Bhattacharyya MH, Wilson AK, Rajan SS, Jonah M (2000) Biochemical pathways in cadmium toxicity. In: Zalup RK, Koropatnick J (eds) Molecular biology and toxicology of metals. Taylor and Francis, London, pp 1–74

Borcea V, Nourooz-Zadeh J, Wolff SP (1999) α-Lipoic acid decreases oxidative stress even in diabetic patients with poor glycemic control and albuminuria. Free Radical Biol Med 26: 1495–1500

Bradl H (2002) Heavy metals in the environment: origin, interaction and remediation, vol 6. Academic Press, London

Briner W (2014) The alchemists approach to metal poisoning: transforming the metal burden. Toxics 2014(2):64–376

Brochin R, Leone S, Phillips D (2008) The cellular effect of lead poisoning and its clinical picture. Georgetown Under Graduate J Health Sci 5:1–8

Brohi RD, Wang L, Talpur HS, Wu D, Khan FA, Bhattarai D, Rehman ZU, Farmanullah F, Huo LJ (2017) Toxicity of nanoparticles on the reproductive system in animal models: A review. Front Pharmacol 8:606. https://doi.org/10.3389/fphar.2017.00606

Bronzetti G, Cini M, Andreoli E, Caltavuturo L, Panunzio M, Croce CD (2001) Protective effects of vitamins and selenium compounds in yeast. Mutat Res 496:105–115

Cano P, Poliandri AHB, Jimenez V, Cardinali DP, Esquifino AI (2007) Cadmium induced changes in Per 1 and Per 2 gene expressions in rat hypothalamus and anterior pituitary: effect of melatonin. Toxicol Lett 172:131–136

Casalino E, Sblano C, Landriscina C (1997) Enzyme activity alteration by cadmium administration to rats: the possibility of iron involvement in lipid peroxidation. Arch Biochem Biophys 346:171–179

Centeno JA, Tchounwou PB, Patlolla AK, Mullick FG, Murakat L, Meza E, Gibb H, Longfellow D, Yedjou CG (2005) Environmental pathology and health effects of arsenic poisoning: a critical review. In: Naidu R, Smith E, Smith J, Bhattacharya P (eds) Managing arsenic in the environment: from soil to human health. CSIRO Publishing Corp., Adelaide, Australia

Centers for Disease Control and Prevention (CDC) (2001) Managing elevated blood lead levels among young children: recommendations from the Advisory Committee on Childhood Lead Poisoning Prevention, Atlanta

Chappell W, Beck B, Brown K, North D, Thornton I, Chaney R, Cothern R, Cothern CR, North DW, Irgolic K, Thornton I, Tsongas T (1997) Inorganic arsenic: a need and an opportunity to improve risk assessment. Environ Health Perspect 105:1060–1067

Chehregani A, Malayeri BE (2007) Removal of heavy metals by native accumulator plants. Int J Agric Biol 9:462–465

Combs GF, Midthune DN, Patterson KY, CanWeld WK, Hill AD, Levander OA, Taylor PR, Moler JE, Patterson BH (2009) Effects of selenomethionine supplementation on selenium status and thyroid hormone concentrations in healthy adults. Am J Clin Nutr 89:1808–1814

Coyle P, Philcox JC, Carey LC, Rofe AM (2002) Metallothionein: the multipurpose protein. Cell Mol Life Sci 59:627–647

Damek-Poprawa M, Sawicka-Kapusta K (2004) Histopathological changes in the liver, kidneys, and testes of bank voles environmentally exposed to heavy metal emissions from the steelworks and zinc smelter in Poland. Environ Res 96:72–78

DeFeo CJ, Aller SG, Unger VM (2007) A structural perspective on copper uptake in eukaryotes. Biometals 20:705–716

Fergusson JE (1990) The heavy elements: chemistry, environmental impact and health effects. Pergamon Press, Oxford

Filipic M, Fatur T, Vudrag M (2006) Molecular mechanisms of cadmium induced mutagenicity. Hum Exp Toxicol 25(2):67–77

Fitzgerald WF, Clarkson TW (1991) Mercury and monomethylmercury: present and future concerns. Environ Health Perspect 96:159–166

Flora SJS, Behari JR, Tandon SK (1982) Protective role of trace metals in lead intoxication. Toxicol Lett 13:51–56

Flora SJS, Kumar D, Gupta D (1999) Interaction of zinc, methionine or their combination with lead at gastrointestinal or post-absorptive levels in rats. Pharmacol Toxicol 68:3–7

Flora SJS, Singh S, Tandon SK (1989) Thiamine and zinc in prevention of lead intoxication. J Int Med Res 17:68–75

Flora SJS, Flora GJS, Saxena G (2006) Environmental occurrence, health effects and management of lead poisoning. In: Cascas SB, Sordo J (eds) Lead: chemistry, analytical aspects, environmental impacts and health effects. Elsevier Publication, Netherlands, pp 158–228

Flora SJS, Mittal M, Mehta A (2008) Heavy metal induced oxidative stress & its possible reversal by chelation therapy. Indian J Med Res 128(4):501–523

Foster CB, Aswath K, Chanock SJ, McKay HF, Peters U (2006) Polymorphism analysis of six selenoprotein genes: support for a selective sweep at the glutathione peroxidase 1 locus (3p21) in Asian populations. BMC Genet 7:56

Franciscato C, Silva LM, Duarte FA, Oliveira CS, Ineu RP, Flores EMM, Dressler VL, Piexoto NC, Pereira ME (2011) Delayed biochemical changes induced by mercury intoxication are prevented by zinc exposure. Ecotoxicol Environ Saf 74:480–486

Friberg L (1948) Proteinuria and kidney injury among workmen exposed to cadmium and nickel dust. J Ind Hyg Toxicol 30:32–36

Friberg L (1950) Health hazards in the manufacture of alkaline accumulators with special reference to chronic cadmium poisoning. Acta Medica Scandinavica 138(suppl 240):1–124

Fulekar M, Singh A, Bhaduri AM (2009) Genetic engineering strategies for enhancing phytoremediation of heavy metals. Afr J Biotech 8:529–535
George V, Kumar D, Suresh P, Kumar R (2015) In vitro protective potentials of *Annona muricata* leaf extracts against sodium arsenite-induced toxicity. Curr Drug Discov Technol 12:59–63
Giugliano D, Ceriello A, Paolisso G (1996) Oxidative stress and diabetic vascular complications. Diabetes Care 19:257–267
Goering PL, Fisher BR, Noren BT, Papaconstantinou A, Rojko JL, Marler RJ (2000) Mercury induces regional and cell-specific stress protein expression in rat kidney. Toxicol Sci 53: 447–457
Goyer RA (1996) Toxic effects of metals. In: Klaassen CD (ed) Casarett & Doull's toxicology: The basic science of poisons. McGraw-Hill, New York, pp 691–737
Goyer RA (2001) Toxic effects of metals. In: Klaassen CD (ed) Cassarett and Doull's toxicology: the basic science of poisons. McGraw-Hill Publisher, New York, pp 811–867
Graeme KA, Pollack CV (1998) Heavy metal toxicity, part I: arsenic and mercury. J Emerg Med 16:45–56
Grandjean P, Budtz-Jørgensen E, White RF (1999) Methyl mercury exposure biomarkers as indicators of neurotoxicity in children aged 7 years. Am J Epidemiol 150:301–305
Grandjean P, Weihe P, White RF (1997) Cognitive deficit in 7-year-old children with prenatal exposure to methylmercury. Neurotoxicol Teratol 19:417–428
Guallar E, Sanz-Gallardo MI, Veer PVT (2002) Mercury, fish oils, and the risk of myocardial infarction. N Engl J Med 347:1747–1754
Gupta R, Flora S (2005) Therapeutic value of *Hippophae rhamnoides* L. against sub chronic arsenic toxicity in mice. J Med Food 8:353–361
Gupta R, Flora S (2006) Protective effects of fruit extracts of *Hippophae rhamnoides* L. against arsenic toxicity in Swiss albino mice. Hum Exp Toxicol 25:285–295
Gupta VK, Sharma B (2015) Environmental hazards due to xenobiotics contamination: growing risk to human health and possible remedies. In: Verma A (ed) Green social work: environmental protection, RPTU-Allahabad
Gupta VK, Singh S, Agrawal A, Siddiqi NJ, and Sharma B (2015) Phytochemicals mediated remediation of neurotoxicity induced by heavy metals. Biochemistry Research International 2015: Article ID 534769. http://dx.doi.org/10.1155/2015/534769
Guzzi G, LaPorta CAM (2008) Molecular mechanisms triggered by mercury. Toxicology 244: 1–12
Halliwell B, Gutteridge JM (1990) Role of free radicals and catalytic metal ions in human disease: an overview. Methods Enzymol 186:1–85
Hartmann A, Peit G (1994) Comparative investigations of the genotoxic effects of metals in the single cell gel assay and the sister chromatid exchange test. Environ Mol Mutagen 23:299–305
Henson MC, Anderson MB (2000) The effects of cadmium on placental endocrine function. Recent Res Dev Endocrinol 1:37–47
Huang C, Costa M, Shi X (2004) Molecular mechanisms of arsenic carcinogenesis. Mol Cell Biochem 255:57–66
Hughes MF (2002) Arsenic toxicity and potential mechanisms of action. Toxicol Lett 133:1–16
Hultberg B, Anderson A, Isaksson A (2001) Interaction of metals and thiols in cell damage and glutathione distribution: potentiation of mercury toxicity by dithiothreitol. Toxicology 156: 93 100
Inada C, Yamada K, Takane N, Nonaka K (1995) Poly (ADPribose) synthesis induced by nitric oxide in a mouse β-cell line. Life Sci 56:1467–1474
International Agency for Research on Cancer (IARC) (1993) Monographs cadmium. Lyon, France
Jamieson JA, Taylor CG, Weiler HA (2006) Marginal zinc deficiency exacerbates bone lead accumulation and high dietary zinc attenuates lead accumulation at the expense of bone density in growing rats. Toxicol Sci 92:286–294
Jomova K, Jenisova Z, Feszterova M (2011) Arsenic: toxicity, oxidative stress and human disease. J Appl Toxicol 31:95–107

Kalia K, Flora SJS (2005) Safe and effective therapeutic measures for chronic arsenic and lead poisoning. J Occup Health 47:1–21

Kim BE, Nevitt T, Thiele DJ (2008) Mechanisms for copper acquisition, distribution and regulation. Nat Chem Biol 4:176–185

Kim S, Dayani L, Rosenberg PA, Li J (2010) RIP1 kinase mediates arachidonic acid-induced oxidative death of oligodendrocyte precursors. Int J Physiol Pathophysiol Pharmacol 2(2): 137–147

Kolb H, Kolb-Bachofen V (1992) Type I insulin dependent diabetes mellitus and nitric oxide. Diabetologia 35:796–797

Kryukov GV, Castellano S, Novoselov SV, Lobanov AV, Zehtab O, Guigo R, Gladyshev VN (2003) Characterization of mammalian selenoproteomes. Science 300:1439–1443

Lanphear BP, Dietrich K, Auinger P, Cox C (2000) Cognitive deficits associated with blood lead concentrations <10 μg/dl in US children and adolescents. Public Health Rep 115:521–529

Leonard SS, Harris GK, Shi X (2004) Metal-induced oxidative stress and signal transduction. Free Radical Biol Med 37(12):1921–1942

Letavayova L, Vlckova V, Brozmanova J (2006) Selenium: from cancer prevention to DNA damage. Toxicology 227:1–14

Lund B, Miller DM, Woods JS (1993) Studies on Hg(II)-induced H_2O_2 formation and oxidative stress in vivo and in vitro in rat kidney mitochondria. Biochem Pharmacol 45(10):2017–2024

Lyons TJ (1991) Oxidized low density lipoproteins: a role in the pathogenesis of atherosclerosis in diabetes? Diabet Med 8:411–419

Mahboob M, Shireen KF, Atkinson A, Khan AT (2001) Lipid peroxidation and antioxidant enzyme activity in different organs of mice exposed to low level of mercury. J Environ Sci and Health: Part B 36:687–697

Manke A, Wang L, Rojanasakul Y (2013) Mechanisms of nanoparticle-induced oxidative stress and toxicity. BioMed Research International 2013: Article ID 942916. http://dx.doi.org/10.1155/2013/942916

Mannino DM, Holguin F, Greves HM, Savage-Brown A, Stock AL, Jones RL (2004) Urinary cadmium levels predict lower lung function in current and former smokers: data from the Third National Health and Nutrition Examination Survey. Thorax 59:194–198

Maret W, Sandstead HH (2006) Zinc requirements and the risks and benefits of zinc supplementation. J Trace Elem Med Biol 20:3–18

Marnett LJ (2000) Oxyradicals and DNA damage. Carcinogenesis 21(3):361–370

Memon AR, Aktoprakligil D, Ozdemir A, Vertii A (2001) Heavy metal accumulation and detoxification mechanisms in plants. Turk J Bot 25:111–121

Miller WH, Schipper HM, Lee JS, Singer J, Waxman S (2002) Mechanisms of action of arsenic trioxide review. Can Res 62:3893–3903

Mocchegiani E, Muzzioli M (2000) Zinc, metallothioneins, immune response, survival and ageing. Biogerontology 1:133–143

Modaihsh A, Al-Swailem M, Mahjoub M (2004) Heavy metal contents of commercial inorganic fertilizer used in the Kingdom of Saudi Arabia. Agric Mar Sci 9:21–25

National Research Council Canada (NRCC) (1978) Effects of arsenic in the environment. National Research Council of Canada, pp 1–349

Nwokocha R, Nwokocha M, Aneto I (2012) Comparative analysis on the effect of *Lycopersicon esculentum* (tomato) in reducing cadmium, mercury and lead accumulation in liver. Food Chem Toxicol 50:2070–2073

O'Halloran TV, Culotta VC (2000) Metallochaperones: an intracellular shuttle service for metal ions. J Biol Chem 275:25057–25060

Ognjanovic B, Pavloic SZ, Maletic SD, Žikic RV, Štajn A, Radojicic RM, Saicic ZS, Petrovic VM (2003) Protective influence of vitamin E on antioxidant defense system in the blood of rats treated with cadmium. Physiol Res 52:563–570

Ogura H, Takeuchi T, Morimoto KA (1996) A comparison of the 8-hydroxyl-deoxyguanosine, chromosome aberrations and micronucleus techniques for the assessment of the genotoxicity of mercury compounds in human blood lymphocytes. Mutat Res 340:175–182

Ong CN, Phoon WO, Law HY, Tye CY, Lim HH (1985) Concentrations of lead in maternal blood, cord blood, and breast milk. Arch Dis Child 60:756–759

Pacyna JM (1996) Monitoring and assessment of metal contaminants in the air. In: Chang LW, Magos L, Suzuli T (eds) Toxicology of metals. CRC Press, Boca Raton, FL, pp 9–28

Paksy K, Rajczy K, Forgacs Z, Lazar P, Bernard A, Gati I, Kaali GS (1997) Effect of cadmium on morphology and steroidogenesis of cultured human ovarian granulosa cells. J Appl Toxicol 17:321–327

Papaconstantinou AD, Brown KM, Noren BT, McAlister T, Fisher BR, Goering PLV (2003) Mercury, cadmium, and arsenite enhance heat shock protein synthesis in chick embryos prior to embryo toxicity. Birth Defects Res. Part B, Dev Reprod Toxicol 68:456–464

Parthiban A, Vijayalingam S, Shanmugasundaram KR, Mohan R (1995) Oxidative stress and the development of diabetic complications antioxidants and lipid peroxidation in erythrocytes and cell membrane. Cell Biol Int 19:987–993

Pearson CA, Prozialeck WC (2001) E-Cadherin, beta-Catenin and cadmium carcinogenesis. Med Hypotheses 56:573–581

Porter AC, Fanger GR, Vaillancourt RR (1999) Signal transduction pathways regulated by arsenate and arsenite. Oncogene 18(54):7794–7802

Pulford I, Watson C (2003) Phytoremediation of heavy metal-contaminated land by trees-a review. Environ Int 29:529–540

Rayman MP (2000) The importance of selenium to human health. Lancet 356:233–241

Rhee HM, Choi BH (1989) Hemodynamic and electrophysiological effects of mercury in intact anesthetized rabbits and in isolated perfused hearts. Exp Mol Pathol 50:281–290

Rin K, Kawaguchi K, Yamanaka K, Tezuka M, Oku N, Okada S (1995) DNA-Strand breaks induced by dimethyl arsenic acid, a metabolite of inorganic arsenics, are strongly enhanced by superoxide anion radicals. Biol Pharm Bull 18:45–48

Rodrigues S, Henriques B, Reis A, Duarte A, Pereira E, Romkens PFAM (2012) Hg transfer from contaminated soils to plants and animals. Environ Chem Lett 10:61–67

Ronis MJJ, Bedger TM, Shema SJ (1998) Endocrine mechanism underlying the growth effects of developmental lead exposure in rat. J Toxicol Environ Health 54:101–120

Rubino FM (2015) Toxicity of glutathione-binding metals: a review of targets and mechanisms. Toxics 3:20–62

Sadeghi A, Bideskan A, Alipour F, Fazel A, Haghir H (2013) The effect of ascorbic acid and garlic administration on lead induced neural damage in rat offspring's hippocampus. Iran J Basic Med Sci 16:157–164

Saleha-Banu B, Danadevi K, Jamil Kaiser, Ahuja YR, Visweswara Rao K, Ishap M (2001) In vivo genotoxic effect of arsenic trioxide in mice using comet assay. Toxicology 162:171–177

Salem HM, Eweida EA, Farag A (2000) Heavy metals in drinking water and their environmental impact on human health. ICEHM2000, Cairo University, Egypt, pp 542–556

Salnikow K, Zhitkovich A (2008) Genetic and epigenetic mechanisms in metal carcinogenesis and cocarcinogenesis: nickel, arsenic, and chromium. Chem Res Toxicol 21:28–44

Satarug S, Baker JR, Urbenjapol S, Haswell-Elkins M, Reilly PE, Williams DJ et al (2003) A global perspective on cadmium pollution and toxicity in non-occupationally exposed population. Toxicol Lett 137:65–83

Satoh M, Koyama H, Kaji T, Kito H, Tohyama C (2002) Perspectives on cadmium research. Tohoku J Exp Med 196:23–32

Shahsavani D, Baghshani H, Alishahi E (2011) Efficacy of allicin in decreasing lead (Pb) accumulation in selected tissues of lead-exposed common carp (*Cyprinus carpio*). Biol Trace Elem Res 142:572–580

Shallari S, Schwartz C, Hasko A, Morel JL (1998) Heavy metals in soils and plants of serpentine and industrial sites of Albania. Sci Total Environ 19209:133–142

Sharma B, Singh S, Siddiqi NJ (2014) Biomedical Implications of heavy metals induced imbalances in redox systems. BioMed Research International 2014: Article ID 640754. http://dx.doi.org/10.1155/2014/640754

Sharma RP, Street JC (1980) Public health aspects of toxic heavy metals in animal feeds. J Am Vet Med Assoc 177:149–153
Shi H, Shi X, Liu KJ (2004) Oxidative mechanism of arsenic toxicity and carcinogenesis. Mol Cell Biochem 255:67–78
Shim JY, Om AS (2008) *Chlorella vulgaris* has preventive effect on cadmium induced liver damage in rats. Mol Cell Toxicol 4:138–143
Shim JY, Shin HS, Han JG (2008) Protective effects of *Chlorella vulgaris* on liver toxicity in cadmium-administered rats. J Med Food 11:479–485
Simeonova P, Wang S, Toriuma W, Kommineni V, Matheson J, Unimye N, Kayama F, Harki D, Ding M, Vallyathan V, Luster M (2000) Arsenic mediates cell proliferation and gene expression in the bladder epithelium: association with activating protein-1 transactivation. Cancer Res 60:3445–3453
Singh N, Gupta VK, Kumar A, Sharma B (2017) Synergistic effects of heavy metals and pesticides in living systems. Front Chem. https://doi.org/10.3389/fchem.2017.00070
Singhal RL, Merali Z, Hrdina PD (1976) Aspects of the biochemical toxicology of cadmium. Fed Proc 35(1):75–80
Smith AH, Hopenhayn-Rich C, Bates MN (1992) Cancer risks from arsenic in drinking water. Environ Health Perspect 97:259–267
Strater E, Westbeld A, Klemm O (2010) Pollution in coastal fog at Alto Patache, Northern Chile. Environ Sci Pollut Res 17(9):1563–1573
Suzuki KT (1997) Equimolar Hg–Se complex binds to selenoprotein P. Biochem Biophys Res Commun 231:7–11
Tchounwou PB, Ayensu WK, Ninashvilli N, Sutton D (2003a) Environmental exposures to mercury and its toxicopathologic implications for public health. Environ Toxicol 18:149–175
Tchounwou PB, Patlolla AK, Centeno JA (2003b) Carcinogenic and systemic health effects associated with arsenic exposure—a critical review. Toxicol Pathol 31(6):575–588
Tchounwou PB, Wilson B, Ishaque A (1999) Important considerations in the development of public health advisories for arsenic and arsenic-containing compounds in drinking water. Rev Environ Health 14(4):211–229
Tchounwou PB, Wilson BA, Abdelgnani AA, Ishaque AB, Patlolla AK (2002) Differential cytotoxicity and gene expression in human liver carcinoma (HepG2) cells exposed to arsenic trioxide and monosodium acid methanearsonate (MSMA). Int J Mol Sci 3(11):1117–1132
Thangavel P, Subbhuraam C (2004) Phytoextraction: role of hyperaccumulators in metal contaminated soils. Proc Nat Acad Sci India, Section B: Biol Sci 70:109–130
Trueba GP, Sanchez GM, Giuliani A (2004) Oxygen free radical and antioxidant defense mechanism in cancer. Front Biosci 9:2029–2044
US Department of Health and Human services, Agency for Toxic substance and Disease Registry (ATSDR) (2007) CERCLA priority list of substances
Valko M, Izakovic M, Mazur M, Rhodes CJ, Tesler J (2004) Role of oxygen radicals in DNA damage and cancer incidence. Mol Cell Biochem 266:79–110
Valko M, Morris H, Cronin MTD (2005) Metals, toxicity and oxidative stress. Curr Med Chem 12:1161–1208
Valko M, Rhodes CJ, Monocol J, Izakovic-Mazur M (2006) Free radicals, metals and antioxidants in oxidative stress-induced cancer. Chem Biol Interact 160:1–40
VanDam PS, VanAsbeck BS, Erkelens DW, Marx JJM, Gispen W, Bravenboer B (1995) The role of oxidative stress in neuropathy and other diabetic complications. Diab Metab Rev 11: 181–192
Varga B, Zsolnai B, Paksy K, Naray M, Ungvary GY (1993) Age dependent accumulation of cadmium in the human ovary. Reprod Toxicol 7:225–228
Vasak M, Hasler DW (2000) Metallothioneins: new functional and structural insights. Curr Opin Chem Biol 4:177–183
Vogt BL, Rossman TG (2001) Effects of arsenite on p53, p21 and cyclin D expression in normal human fibroblasts—a possible mechanism for arsenite's comutagenicity. Mutat Res 478(1–2):159–168

Waalkes MP, Liu J, Diwan BA (2007) Transplacental arsenic carcinogenesis in mice. Toxicol Appl Pharmacol 222(3):271–280

Waalkes MP, Rehm S (1992) Carcinogenicity of oral cadmium in the male Wistar (WFNCr) rat: effect of chronic dietary zinc deficiency. Fundam Appl Toxicol 19:512–520

Waalkes MP, Berthan G (eds) (1995) Handbook on metal-ligand interactions of biological fluids, vol 2. Marcel Dekker, New York, pp 471–482

Waalkes MP, Liu J, Ward JM, Diwan BA (2004) Mechanisms underlying arsenic carcinogenesis: hypersensitivity of mice exposed to inorganic arsenic during gestation. Toxicology 198:31–38

Waalkes MP, Misra RR, Chang LW (eds) (1996) Toxicology of metals. CRC Press, Boca Raton, FL, pp 231–244

Wang Y, Fang J, Leonard SS, Rao KMK (2004) Cadmium inhibits the electron transfer chain and induces reactive oxygen species. Free Radical Biol Med 11:1434–1443

Whagner PD (1992) Selenium in the treatment of heavy metal poisoning and chemical carcinogenesis. J Trace Elem Electrolytes Health Dis 6:209–221

Williams PL, Sergeyev O, Lee MM, Korrick SA, Burns JS, Humblet O, DelPrato J, Revich B, Hauser R (2010) Blood lead levels and delayed onset of puberty in a longitudinal study of Russian boys. Pediatrics 125(5):1088–1096

Wilson DN (1988) Association cadmium. Cadmium—market trends and influences. In: Cadmium 87 Proceedings of the 6th international cadmium conference, London, pp 9–16

Wuana RA, Okieimen FE (2011) Heavy metals in contaminated soils: a review of sources, chemistry, risks and best available strategies for remediation. ISRN Ecology 2011: Article ID 402647. http://dx.doi.org/10.5402/2011/402647

Yamanaka K, Takabayashi F, Mizoi M, An Y, Hasegawa A, Okada S (2001) Oral exposure of dimethylarsinic acid, a main metabolite of inorganic arsenics, in mice leads to an increase in 8-oxo-2′-deoxyguanosine level, specifically in the targetorgans for arsenic carcinogenesis. Biochem Biophys Res Commun 287:66–70

Yedjou GC, Moore P, Tchounwou PB (2006) Dose and time dependent response of human leukemia (HL-60) cells to arsenic trioxide. Int J Environ Res Public Health 3(2):136–140

Yedjou GC, Tchounwou PB (2007) In vitro cytotoxic and genotoxic effects of arsenic trioxide on human leukemia cells using the MTT and alkaline single cell gel electrophoresis (comet) assays. Mol Cell Biochem 301:123–130

Yee S, Choi BH (1996) Oxidative stress in neurotoxic effects of methyl mercury poisoning. Neurotoxicology 17:17–26

Yoshizawa K, Rimm EB, Morris JS (2002) Mercury and the risk of coronary heart disease in men. N Engl J Med 347:1755–1760

Yun H, Kim I, Kwon SH, Kang JS, Om AS (2011) Protective effect of *Chlorella vulgaris* against lead-induced oxidative stress in rat brains. J Health Sci 57:245–254

Zadorozhnaja TD, Little RE, Miller RK, Mendel NA, Taylor RJ, Presley BJ, Gladen BC (2000) Concentrations of arsenic, cadmium, copper, lead, mercury, and zinc in human placentas from two cities in Ukraine. J Toxicol Environ Health 61:255–263

Zalups RK, Koropatnik DJ (2000) Molecular biology and toxicology of metals. Taylor & Francis, London

Zalups RK (2002) Molecular interactions with mercury in the kidney. Pharmacol Rev 52:113–143

Zhang P, Xu Y, Sun J, Li X, Wang L, Jin L (2009) Protection of pyrroloquinoline quinone against methyl mercury induced neurotoxicity via reducing oxidative stress. Free Radical Res 43: 224–233

Index

M. Rai et al. (eds.), *Biomedical Applications of Metals*,
https://doi.org/10.1007/978-3-319-74814-6

The manufacturer's authorised representative in the EU is Springer Nature Customer Service Centre GmbH, Europaplatz 3, 69115 Heidelberg, Germany. If you have any concerns regarding our products, please contact ProductSafety@springernature.com

Printed and bound by CPI Group (UK) Ltd, Croydon, CR0 4YY

25/09/2026

02222855-0015